Nuclear Medicine Applications and their Mathematical Basis

Nuclear Medicine Applications and their Mathematical Basis

MICHAEL GORIS

Stanford University, USA

World Scientific

NEW JERSEY · LONDON · SINGAPORE · BEIJING · SHANGHAI · HONG KONG · TAIPEI · CHENNAI

Published by

World Scientific Publishing Co. Pte. Ltd.

5 Toh Tuck Link, Singapore 596224

USA office: 27 Warren Street, Suite 401-402, Hackensack, NJ 07601

UK office: 57 Shelton Street, Covent Garden, London WC2H 9HE

British Library Cataloguing-in-Publication Data
A catalogue record for this book is available from the British Library.

NUCLEAR MEDICINE APPLICATIONS AND THEIR MATHEMATICAL BASIS

ISBN-13 978-981-283-734-9
ISBN-10 981-283-734-5

Typeset by Stallion Press
Email: enquiries@stallionpress.com

Printed by Fulsland Offset Printing (S) Pte Ltd. Singapore

Contents

Introduction   1

1. Renography   3

    1.1.   Short Overview   3
        1.1.1.   Purpose of Renography   3
        1.1.2.   Indications   3
        1.1.3.   Tracers   4
    1.2.   The Model   5
        1.2.1.   Plasma Clearance   5
        1.2.2.   The Renogram   6
    1.3.   Semiotics   8
    1.4.   The Diagnosis of Renovascular Hypertension   10
    1.5.   Diuresis Renography: The Differential Diagnosis
        of Obstruction   18
        1.5.1.   Basic Principle   18
        1.5.2.   Indications   19
        1.5.3.   Procedure   19
            1.5.3.1.   Preparation   19
            1.5.3.2.   Renographic technique   20
        1.5.4.   Interpretation   21
    1.6.   The Application of Renography in Renal Transplantation . . .   27
    1.7.   Glomerular Filtration Rate   29
        1.7.1.   Background   29
        1.7.2.   Single Injection Method   31
        1.7.3.   Conclusion   36
    References   36

2. Ventilation Perfusion Imaging   43

    2.1.   Ventilation and Perfusion Comparisons   43
           2.1.1.   Basic Paradigm   43
           2.1.2.   Pulmonary Perfusion Imaging   43
           2.1.3.   Pulmonary Ventilation Imaging   44
                    2.1.3.1.   Pulmonary ventilation imaging with
                               xenon-133 (^{133}Xe)   44
                    2.1.3.2.   Pulmonary ventilation imaging with
                               krypton-81m   46
                    2.1.3.3.   Pulmonary ventilation inhalation imaging   48
    2.2.   Pulmonary Embolism   50
           2.2.1.   Interpretation   50
           2.2.2.   PIOPED   51
           2.2.3.   Worsley   52
           2.2.4.   Freitas   54
           2.2.5.   The Society of Nuclear Medicine   55
                    2.2.5.1.   High probability ($\geq$80% probability
                               of PE)   55
                    2.2.5.2.   Intermediate probability (20%–79%) . . .   56
                    2.2.5.3.   Low probability (<19%)   56
                    2.2.5.4.   Normal   56
                    2.2.5.5.   Gestalt interpretation   56
                    2.2.5.6.   McNeil   57
                    2.2.5.7.   Stanford   58
           2.2.6.   PIOPED II and PIAPED   60
    2.3.   Ciliary Function and Epithelial Permeability   62
    2.4.   Detecting Right to Left Shunting   63
    2.5.   Monitoring Pulmonary Blood Flow Distribution   64
    References   66

3. Renal Imaging with DMSA and the Generation of 3D Regions
    of Interest in Volume Images   71

    3.1.   Clinical Context   71
    3.2.   Analyzing Images as Truly Three-Dimensional   76
           3.2.1.   Material and Methods   77
                    3.2.1.1.   Patient population   77
                    3.2.1.2.   SPECT data   78
                    3.2.1.3.   3D regions of interest   78

      3.2.2. Results 78
  3.3. Discussion and Conclusion 81
  References 83

4. Therapy with Radionuclides   87
  4.1. Introduction 87
  4.2. Dosimetry: Internal Radiation Dosimetry 88
      4.2.1. Radiation Depends on the Amount of Radioactivity
              and the Length of the Exposure: Cumulative
              Activity 88
      4.2.2. Radiation Depends on the Energy Emitted Over
              the Cumulative Time: Equilibrium Absorbed
              Dose Constant 89
      4.2.3. Emitted Dose and Absorbed Dose (Φ) 91
      4.2.4. Actual Application 92
  4.3. Therapy 94
      4.3.1. Introduction and Survey 94
      4.3.2. Radioimmunotherapy in Lymphomas 96
      4.3.3. Predicting Outcome 100
          4.3.3.1. Background: Fusion 101
          4.3.3.2. Results 103
  4.4. Releasing Patients Treated with Radioactive Agents 103
      4.4.1. Background 103
      4.4.2. Basis for Occupancy Control: Kinetics 104
      4.4.3. The Case of Thyroid Treatment without
              Measured Kinetics 106
  References 108

5. Myocardial Imaging Studies   111
  5.1. Indications 111
  5.2. Tracers 112
      5.2.1. Flow Tracers 112
          5.2.1.1. Potassium analogues 112
          5.2.1.2. Membrane affinity 113
      5.2.2. Metabolic Tracers 113
      5.2.3. Cell Damage Tracers: Antimyosin 114
  5.3. The Central Paradigm of Myocardial Perfusion Studies 115
      5.3.1. Paradigm Shift 116

5.4.   Procedures and Techniques 117
        5.4.1.   Imaging 117
        5.4.2.   Stress Testing 118
        5.4.3.   Pharmacological Challenge 118
                  5.4.3.1.   Dipyridamole 118
                  5.4.3.2.   Adenosine 119
                  5.4.3.3.   Regadenoson (Lexiscan™) 120
                  5.4.3.4.   Dobutamine 120
5.5.   Data Analysis 121
        5.5.1.   Visual Interpretation 121
        5.5.2.   Polar Transformation (Circumferential Profile) . . . 121
        5.5.3.   3D Polar Transformation (Bull's Eye) 123
        5.5.4.   Non-Rigid Registration 124
5.6.   Conceptual Detours 125
        5.6.1.   The Points to Remember 127
        5.6.2.   In Addition 127
        5.6.3.   Eventually People Started to Accept Two Things . . 128
        5.6.4.   Modified Semiotics 128
5.7.   Operating Characteristics: The Detection of Coronary
        Artery Disease 129
        5.7.1.   The Arteriogram as the Defining Standard 129
        5.7.2.   Methodological Problems 130
        5.7.3.   Identification of Individual Vessels 130
        5.7.4.   Type of Stress 133
        5.7.5.   Wall Thickening 134
5.8.   Prognostic Significance 138
5.9.   Peri-Operative Risk 140
5.10.   Defining Viability 142
5.11.   Incidental Findings 147
References 148

6. Ventriculography   161

6.1.   Introduction 161
6.2.   Scintigraphic Evaluation of Ventricular Function 162
        6.2.1.   Physics, Physiopathology and Analysis 162
        6.2.2.   First Pass Nuclear Angiocardiography (FPNA) . . . 163
        6.2.3.   Equilibrium ECG-Gated
                  Angiocardiography (EGNA) 164

6.2.3.1. Global function 164
6.2.3.2. Regional wall motion (phase analysis) . . 170
6.2.4. Clinical Applications 171
6.2.4.1. Early validations 171
6.2.4.2. Detection of coronary artery disease . . . 172
6.2.4.3. Prognostic significance 173
6.2.4.4. Other applications 174
6.3. Conclusion 175
References 175

7. Bayes' Theorem and Related Problems   181

7.1. Bayes' Theorem: A Tautology 181
7.2. Using the Likelihood Ratio 183
7.3. Two by Two Contingency Tables 184
7.4. Accuracy 186
7.5. Verification Bias 186
7.5.1. Eliminating Verification Bias by Applying
the Positive and Negative Predictive Values
to the Population as a Whole (10, 11, 19) 187
7.5.2. Validation of Diagnostic Procedures
on Stratified Populations (24) 189
7.6. Heterogeneous Populations 189
7.7. Multiple Signs and Symptoms 190
7.8. Quantitative Symptoms and Receiver Operating
Characteristics Function (Roc Function) 191
References 193

8. Compartmental Systems   197

8.1. Tracer Kinetics and Compartmental Systems 197
8.2. Single Compartmental Systems and Radioactive Decay 199
8.2.1. Single Compartment Systems 199
8.2.2. Radioactive Decay 201
8.2.3. Half-Life and Effective Half-Life 202
8.2.4. Average Life 203
8.2.5. Semi-Logarithmic Plots 203
8.2.6. A Simple Application: Liver Blood Flow 204
8.3. Constant Infusion Model 205

8.4.   Catenary Systems 207
        8.4.1.   Generators and the Bateman Equation 209
        8.4.2.   Multiple Compartments with Identical
                  Fractional Transfer Rates 211
8.5.   Two-Compartmental Systems 214
        8.5.1.   The System 214
        8.5.2.   Integral Solution 215
        8.5.3.   Observed Values 218
        8.5.4.   Effect on the Exponentials 218
        8.5.5.   Another View: Looking at Compartment 2 219
        8.5.6.   When α_{13} is Equal to Zero 223
        8.5.7.   A Special Case: Two Compartments Connected
                  to Common Compartment with no Return 224
        8.5.8.   A Special Case: Two Compartments Connected
                  to Common Compartment with Return 226
References 228

9. Non-Compartmental Models   229

9.1.   Density Distribution of Transit Times 229
        9.1.1.   Sampling the Output Function 229
        9.1.2.   Compartmental Analog 232
        9.1.3.   Residency Times: Sampling the Compartment 233
        9.1.4.   Compartmental Analog 234
                  9.1.4.1.   Single compartment 234
                  9.1.4.2.   For the two-compartment system 234
9.2.   Gastric Emptying 235
9.3.   Red Blood Cells Survival Times 239
9.4.   The Patlak Method Applied to Kidneys 241
9.5.   Stewart Hamilton and the Cardiac Output 243
9.6.   Competitive Systems 245
References 245

10. Mathematical Techniques   247

10.1.   Matrix Algebra 247
        10.1.1.   Formalism 247
        10.1.2.   Channel Crosstalk 249
10.2.   Logarithms and Exponentials 250
        10.2.1.   Plotting Exponential Functions in Semi-Log Plots . . 251
        10.2.2.   The Gamma Function 252

10.3. Partial Derivative 253
10.4. Averages 253
10.5. Conjugate Counting 254
10.6. Fourier Series 256
10.7. Linear Transforms 257
    10.7.1. Laplace Transform 257
    10.7.2. Fourier Transform 259
    10.7.3. Convolution 261
    10.7.4. Smoothing and Filtering 263
    10.7.5. Modulation Transfer Function 264
    10.7.6. Lag Normal Function 265

Index   269

Introduction

This book is, in part, a reaction to a number of irritants.

First, textbooks in Nuclear Medicine tend to have the "basic" sciences in the first few chapters, but their content is never explicitly reused in the following clinical chapters. Bayes theorem may have been mentioned, with an emphasis on the difference between operating characteristic and predictive values, but results of clinical studies are too often expressed as accuracy or predictive values, without reference to prevalence.

In addition, many texts suffer from excessive empiricism. Chesterton is quoted as saying: "If the data do not fit the theory, check the data."[a] The third part of the renographic curve continues to be referred to as expressing renal excretion, while it does necessarily also reflects plasma clearance. The example of the Bateman equation is not used to explain the renogram.

Finally, there is a fundamental difficulty in understanding hand-waving explanations, at least to progress. In my experience, the hard explanation is the useful one.

Therefore, the book was structured as follows: the basic mathematical "techniques" needed to fully understand the derivations of the physiological problems, are explained in the last chapters, but referred to whenever they are likely to clarify a particular point. I am assuming that the reader is primarily interested in the physiological aspects, and would not readily struggle through basic mathematical techniques, without knowing their purpose.

Finally, when reviewing clinical literature, I have rendered the results (painstakingly) as operating characteristics.

---

[a]In this he was incorrect, except in the sense that data are not information unless they are understood in a framework.

Renography

1.1. SHORT OVERVIEW

1.1.1. *Purpose of Renography*

The purpose of renography is to estimate the global and individual renal function:

a. Global and individual renal cortical perfusion (ERPF)[a].
b. Global and individual renal glomerular function (GFR)[b].
c. Individual renal excretion rate.

1.1.2. *Indications*

a. The diagnosis of renovascular hypertension by demonstrating a renal ischemic response. The ischemic (underperfused) kidney can be shown to have a lower effective plasma flow than the heterolateral one, and simultaneously to conserve water. A challenge of an ischemic kidney with an ACE inhibitor (captopril) results in lower GFR, without much change in ERPF; captopril increases the transit time (see Section 1.4).
b. The differential diagnosis of dilatation of the collecting system versus obstruction, where obstruction is defined as increased resistance (pressure) when the urine flow increases. Urine flow cannot be increased beyond the point where pressure equals filtration pressure (cf. Whitaker test[c]) (see Section 1.5).
c. The evaluation of transplanted kidneys for the differential diagnosis of obstruction: (dilated collecting system, ERPF plus or minus maintained, excretion low), ATN (ERPF low, no excretion), acute rejection (ERPF and excretion

---

[a]Effective Renal Plasma Flow. The term effective accounts for the fact that all renal tubular tracers do not have the same extraction efficiency.
[b]Glomerular filtration rate.
[c]See Ref. 48.

proportionally decreased), chronic rejection (ERPF decreased, excretion normal to low) and verification for leakage.

d. The evaluation of drug toxicity affecting the GFR, e.g. in oncology.

e. The evaluation of renal scarring.

1.1.3. *Tracers*

One should define renal tracers as tracers which may diffuse freely in different tissues, but are extracted from the plasma mainly or exclusively by the kidneys. There are three types of renal tracers classified according to the mechanism of transit through the kidney (uptake and excretion). The classification could also have been made according to the type of observation they are used for, i.e. imaging or blood sampling, but we are mainly interested in imaging except for the GFR that will be described as a blood sampling technique.

1. Tubular tracers that are not excreted, but retained in the tubular cell. The prototype is DMSA (Dimercaptosuccinic acid) labeled with 99m-technetium (^{99m}Tc). The tracer is cleared from the plasma by the proximal renal tubular cells, where the tracer remains (1, 2).

2. Tubular tracers that are secreted from the tubular cell to the tubular lumen and excreted. The prototype is hippuran, or iodo-ortho-hippurate (IOH), labeled either with 131-Iodine or 123-Iodine (^{131}I and ^{123}I), now replaced by MAG3 (mercaptoacetyltriglyceride) labeled with ^{99m}Tc. Both tracers are equivalent except that plasma clearance is slower for MAG3 and protein binding is higher (3–9). The time spent by those tracers in the kidney is defined by the flow of nascent urine[d] in the tubular lumen. The renal tubular tracer ^{99m}Tc-L, L-EC, also equivalent to IOH (10) never conquered the market (Figure 1.1).

3. Glomerular tracers cleared from the plasma to the kidneys exclusively through glomerular filtration. The most common is diethylenetriaminepentaacetic acid (DTPA) labeled with ^{99m}Tc, used for imaging or Glofil® or sodium iothalamate labeled with 125-iodine (^{125}I) used for GFR determination by blood sampling. It should be noted that all those tracers, including the tubular ones, are relatively small molecules, such that a fraction (about 15%) of the tubular agents also enter the kidney by glomerular filtration.

---

[d]The nascent urine is the GFR at the glomerular level; the urine (after water reabsorption) at the collecting system level.

1.2. THE MODEL

1.2.1. *Plasma Clearance*

If one were to sample plasma from the renal artery and the renal vein simultaneously, one would observe that the tracer concentration is lower in the renal vein plasma. The difference was extracted by the kidneys. This concentration difference divided by the arterial concentration defines the extraction ratio, or extraction efficiency. If the extraction efficiency and plasma flow remains constant, the plasma clearance is a first order process (see Section 8.1). The matter is complicated by the fact that the tracers are also exchanged between the extravascular or extracellular space and the plasma. However, the kinetics of the tracer in the plasma are fairly accurately described by a two compartmental system (see Section 8.5). They are described by a sum of two exponentials: The total plasma activity is influenced by the activity leaving towards the kidneys (and not returning) and the activity mixing (and returning) to the extravascular spaces. The total plasma activity is well described by two exponentials:

$$TA_t = Ae^{-at} + Be^{-bt},$$

where TA_t is the total activity at time t and $A + B$ is the activity at $t = 0$ or the injected dose. If the total effective renal plasma flow is FT, and the plasma volume is V_p, the fractional plasma activity to the kidneys is $FT/V_p = \alpha_{13}$. The fractional

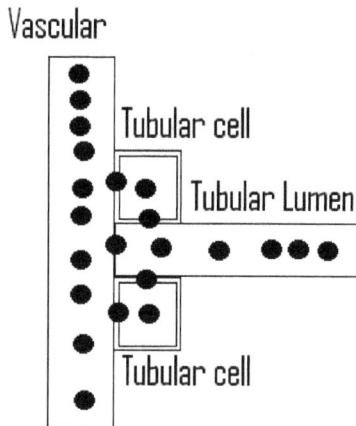

Figure 1.1 The renal model is illustrated schematically: The renal tracer in the vascular system is picked up by the tubular cells or filtered by GFR directly in the tubular lumen. The tracer is pushed downstream by the nascent urine.

transfer rate "α_{13}" represents the fraction of the total activity in plasma that is extracted from the plasma by the kidneys per unit of time.[e]

From the analysis of two compartmental systems, we know that α_{13} is derived from the two intercepts (A and B), and the two exponents (a and b):

$$\alpha_{13} = \frac{ab(A + B)}{Ab + Ba}. \text{ equation } 8.37^{f}$$

This value multiplied by the appropriate volume, depending on the tracer, is the effective renal plasma flow (ERPF) or the GFR (Section 1.7).

1.2.2. *The Renogram*

The renogram is the time activity function observed when one measures the activity in the kidneys after the injection of a dose of radiolabeled renal tracer. Although there are alternative descriptions in this exposition, we will look at the renogram as composed of two phases: first an accumulation phase, then an excretion phase. A typical normal renogram is shown in Figure 1.2.

- The rate of plasma clearance (fraction taken up by both kidneys per unit of time) increases with increased ERPF or GFR. Early on, the proportion of tracer in each kidney (prior to any excretion[g]) relative to the other kidney, is equal to the proportion of GFR or ERPF to each kidney (11); (Section 8.5.7). However, in the direct estimation of relative renal blood flow in dogs' curve, slope ratios correlated well with measured flow ratios with and without background correction, while 1- to 2-minute uptake ratios correlated well only when corrected for background (12). This finding explains, in part, the amount of reports on the determination of regions of interest (ROI) (13–16) (Section 1.5.3.2).
- The transit time or retention time in the kidney is inversely proportional to the nascent urine flow (F)t = V/F.[h] The nascent urine flow, proximally, is the GFR (ml/min) and distally, is the GFR minus the reabsorbed water (in the loop of Henle).
- The time of peak activity is the time at which exit from the kidney equals uptake by the kidney; it comes later when the transit time becomes longer.

---

[e]Assuming that the tracer is a true renal tracer and leaves the plasma only to mix in the extravascular pools, or to be irreversibly accumulated by the kidney.

[f]See Section 8.5.3.

[g]In adults, that would be within 4 minutes, whereas in children it would probably be within 3.

[h]See Sections 8.2.4 and 10.4.

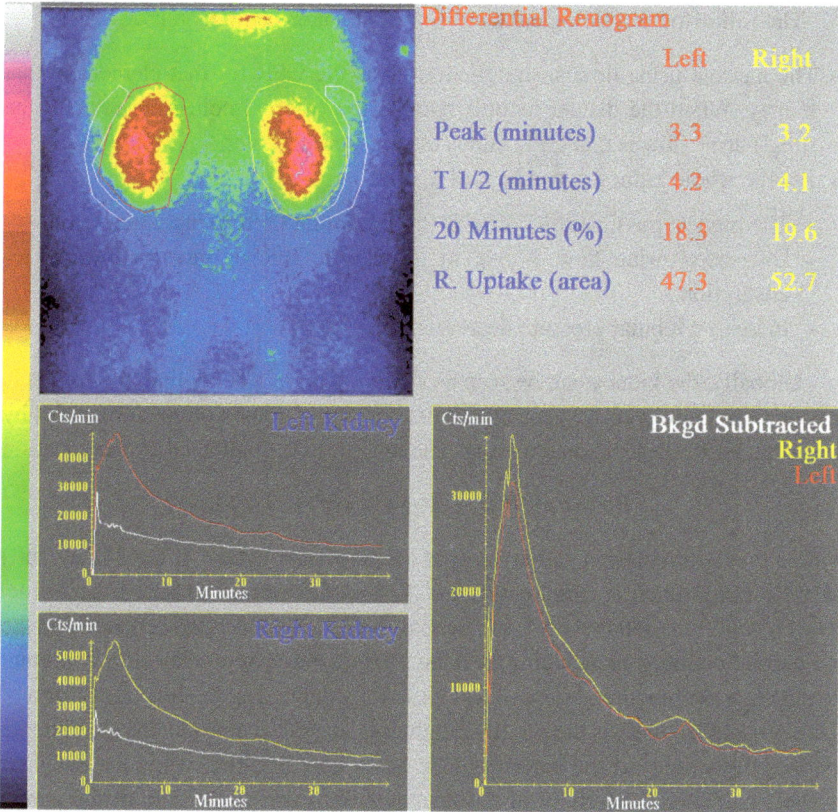

Figure 1.2 Normal renogram: The two curves (lower right quadrant) represent the net renal activities over time. There is a sharp increase of activity (soon), followed by a relatively steep decrease in activity. Descriptive parameters of the curve are the uptake ratio (left: 47.3 vs. right: 52.5), the time of peak activity (3.3 vs. 3.2 minutes) and the half-emptying time (4.2 vs. 4.1 minutes). The relative uptake or relative ERPF is proportional to the activity for only as long as when no activity is excreted (in a normal case, the excretion does not begin within the first 3 minutes).

- A decrease in the steepness of the curve in the excretion phase may reflect a longer transit time, but it also reflects slower plasma clearance if there is an element of global[i] renal insufficiency (see Sections 8.4 and 8.4.1).
- An abrupt increase in tubular flow of nascent urine will also increase the slope of the excretion component of the renogram.

---

[i]The term global is significant because both kidneys interact with the same plasma.

The following physiological factors must be taken into account:

- The nascent urine flow at the glomerulus is the GFR for that element in that kidney. When the distant tubulus reaches the external collecting system, the (final) urine flow is that GFR minus the reabsorbed water.
- For the whole kidney, it can be said that:
  - The highest possible urine flow is the maximum GFR to that kidney.
  - Decreased urine flow is due to decreased GFR or increased water re-adsorption.
  - Increased tubular pressure decreases GFR (as in obstruction).

Globally, the kidney can be seen as a delay line; in a delay line, the first in is the first out. However, because all tubules are not of equal volume, or are fed by the same GFR, there is some mixing. The renogram is dominated by the equation

$$R(t) = a_{13}P(t) - m(t) * a_{13}P(t - TTT),$$

where $P(t)$ is the plasma activity, α_{13} is the fractional uptake in the kidney, $m(t)$ is the mixing function (Figure 1.3) and TTT is the average tubular transit time. The convolution (denoted by *, see Section 10.7.3) of the mixing function and the accumulation function including the delay, defines the excretion rate. It is important to note that the functional form of $R(T)$ is mainly defined by the functional form of $P(t)$. A useful analogy is the parent–daughter relationship in which the slowest rate defines the system. If the parent isotope has a long half-life, while the daughter a short half-life, the activity of the daughter decreases at the rate of the parent (see Section 8.4.1). If plasma clearance (parent) is slow, the excretion part of the renogram (daughter) is sluggish (Figure 1.3).

General descriptions of the renogram abound (17), however, not all are specific in their indication. Brock (18) and Bueschen (19) describe it as the functional equivalent of excretion urography. Peters (20) applies the method to physiological measurements not specific diagnostic problems. The DeGrazia (21) model is more specific in the metrics and semiotics.

1.3. SEMIOTICS

a. Relative renal activity is equal to relative ERPF only before any activity has left the kidney (<3 minutes) (22).
b. If the excretion phase is slow, and the peak does not come late, the global renal function is likely to be abnormal. However, in cases of poor global renal function, the slowness of the excretion phase must be bilateral if there are two

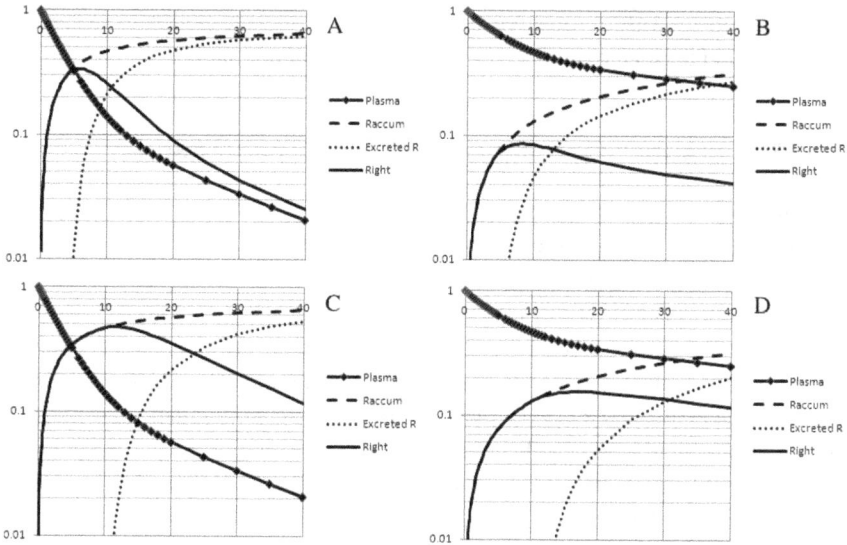

Figure 1.3   The figure illustrates three cases; in all cases, the plasma activity and the right (R) renal activity is plotted. In addition, the accumulation curve in the R kidney is plotted; the accumulation curve is distorted by the mixing function and delayed by the average tubular transit time (TTT). The actual renal activity is the accumulation function minus the distorted and delayed accumulation function. In panel A, the ERPF = 600 ml/min with a the TTT = 4 minutes. On the logarithmic scale, it is clear that the renographic downslope is close to parallel with the plasma curve. In panel B, the ERPF = 100 ml/min with a TTT = 4 minutes. The renographic excretion phase is sluggish, but again closely parallels the plasma curve; T_{max} comes early. In panel C, ERPF = 600 ml/min, but the TTT is 30 minutes. The excretion phase does not parallel the plasma curve and T_{max} is larger than 10. In panel D, ERPF = 100 ml/min and TTT = 30 minutes; again T_{max} is much delayed, compared to the case in panel B. The first pass uptake is not included in the analysis (14) although it provides a nice application for the Patlak plot (15, 16) (see Section 9.4).

kidneys. On the face of it, Kempi's (23) statement that the renographic curves obtained from IOH and DTPA are not significantly different cannot be correct. Since the plasma clearance of DTPA is slower than that of hippuran (considering GFR is only 15% of ERPF), the functional shapes have to be different.

c. If the peak comes late, whether or not the excretion phase is slow, there must be decreased tubular flow.

    i. Consider a decrease in GFR (e.g. obstruction).

    ii. Consider increased water readsorption.

d. Unilateral increased water readsorption would be associated with decreased ERPF, and thus, an earlier decrease in uptake (proportionally).

1.4. THE DIAGNOSIS OF RENOVASCULAR HYPERTENSION

The model for renovascular hypertension is the ischemic kidney model proposed by Stamey (24), in which the affected kidney is less perfused, and responds by increasing water readsorption[j] (24). The reference measurement is the constant infusion test, in which PAH (para-aminohippurate) or inulin is infused at a constant rate, while the ureters are cannulated individually. Over the cannulation interval, the proportion of the total amount of infused substance collected from each ureter is proportional to the effective renal plasma flow (the amount supplied to the kidneys by the plasma, multiplied by the extraction efficiency). Since the plasma concentration is identical for both kidneys, paraaminohippurate (PAH) or inulin will be more concentrated on the side with the higher water re-adsorption (25, 26).

The functional equivalent in renography is that the ischemic kidney has a proportionally lower accumulation function, either because of a lower ERPF (with IOH analogues) or because of a lower GFR (with DTPA or a glomerular agent) and a longer transit time. The longer transit time would be even more pronounced if the vascular stenosis results in a drop of the glomerular filtration rate (which does not always happens due to efferent vasoconstriction).

If the unilateral ischemic kidney is characterized by ipsilateral decreased accumulation and prolonged transit times, the same is not necessarily true in the case of bilateral renal artery stenosis. If the stenoses are equal, the accumulation functions would be equal, and in addition, bilateral increased water re-adsorption could not be sustained. In other words, a well-balanced bilateral stenosis may not be detectable directly by renography. In addition, decreased unilateral ERPF, with decreased glomerular filtration (and therefore prolonged transit times) are also characteristics of obstruction and acute tubular necrosis (ATN).[k]

In what follows, it is important to distinguish between glomerular tracers (usually DTPA) and tubular tracers (IOH or MAG3), because the effect of captopril (or ACE inhibitors) is an additional decrease of GFR (with lesser DTPA uptake), and a prolongation of the transit time (affecting both DTPA and IOH) or MAG3.

---

[j] In the absence of diuretics, a necessary condition for a baseline study. The diuresis renogram which was proposed by a few (Radó, 1971) in this context never caught on.

[k] In other words, if the semiotics for an ischemic kidney are unique, an ischemic kidney is not unique for the semiotics.

Increased sensitivity and specificity is obtained through the use of ACE inhibitors, or the introduction of captopril renography. Captopril is an angiotensin-converting enzyme (ACE) inhibitor. In the ischemic kidney, maintenance of glomerular filtration depends, in part, on angiotensin II-mediated efferent arteriolar constriction. ACE inhibitors reduce this constriction, and therefore the pressure distal of the renal artery stenosis in the glomerular vessels, thus reducing filtration (27). The reduction in glomerular filtration has two effects: It decreases the renal accumulation rate of glomerular agents (28), and prolongs the tubular transit time of all excreted agents, because the flow of nascent urine is decreased. The decrease in glomerular filtration can be augmented by dehydration triggered by diuretics.

In what follows, captopril renography is usually compared to the baseline renogram, and the criteria are: partially baseline or intervention (captopril) abnormalities, or provoked or increased abnormalities under intervention.

In rats, Kopecky (29) found that, with DTPA, the effect of captopril was enhanced with volume depletion obtained by furosemide. De Zeeuw (30) found that the effect of captopril was minimal on the unaffected side (in clipped arteries in dogs).

However, captopril increases the sensitivity of the renogram when the transit time is used as a criterion. He found no effect on IOH uptake to the affected kidney, with a slight increase on the unaffected side, suggesting that tubular flow may be increased to some extent. With captopril, the sensitivity was increased in 10 dogs from 50% to 100%; with IOH, the sensitivity in patients was increased from 87% to 93% while that with DTPA, increased from 60% to 86%.

One can conclude that the effect of captopril on the uptake of tubular agents by the kidneys, or on ERPF, is unclear or minimal when tubular tracers are being used. On balance, the accumulation function is not much affected,[1] but the transit time is, since the progression through the tubular lumen is entirely passive and due to nascent urine flow.

In rats, Lee (31) found a slight increase with captopril in the plasma to renal clearance of IOH and MAG3 in normal rats, the same increase in the heterolateral side in rats with renal arterial clamps (also confirmed by McAfee (32)), with a significant decrease on the affected side, and a slight decrease in bilaterally clamped rats.

While the renal uptake of tubular agents in the ischemic kidney is not very much affected by captopril, DTPA uptake is profoundly affected (32), since the GFR

---

[1]On the affected side, a decrease in the filtered fraction would be partially compensated by an increase in tubular flow.

decreases. With glucoheptonate, the effect of captopril (in experimental studies on rats with unilateral clamped renal arteries) is a decreased uptake (33), suggesting that the glomerular filtration fraction of this agent is important.

In what follows, we codify the interpretation of the renogram for the diagnosis of renovascular hypertension as follows:

α. Asymmetry in renal uptake (when t < 3 minutes), in the baseline study, for glomerular and tubular tracers.

α1. A differential uptake difference larger than 10 points.

α2. Renal blood flow as a fraction of cardiac output lower than 0.088 on the left or lower than 0.077 on the right (34).

β. Delayed transit, or delayed time of peak activity, for glomerular or tubular tracers in the baseline.

β2. The transit time is evaluated by looking at the downslope (or excretion rate part) of the renographic curve.[m]

γ. Abnormality triggered or increased by ACE inhibitor.

γ1. An increase in the asymmetry of uptake with glomerular agents.

γ2. An increased delay of the time of peak activity, independently of the tracer.

γ3. A prolongation of the transit time, computed by deconvolution of the plasma input function, independently of the tracer.

γ3a. The transit time is evaluated by looking at the downslope (or excretion rate part) of the renographic curve and $T_{1/2}$ is longer.

γ4. An absolute decrease in GFR mainly in bilateral disease.

The asymmetry in renal uptake must be measured before renal excretion affects any of the renographic curves. Peak activity ratios cannot be used. Nally (35–36), still with DTPA, confirmed this in a study of experimental renovascular hypertension in dogs; he also confirmed that the time to maximum is longer and the excretion rate is slower on the affected side. Unfortunately, he does not separate measurements of transit times from measurements of flow in his analysis of the IOH renogram.

Theoretically, one should not expect the flow abnormalities or asymmetries to be highly specific since they would be present in any other type of renal malfunction, as well as in small congenital kidneys. The findings by Peters (34) confirm this

---

[m]This is dangerous, if global renal function is not factored in.

suspicion. Higher specificities will (of course) be found if the population has either no renal abnormality or renovascular hypertension (see Section 7.6).

Nally (36) proposed an analysis in which a positive finding was a decreased uptake, a delay in peak time, or a slower excretory phase on one side. All criteria of abnormalities are combined as one (in an logical OR combination).[n] (see Section 7.7).

Fommei (37) presented data (using DTPA) which can be reanalyzed as follows: if the lower limit of uptake in one kidney is set at 42%, 7 out of 10 positive arteriograms (criterion not further specified) are detected by the baseline renogram, but 2 out of 8 cases are falsely abnormal. After captopril, the pick-up rate is 10 out of 10 and there are 0 out of 8 false positives. A decrease with captopril in unilateral uptake of more than 5% is present in 8 out of 10 of the positive arteriograms and in none of the kidneys with normal renal arteries. If the limit is set at 44%, the baseline renogram has a sensitivity of 8 out of 10 and a specificity of 5 out of 8, but the captopril renogram has a sensitivity of 10 out of 10 and a non-specificity of 2 out of 8. It is obvious that the criterion $\gamma 1$ is the best discriminator, mainly by an increase in specificity.

Also using DTPA and captopril-enhanced renal scintigraphy, Dondi (38) found that he could increase the sensitivity from 49 to 94%. His criteria are worth mentioning, because he measures relative flow and prolonged transit time:

- Normal renal uptake symmetry is defined as within the 44–56 brackets.[o]
- T_{max} is prolonged >5 minutes under captopril
- The up-slope of the curve is "abnormal".[p]
- A prolonged transit time by input function deconvolution[q] (see Section 10.7.3).
- A positive captopril effect is an increase in the degree of abnormality for any criterion.

He uses the criteria in a logical *OR* combination, hence a normal result assumes normality in all criteria.

---

[n]In a logical OR, any abnormality by any criterion, makes the case positive.
[o]Derived from renal net counts between 90 and 150 seconds (see Section 1.2.2).
[p]Since the renograms are not absolutely scaled, one assumes that this change in upslope shape reflects a later peak activity time.
[q]In cases in which a transit time is measured (in seconds), he finds (B: Basal, C: Captopril):

Type	Normal	>50% Stenosis
B	313.7 ± 33.6	331 ± 59.0
C	270.7 ± 39.5	406.4 ± 47.8

In 1991, Dondi (39) repeated the study using MAG3. In this paper, he refined the criteria for a positive captopril response (γ), which was considered positive if any two of the following occurred:

γ1. A decrease of more than 5% of the relative flow symmetry ratio, or a transition from within to without the normal bracket. This is unlikely for a tubular agent since tubular flow is not affected.

γ2. An increase in the peak time of more than 300 seconds.

γ3. An increase in the transit time of more than 20%.[r]

We give the results for the individual criteria in Table 1.1. For the combination, the sensitivity should be lower than 81%, but Dondi reported 89%, with a specificity of 91%.[s] Pedersen (40) gives valuable information, using DTPA for baseline and captopril renography on patients with unilateral and bilateral renal artery stenosis. The stenosis is variable and never exactly balanced, but the most affected site has less than 40% residual diameter. The measurements are the individual kidneys glomerular filtration rate and mean transit time. The data are beautifully tabulated and allowed for the derivation of the following criteria:

α. Asymmetry in renal uptake (when t < 3 minutes), in the baseline study, for glomerular and tubular tracers (less than 44% of uptake on the affected side).

β. Delayed transit, or delayed time of peak activity, for glomerular or tubular tracers in the baseline (transit time > 3.0 minutes).

γ. Abnormality triggered or increased by ACE inhibitor.

$\quad$ γ1. An increase in the asymmetry of uptake, more pronounced for glomerular agents (> 5%).

$\quad$ γ3. A prolongation of the transit time independent of the tracer (> 20%).

$\quad$ γ4. An absolute decrease in GFR (> 5 ml/min).

---

[r]With MAG3, the transit time does not differ very much from the one found with DTPA:

Type	Normal	> 50% Stenosis
B	243 ± 46	334 ± 93
C	271 ± 95	468 ± 96

[s]The combination of two criteria is an intersection, which cannot be larger than any individual criterion.

In the cases presented, bilateral stenosis, when present, was rarely symmetrical, and the cases had a higher likelihood of being detected, perhaps because the disease was more advanced.

Setaro (41) reviewed the renogram in relation to the arteriogram (criterion is >75% stenosis, or between 50% and 75% if followed by a post-stenotic dilatation, for fibromuscular displasia, the criterion is moderate or severe), and the results of surgery. The renographic criteria were as follows:

α. Asymmetry in renal uptake (when t<3 minutes), in the baseline study, for glomerular and tubular tracers (normal bracket is a 40–60 split).

β. Delayed transit, or delayed time of peak activity, for glomerular or tubular tracers in the baseline ($T_{max} > 11$ minutes).

γ. Abnormality triggered or increased by ACE inhibitor.

$\gamma1$. Asymmetry of uptake, more pronounced for glomerular agents (normal bracket is a 40–60 split).

$\gamma2$. An increased delay of the time of peak activity, independent of the tracer ($T_{max} > 11$ minutes).

The tracer is DTPA. Patients with renal insufficiency are included, an important application since hypertensive azotemic patients can sometimes be helped by vascular intervention.

Roccatello (42) using MAG3, IOH or DTPA used the following criteria, where a baseline abnormality was used to select the patients for a captopril renography:

Six hundred and sixty-seven hypertensive patients were analyzed by captopril-enhanced scintigraphy.

β. $T_{max} \geq 5$ minutes using ^{99m}Tc-diethylenetriaminepentaacetic acid (DTPA) or ≥ 3 minutes with 123I-o-iodohippurate (IOH) and ^{99m}Tc-mercaptoacetyl-triglycine (MAG3) and washout time ≥ 15 minutes.

$\gamma2$. Increased $T_{max} \geq 5$ minutes with ^{99m}Tc-DTPA or ≥ 3 minutes with 123I-IOH and ^{99m}Tc-MAG3.

Based on these criteria, 58 out of 667 (8.7%) scintigrams were found to be abnormal. Thirty-five of these 58 patients and 32 of the remaining 609 scintigraphically negative cases underwent additional arteriographic examinations.

Using asymmetry of either flow (ERPF) or GFR as the only criterion (for renovascular hypertension) results in a lower specificity because any renal dysfunction could have that effect. The specificity comes mainly from the captopril effect.

The evaluation of the transit time by looking at the so-called renal clearance part of the curve ($\gamma2a$) is fraught with danger. As we have seen, the excretory phase of the renogram also reflects plasma clearance. This is well illustrated by the work of Erbsloh-Moller (43). He looks at the residual cortical activity at 20 minutes, as a fraction of the maximum activity. The measure is a measure of washout. In patients with normal renal function and no RVH, the value is on average 15.2% (range 4–30). Only 1 out of the 14 patients has a value above 25%. In patients

Table 1.1 In this table, the greek letters are the metrics, as described in the text. G stands for a glomerular tracer (usually DTPA) and T for a tubular tracer (Hippuran or MAG3). B indicates the baseline, C indicates captopril or an equivalent ACE inhibitor. ARG stands for arteriography. The associated percentage value is the criterion for positivity. Reference 44 is special because the interpretation is visual: the first line is all cases, the second unilateral disease and the third bilateral disease.

Reference	Type	Tracer	Metric	Sensitivity	#	Specificity	#	Criterion
36	B	G	any	0.64	11	0.8	5	ARG+
36	B	T	any	0.77	9	0.8	5	ARG+
36	C	G	any	1	11	0.8	5	ARG+
36	C	T	any	1	8	0.8	5	ARG+
37	B	G	α	0.7	10	0.75	8	ARG+
37	C	G	α	1	10	1	8	ARG+
37	C vs. B	G	$\gamma 1$	0.8	10	1	8	ARG+
38	B	G	$\alpha\beta\gamma$	0.49	49	0.98	159	>50%
38	C	G	C	0.94	49	0.98	159	>50%
39	C vs. B	T	$\gamma 1$	0.65	34	0.94	128	>50%
39	C vs. B	T	$\gamma 2$	0.68	34	0.85	128	>50%
39	C vs. B	T	$\gamma 3$	0.81	34	0.86	128	>50%
40	B	G	α	0.71	14	0.91	11	>50%
40	B	G	β	0.57	14	0.91	11	>50%
40	C vs. B	G	$\gamma 1$	0.5	14	1	11	>50%
40	C vs. B	G	$\gamma 3$	0.86	14	1	11	>50%
40	C vs. B	G	$\gamma 4$	0.93	14	0.91	11	>50%
41	C vs. B	G	$\alpha\beta\gamma$	0.91	58	0.87	55	ARG+
42	C vs. B	G & T	β and $\gamma 2$	0.92	36	0.93	31	>50%
43	C	T	$\gamma 2a$	0.93	14	0.93	14	ARG+
45	C	G	$\alpha 1$	0.74	31	0.44	109	ARG+
45	C	T	$\alpha 1$	0.71	31	0.41	109	ARG+
44	C		visual	0.91	58	0.72	18	cure
44	C		visual	0.95	37			
44	C		visual	0.86	21			

with normal renal function, but with RVH, the average (with captopril) is 70.6%, with a range from 18–100. Thirteen of 14 patients have a value larger than 30%. In patients with abnormal renal function, the averages (and ranges) are 36 (5–74) and 93.7 (48–100) respectively. The specificity is recovered in the azotemic patients by comparing the captopril renogram with a baseline renogram. The problem of the evaluation of renal clearance in patients with poor renal function will be revisited under the diuresis renogram.

Captopril allows one to detect bilateral, but not necessarily well-balanced renal artery stenosis (44).

Some cases are dramatic (45): In a 56-year-old man with severe familial hypertension and unilateral renal artery stenosis, captopril induced striking changes in the renograms of the affected kidney. After injection of ^{131}I-IOH, the percentage uptake was unchanged but the curve showed continuous accumulation even after 21 minutes. In contrast, the uptake of DTPA was zero. These changes demonstrate a cessation of filtration and maintenance of renal blood flow. After balloon dilatation of the stenosis, the blood pressure became lower, and these changes could no longer be demonstrated.

There are some reservations. de Zeeuw (30) finds that the renogram does not predict the good result of surgery perfectly (8/15 total response, 5/15 partial response, 2/15 no response) but the physical result of the surgery is not considered. Svetkey (46) also has disappointing results, but does not explicitly refer to changes between baseline and intervention. An interesting case of acquired and recurrent fibromuscular dysplasia diagnosed and monitored by captopril renography is presented by Thorstad (47). A synopsis of the results is given in Table 1.2 and illustrated in Figure 1.4; for the symbols and definitions for the operating characteristics, see Section 7.1.

Table 1.2 The table aggregates the results tabulated in Table 1.1. The symbols are the same. In addition, likelihood ratios are shown. The best results (highest likelihood ratio) is from the comparison of captopril renography with basal renography.

		P(S+|D−)	P(S+|D+)	LR
C vs. B	**ALL**	0.07	0.75	10.90
ALL	**G**	0.12	0.77	6.54
ALL	**ALL**	0.14	0.77	5.45
B	**All**	0.14	0.65	4.56
ALL	**T**	0.20	0.75	3.78
C	**All**	0.23	0.90	3.85

1.5. DIURESIS RENOGRAPHY: THE DIFFERENTIAL DIAGNOSIS OF OBSTRUCTION

1.5.1. *Basic Principle*

Contrast intravenous urography, ultrasonography and conventional radionuclide renography cannot reliably differentiate obstructive from non-obstructive causes of hydronephrosis (HN) and hydroureteronephrosis (HUN) (distension of the pelvi-calyceal system and ureter).

The pressure perfusion study or Whitaker test (48), which measures collecting system pressure under conditions of increased pelvic infusion rates, is relatively invasive but defining. The test defines "obstruction" as resistance to increased flow (Figure 1.5).

While the evaluation of function in the presence of obstruction does not give reliable indication of potential for recovery following surgical correction, high pressure in the collecting system results in reduction of renal blood flow and function. If the pressure exceeds the oncotic pressure at the glomerular level, glomerular filtration is stopped.

The purpose of diuretic renography is to differentiate a true obstruction from a dilated non-obstructed system (stasis) by serial imaging after intravenous administration of furosemide (Lasix).

A particular situation arises where anatomical imaging (often intra-uterine ultrasonography) reveals an enlarged collecting system or hydronephrosis connoting, but not always due to obstruction. Hydronephrosis detected *in utero* may resolve spontaneously and is related to physiologic change during early development. The question is whether there is a dilated (partially intrarenal) collecting system, or whether there is obstruction. The diagnosis of obstruction often requires sequential scintigraphic examinations.

We need to underscore a simple physical relation: the ratio of distance over velocity defines the time. In the same way, the ratio of volume over flow defines the time: $\bar{t} = V/F$ (see Section 9.1.1). Long transit times through the kidneys are either due to decreased nascent urine flow (F) or an increase of the total volume through which the urine flows. It is necessary to consider V carefully, and some have evaluated the ureter volume explicitly (49, 50). To follow the approach we first need to define obstruction. The common and radiological gestalt for obstruction is actually (eventually partial) occlusion. This leads to the terminology of sub-obstruction, but that approach is wrong.

Obstruction well understood is resistance to increased flow (48). One metaphor comes to mind. Early in the morning (at 6:00 a.m.), my commute to work takes

20 minutes, mostly over a four-lane freeway. At 8:00 a.m., the commute requires 40 minutes. It does not come to mind that the transit authorities managed to eliminate 2 of the 4 lanes between 6:00 and 8:00 a.m. What happened is that the flow of traffic increased but that the capacity of the freeway was reached.

In the case of the kidneys, we will start by saying that the collecting system does not have to accommodate any urine flow. The highest urine flow one can expect is one equal to the GFR. Testing how much flow can be accommodated is immediately done with the Whittaker test.

In renography, the same test is performed, but indirectly. To increase the flow, one uses Lasix (furosemide 1.0 mg/kg with a usual maximum dose of 40 mg). This suppresses water re-absorption and should increase tubular flow. If tubular flow is increased, the injection works as a flush, and the slow excretion of the injected tracer is (abruptly) accelerated (Figure 1.6). If there is resistance to flow, the pressure increases, and partially or totally counteracts the filtration pressure; GFR decreases or approaches zero, hence urine flow decreases. The system works as a negative feedback. In fact, Jacobsen (51) found that in confirmed obstruction: "Obstruction was found at the pressure flow studies in 7 of 14 patients (50%), while an obstructive pattern was found at diuresis renography in 12 of 13 patients (92%)". Due to a very low glomerular filtration rate, diuresis renography was equivocal in one case. Based upon these results, diuresis renography seems to be superior to pressure flow studies in cases with upper urinary tract obstruction.

1.5.2. *Indications*

- Ureteropelvic or ureterovesical obstruction.
- Prenatal ultrasound diagnosis of hydronephrosis.
- Postsurgical evaluation of a previously obstructed system.
- Distension of pelvicalyceal system as an etiology of back pain.

1.5.3. *Procedure*

The renogram is started as always, usually with the patient supine and the detector facing his back (under the table). The tracer is injected intravenously and after 12 minutes (this time varies), the furosemide is injected. At the end of the acquisition the data are analyzed.

1.5.3.1. *Preparation*

- Hydration: If the patient is not going to receive intravenous fluids, oral hydration is encouraged prior to arrival and while in the department.

- IV access: In all patients being evaluated for obstruction, an indwelling venous catheter should be inserted to maintain sufficient hydration for a good diuretic effect and obviate the necessity for repeated traumas from multiple percutaneous venous injections.
- Bladder catheterization: More controversial is the bladder catheterization. Reflux could act as an obstruction, so could a full bladder in some anatomical configurations. The advice to be careful in the presence of HUN and not to use a balloon catheter is welcome. Still, bladder catheterization is not without risk and is traumatic. In our service, all diuresis renograms referred from Pediatric Urology are performed with a bladder catheter in place to avoid false positive cases due to reflux or increased bladder pressure. If the urologist wants the catheterization to be omitted, the requisition will explicitly state this.[t]
- Sterile ureteral catheterization should be performed with the largest size Foley or feeding catheter that will comfortably pass the meatus: a 2.6-mm diameter catheter (French #8) for most patients and 1.8-mm diameter (French #6) for infants. A French #8 feeding catheter may also be used for continual bladder drainage.
- Continual drainage by catheterization of bladder is required in patients with hydroureter, vesicoureteral reflux, neurogenic bladder, a small capacity bladder, dysfunctional bladder or posterior ureteral valves.

1.5.3.2. *Renographic technique*

- Tracer: Using a tubular agent is recommended because plasma clearance is faster and in unobstructed cases as response to furosemide, so is the excretion phase.
- ROI: The authors recommend a renal ROI including the collecting system. We favor a renal ROI matching the renal parenchyma in the first 2 minutes of the renogram. They also defined the background as 2 pixels wide, although a pixel is not exactly part of the cgs system (Figures 1.2 and 1.6).
- Diuretic phase: The authors recommend a resetting of the ROIs. Our alternative is to analyze with multiple ROIs (Figure 1.7).
- Data analysis: The differential renal function corresponds to the net renal count ratio before excretion has taken place. Waiting for the appearance of activity in the collecting system may be late.
- Excretion phase: The excretion phase is used to evaluate the tubular transit time. There are different approaches, including the time at which furosemide

---

[t]This is actually very controversial and is more common in the US than Europe, where bladder catheterization is avoided.

is administered. We favor an injection at 12 minutes, because the effect of furosemide is well illustrated in normal cases, and the normal kidney is usually not emptied from radioactivity. If the emptying rate is estimated by a ratio, there is a *proviso*: The ratio of peak counts to counts at 20 minutes is a strange parameter. Peak counts may be reached before or after the furosemide injection. The question is "how does the normal kidney excretes, and what is the effect of furosemide". For the former, the 20% peak ratio is a fair measure; for the latter, it should be 20 minutes after furosemide injection or response and the ratio should be activity "20 minutes after overactivity at furosemide injection time".

1.5.4. *Interpretation*

The interpretation involves the same parameters discussed above. Descriptive parameters of the curve are the uptake ratio (in this case, nearly equal (47.3 vs. 52.5)), the time of peak activity[u] (3–4 minutes) and the half-emptying time (< 9 minutes). The time of peak activity is irrelevant, because whether the abnormality is obstruction or dilatation, if the transit time is prolonged, the peak time will be

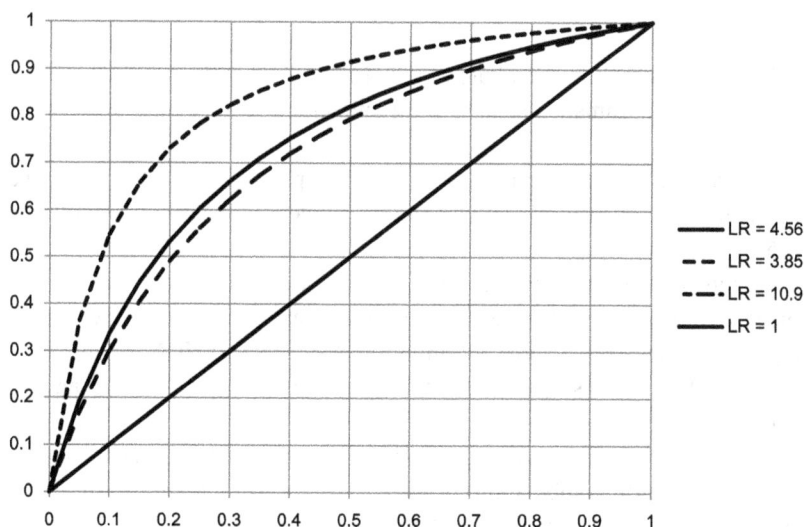

Figure 1.4 The figure illustrates Table 1.2, in which the likelihood ratio is shown for all tracers and all methods and separately for tubular or glomerular tracers and for basal, captopril and combined renography. The x-axis is the prevalence, the y-axis is the posterior probability for the LR values shown (see Section 7.2).

---

[u]The T_{max} is irrelevant if excretion is delayed before the administration of furosemide.

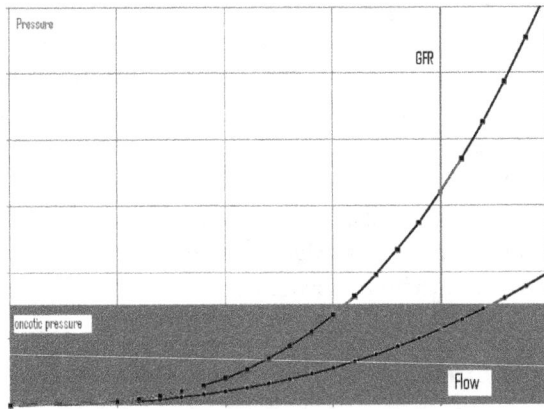

Figure 1.5   In the Whitaker test (48), a needle is placed in the collecting system, connected to a graduated flow pump and a pressure probe. Flow is gradually increased while pressure is monitored. If pressure increases at a rate well below the physiological urine rate (or GFR), there is obstruction (resistance to flow). If flow rates higher than physiological rates can be obtained, with a pressure below the filtration pressure (oncotic pressure) at the glomerular, there is no obstruction. The x-axis is flow, the y-axis is pressure.

late. The renal curve may continue to rise, but soon after the injection of Lasix, there should be a dramatic change almost amounting to a flushing of the system (Figure 1.4).

To further analyze the method, we will use the paper generated as a consensus paper by the Society of Fetal Urology and the Nuclear Medicine Pediatric council (52, 53).

The introduction starts by noting that perinatal HN and HUN[v] are now recognized five times more frequently than in the past because of the use of pre- and post-natal ultrasonography. But in most cases, HN and HUN do not connote obstruction. In some cases, anatomical imaging can identify an underlying cause. One cause could be vesicoureteral reflux.

The advantage of diuresis renography is that it evaluates both renal function and obstruction, both (in combination) of which are a basis for surgical intervention. The method has potential pitfalls, both in execution and interpretation.

Some authors propose a prior ultrasonography and cystouretrography (radiological?) to exclude anatomical abnormalities. A vesicoureteral reflux could act as an obstruction (see Section 1.5.3.1). They claim that the patient should be at least 1 month old, because GFR is low in newborns (54). It is interesting to note

---

[v]Hydronephrosis and hydrourethronephrosis.

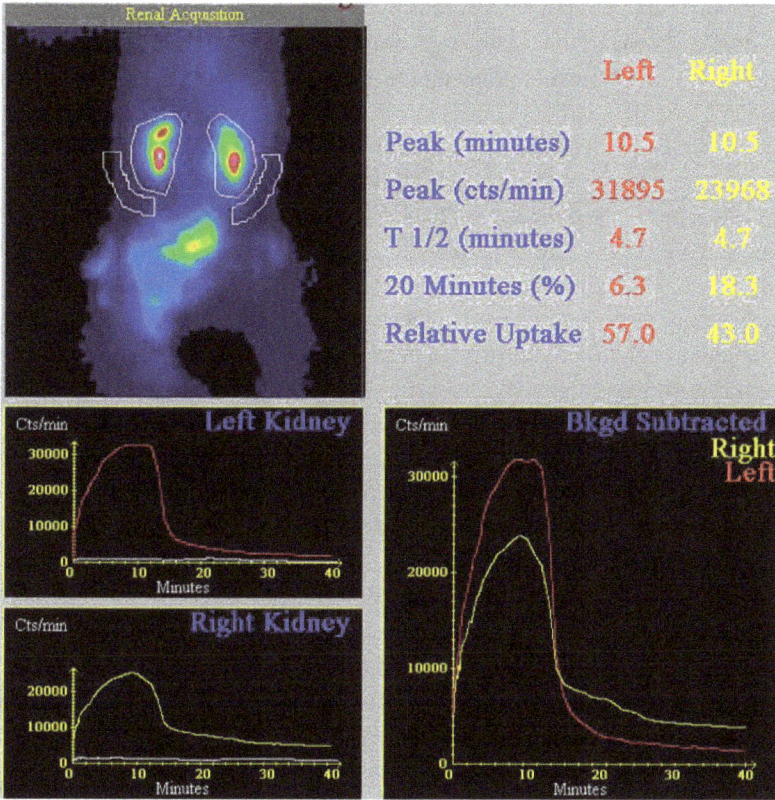

Figure 1.6 Diuresis renography: Lasix is administered 12 minutes into the renogram. The response is an abrupt clearance of the tracer from the kidneys. There is no obstruction.

that the basis for the assertion is that the heterolateral kidney without HN or HUN in infants less than a month old has a half emptying time of more than 9 minutes with furosemide, again illustrating that the "excretion phase" of the renogram also reflects plasma clearance (see Figure 1.6). Poor renal function decreases the rate of tracer excretion from the kidneys. However, a degree of obstruction (resistance to increased flow) can still be assumed if one kidney has a slower excretion than the other, since both kidneys "see" the same plasma (Section 8.4.1).

The authors also recommend excluding azotemia, again because low renal function would slow the excretion curve. This could partly be due to insensitivity to furosemide, but that was not demonstrated (55).

The relation between the downslope and renal function has been exhaustively preached by some (56–59) and a deconvolution of the plasma curve from the renographic curve has been proposed to overcome it. In fact, the technique was empirically shown by the direct injection of a tracer in the collecting system. Regardless of renal function, furosemide accelerated the excretion (60, 61) (Sections 8.4.1 and 10.7.3).

Nevertheless, as a parameter or metric of excretion rate we prefer the slope or $T_{1/2}$ of the steepest fit of an exponential, either after furosemide, or after the maximum is reached in the normal case. In fact, Zechman (62) considers an exponential response a sign of positive response. Rossleight (63) makes an implicit point that a well-functioning kidney may not appear to respond to furosemide, because it is already empty. If the heterolateral kidney appears normal, we start the exponential fit search not after the administration of furosemide, but at T_{max} (Section 10.2).

Even if one can sample plasma activity with fair accuracy, the deconvolution technique remains difficult, and much influenced by noise in the data. An alternative method is to derive what the renal curve would have been had there been no excretion. This is easily done by scaling an integral of the first derivative of the plasma clearance curve to the first part of the renogram (before excretion starts). This curve will diverge from the actual renographic curve when excretion starts. The divergence will be large and fast when there is no obstruction, and small and late when there is. The distinction between poor global renal function and obstruction becomes obvious (Figure 1.3), but is not exactly quantifiable. This technique is based on the same principle as the excretion index proposed by Tauxe discussed in the next section (see Section 1.6).

A number of renographic patterns are proposed: a normal, immature, stasis or obstruction or poor function. The immature response could be the result of late filling of a large and compliant collecting system (Figure 1.7). O'Reilly (64) also looked at patterns, but performed a standard renogram 4 minutes after the diuretic. Koff (61) also described typical patterns, but did look at the collecting system separately.

The relationship between renal function and the response to furosemide needs to be underscored. Of course, a decrease in GFR would occur in bilateral obstruction, but barring that, GFR and creatinine clearance correlated with the urine flow 3–6 and 15–18 minutes after furosemide injection (65). The urine flow rate is higher after 15–18 minutes than after 3–6. This is, in part, the rationale for the F-15 versus the F + 20 injection of furosemide. In the well-tempered renogram, furosemide is injected at 20 minutes, which appears late for a 30-minute renogram, considering that the response may be delayed. We acquire for 40 minutes, and administer furosemide at 12 minutes.[W] But a pre-injection 15 minutes before the injection of the tracer has been suggested to yield less ambiguous results because of the potential late response (65) to furosemide. Another rational for the F-15 method (66) is to avoid false negatives if there is a large, empty and compliant collecting system (Figure 1.7). The importance of analyzing the pelvis and the ureters is underscored by Jamar (67).

Lupton (68, 69) validated the method by pathological analysis of anatomical specimens and by the results of corrective surgery. The result of the latter validation deserves to be noted. Of the 21 cases diagnosed as obstructed by diuresis renography, 20 were non-obstructed after surgery. Two equivocal cases before, were normal after.

Lupton (70) compared parenchymatic transit times (obtained by deconvolving the plasma input curve from the renal output function) and classic diuresis renography.[X] There were 36 patients (46 kidneys) with urographically demonstrated renal pelvic dilatation. The mean transit times obtained by deconvolution

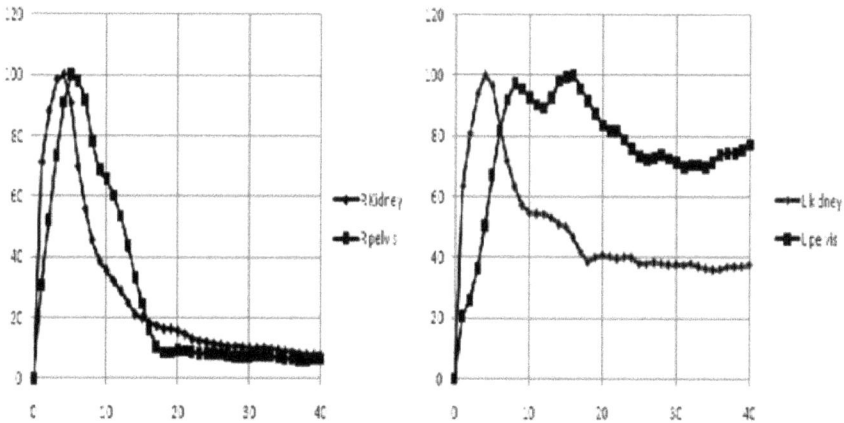

Figure 1.7   Filling of a compliant or empty collecting system with a partial or incomplete response of the left kidney. In the normal R kidney (seen in the left panel), the filling and emptying of the pelvis follows but mimics the renal parenchyma. In the left kidney (seen in the right panel), the parenchyma seems to empty, but as the collecting system fills, the emptying of the parenchyma slows down.

[W]The disadvantage is that we do not know if the diuretic injection was really necessary, because it is difficult to visually evaluate if there is tracer retention in the collecting system.
[X]The parenchymatic transit time would, thus, be independent of plasma clearance rates and global renal function.

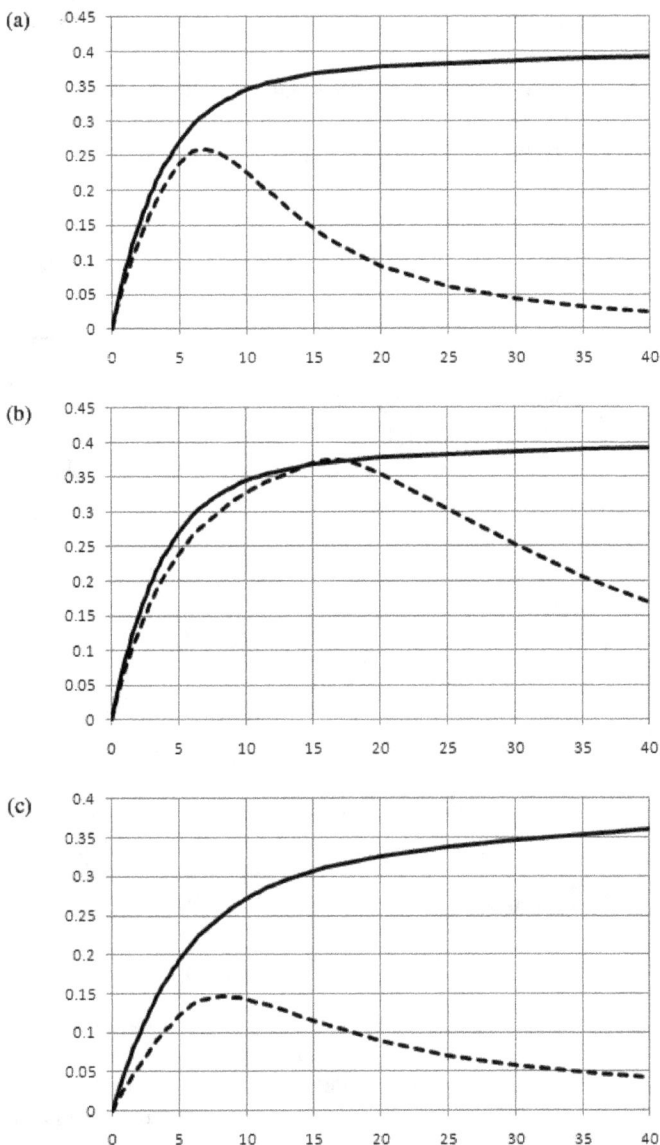

Figure 1.8   In panel A, a normal renogram is shown. The fitted curve is the integral of the plasma clearance curve, scaled to the renographic upslope prior to excretion. In panel B, a case of obstruction is shown: T_{max} comes late, and the area between the fitted curve and the renographic curve is relatively smaller. In panel C, a case of decrease global renal function, the downslope rate of the renal curve is slower, but the area between renal and fitted curve is still large.

analysis of the parenchymal renograms of eight normal volunteers had a mean value of 2.8 ± 0.6 (S.D.) minutes, and the upper limit of normal was thus established as 4 minutes. Twenty-two of 29 kidneys (76%) with non-obstructive diuresis renograms had parenchymal mean transit times of 4 minutes or below. Fourteen out of 17 kidneys (82%) with obstructive diuresis renograms had parenchymal mean transit times above 4 minutes.

It is not easy to come up with hard and fast normal values. Carlsen (71) gives the IOH and presumably MAG3 L/R split as $0.51 \pm 0.03 / 0.49 \pm 0.03$ and a plasma clearance for hippuran of 518 ± 142 ml/min/1.73m^2. The renal transit time is 4.2 minutes. Erbslöh-Möller (43) finds that renovascular hypertension is unlikely if the T_{20min} value was less than 30% (with IOH). The parenchymatic transit time in the normal kidney was bracketed between 243 ± 46 and 271 ± 95 seconds (± 4.5 min) by Dondi (39). Koff (54) seems to be setting the upper limit of normal for $T_{1/2}$ at 9 minutes, at least for normal global function. Lupton (70) sets the maximum parenchymatic transit time at 4 minutes. Normal T_{max} was below 5 minutes for DTPA and below 3 minutes for IOH according to Rocatello (42). For Rossleigh (63), $T_{1/2}$ is less than 9.8, with MAG3 with an average of 3.4 minutes.

In kidneys of children without dilated collecting system and good function with MAG3, we found T_{max} to be less than 3.2 and $T_{1/2}$ (by exponential fit) to be less than 5.5. If $T_{1/2}$ is more than 6 or 8 minutes and the heterolateral side is less than 5.5, we call the study positive for obstruction, understood as resistance to increased physiological urine flow.

1.6. THE APPLICATION OF RENOGRAPHY IN RENAL TRANSPLANTATION

In general, after renal transplantation there are four situations that may require intervention: acute rejection, vascular injury (e.g. obstruction), urine leak and outflow tract obstruction. In addition, one has to deal with the possibility of acute tubular necrosis (ATN). The semiotics of the renogram are not very complex, as we have seen before. Acute rejection, ATN, and vascular injury would all be associated with poor tracer uptake and prolonged transit times, as would acute obstruction. Only urine leaks are generally easy to detect.

Attempts were made to refine a differential diagnosis. Anaise (72) proposed the cortical perfusion index. The index is based on observations during the arterial phase of a bolus injection of ^{99m}Tc-DTPA. The index is based on a ratio of the area under the arterial curve from $t = 0$ to $t = T_{max}$ of the bolus, divided by the ratio of the renal activity in the same time interval. Lower renal (capillary) flow results in a higher ratio or perfusion index. The ratio is calculated for three regions of interest, one global renal, one cortical and one medullary.[y] He found that the increase in this ratio (from a previous renogram in the normal state) effectively differentiated acute rejection from (drug or viral) nephropathy and obstruction; the index increased only for acute rejection. The best discriminator was the cortical index, with a sensitivity of 94% and a specificity of 94%. However, a binary limit was not given and a differential with ATN was not considered (see also Pattak plot in Section 9.4).

Ash (73) seems to refine the method, introducing two observational variations: one a correction for kidney depth, one a "search" for the best location for the vascular ROI (in this case aortic). The vascular bolus is fitted by gamma fit and integrated (Section 10.7.6). The maximum upslope of the renal (arterial) curve is also fitted. Normalization is obtained on the basis of the relative values of the maximum upslope of the renal and gamma curves. The cardiac output is derived from the integrated aortic gamma function and the total injected dose (both in cpm). The resulting metric is the renal blood flow as a percentage of the cardiac output (Section 9.5). The results are characterized by two facts: the differential diagnosis considers only normal or rejection, but differentiates between chronic, mild or severe. Both authors cited here do not explicitly consider the influence of the size of the ROI (kidney versus vascular).

Hilson (74), however, does. His approach is otherwise not different from that of Anaise. He adds a statistical weight to the perfusion index based on the counts in the area. He shows that the perfusion index is highest (on average) in patients with rejection, but also increases (but less) in ATN and renal artery stenosis.

If it is true that the renogram's semiotics are too reduced for complex differential diagnoses, the general approach discussed here is even more reductive. A more sophisticated approach originated with Tauxe (75, 76, 77) and Yester (78) and was explicitly applied to the differential diagnosis in transplantation by Dubovsky (79).

The first step is to determine the global function, as expressed by the effective renal plasma flow. This can be done (see Section 1.7) by the single injection method and multiple plasma sample counting. Tauxe (75, 76) introduced an approach (for hippuran) with a single plasma sample, taken at 44 minutes (Section 8.4). The formula is entirely empiric, and was derived from a large spectrum of patients, including healthy volunteer kidney donors. The parameters are: the expected maximum effective renal plasma flow F_{max}, a slope α, an intercept V_{lag} and a theoretical distribution volume at 44 minutes:

$$ERPF = F_{max}(1 - e^{-\alpha(V_t - V_{lag})}).$$

---

[y]The idea that in planar (projection) images one can separate cortex from medulla is quaint, if generally accepted out of necessity.

Table 1.3   The actual graph is available in Ref. 79.

	ERPF	EI
Normal	Normal	Normal
Chronic rejection	Low	Low
Chronic rejection	Moderate	High
Acute rejection	Proportionally moderate	
ATN	Moderate	Very low

The normal value would be larger than 300 ml/min/1.73 m^2.

The next step is to define an expected excretion (77, 78). The approach is not fundamentally different from that described above (diuresis renography): If the transit times are normal, the uptake of the tracer by the kidney must predict the excretion to the bladder with a fixed transit time. Yester found that the expected excretion at 35 minutes, expressed as a percentage of the dose (ED%) was related to the ERPF as:

$$ED\% = 79.3[1 - e^{-0.00479 \times ERPF}]^z.$$

If the actual excretion (amount in the voided urine + residual activity in bladder) is X, the excretion index EI is X/ED%. The normal value would be close to 1.

First, since in general there is only one kidney functioning in the case of transplants, the global parameters (ERPF and EI) apply entirely to the transplanted kidney.[aa] There are now two parameters. Dubovsky (79) looked at the vectorial distribution of those parameters in five states and found the results shown in Table 1.3.

1.7. GLOMERULAR FILTRATION RATE

With Hongyun J. Zhu, MD and Jagruti Shaw, MD.

1.7.1. *Background*

In the two-compartmental method used to measure the glomerular excretion rate (GFR) with sodium iodothalamate I-125, the primary metric is the fractional

---

[z]See Section 8.5.4 and Figure 8.7.

[aa]This is not always true. We have seen some cases where the native kidneys contributed significantly to the global renal function. The distribution of the ERPF to each kidney can easily be obtained from regions of interest. The contribution to urine is harder, unless the tubular transit times are calculated for each kidney.

excretion rate (a_{13}) from compartment I. The GFR is derived by multiplying this value by the distribution or dilution volume (DV). The GFR is then normalized (nGFR) on the basis of body surface area. This normalization does not, however, maintain a strict congruency between a_{13} and nGFR if the relation between BSA and DV is not linear. This creates a problem since clinicians require the results under the form of nGFR and not as a fractional excretion rate.

The clinical custom to express glomerular filtration rates (GFR) as milliliter per minutes, normalized to a body surface area (BSA) results from the original methods to measure GFR.

In the original method, the plasma concentration $c(t)$ (g/ml), during an interval 0–T (min), of a filtered substance, is compared to the total amount Q (g) recuperated over the time T (min). Explicitly,

$$Q_T = GFR \int_0^T c(t)dt,$$

although the integral is often replaced by an average multiplied by the time interval:

$$\int_0^T c(t)dt = \bar{c} \times T,$$

and therefore,

$$GFR = \frac{Q_T}{\bar{c} \times T}.$$

The resulting units are therefore:

$$GFR = Q_t(g) \times \frac{1}{\bar{c} \times T} \left(\frac{ml}{g \times min} \right),$$

that reduces to:

$$\frac{g \times ml}{min \times g} = \frac{ml}{min}.$$

With the constant infusion method, if the rate of infusion is k (g/min) when the plasma concentration becomes constant ($c(\infty)$ g/ml), GFR is equal to k/ $c(\infty)$, therefore $\frac{g}{min} \div \frac{g}{ml} = \frac{g \times ml}{min \times g}$ g or again ml/min (Section 8.3).

Normalization is necessary, since the physiological relevant value is the fraction of the tracer in the distribution volume DV (assumed to be a measure of part of the extracellular fluid volume or ECF) that is cleared or filtered per unit of time. Larger volumes in larger subjects require larger GFR values (a normal value for an elephant would not be a normal value for a mouse.

1.7.2. *Single Injection Method*

In contradistinction, the single injection two-compartmental model (Sections 8.5 and 8.5.3) proposed by Sapirstein (80) and used by Blaufox (81) yields a fractional rate directly. The two-compartmental model yields a function composed of two exponentials:

$$c(t) = C_A e^{-\alpha t} + C_B e^{-\beta t}.$$

The observables are the concentrations in the plasma samples. C_A and C_B are the extrapolated intercepts for the fast and slow exponential fit. The injected dose (D) divided by the sum of the concentrations $A + B$ defined the plasma volume or compartment 1. The fractional excretion rate a_{13} of the first compartment is defined by,

$$a_{13} = \frac{\alpha\beta(C_A + C_B)}{C_A\beta + C_B\alpha}.^{bb}$$

This is the approach we have used: The tracer was iodine-125-labeled Glofil,[cc] while the dose was $50\,\mu$Ci. Blood samples were taken at 5, 15, 25,120, 180 and 240 minutes, and the plasma concentration expressed as counts per minute (cpm). The injected dose was also expressed as cpm. The two exponentials were fitted by curve peeling and linear regression after a logarithmic transformation. The derivation of a_{13} was done according to the formulation in the introduction.

The fractional excretion rate a_{13} does not require normalization, and has units 1/min independently of the distribution volume. It defines the fraction of tracer leaving compartment 1 through the kidneys per unit of time. However, since clinicians are not familiar with this metric, the GFR is obtained by multiplying a_{13} $\min^{-1}$ by the distribution volume (DV), given by dividing the injected dose (D) by the initial (extrapolated) concentration (in this case $DV = D/(C_A + C_B)$ ml). The resulting value for GFR then requires normalization, since it is volume dependent. The usual normalization is by body surface area (BSA) expressed in m^2.

$$nGFR = measured\ GFR \frac{1.73}{patient\ BSA} ml/min/1.73\,m^2.$$

Implicitly, this normalization assumes that the BSA is a good predictor of the distribution volume (DV) or the extracellular fluid (ECF) volume. *A priori* the assumption can be faulted on two counts: in children that may not apply (82, 83), and in individual patients with a variety of pathologies, the ECF volume may be abnormal.

[bb] See Section 8.5.3.
[cc] Sodium Iothalamate I-125, Questor pharmaceutical.

Table 1.4   BSA computations.

---

a. Gehan

$$BSA = 0.02350 \cdot H^{0.42246} \times W^{0.51456} \text{ m}^2$$

b. Dubois & Dubois

$$BSA = 0.007184 \cdot H^{0.725} \times W^{0.425} \text{ m}^2$$

c. Haycock

$$BSA = 0.024265 \cdot H^{0.3964} \times W^{0.5378} \text{ m}^2$$

d. Mosteller

$$BSA = \sqrt{\frac{H \times W}{3600}} \text{ m}^2$$

a. Boyd (W in g)

$$BSA = 0.0003207 \times H^{0.3} \times 1000 \times W^{(0.7285 - 18.8 \ln(W))} \text{ m}^2$$

The problem is unrelated to the BSA calculation. There are a number of formulae to calculate BSA. The derivation by Gehan (84), Dubois and Dubois (85), Haycock (86), Mosteller (87) and Boyd (88) all yield very much the same results (Table 1.4), at least for the patients we studied. The problem therefore does not lie with the BSA. What is surprising, however, is that the BSA is used for normalization for what is in essence a volumetric normalization.

Since a_{13} does not require normalization, if the normalization by BSA were correct, there would be a one to one correspondence between a_{13} and the normalized nGFR. In fact, there is not; the standard error of the estimate (SEE) is equal to 28 ml/min or 25% of the average value of 109 ml/min, large enough to change a normal value to an abnormal one or vice-versa (Figure 1.9). The regression between a_{13} and the normalized nGFR is nGFR $= 20.4 + 6256 \times a_{13}$ (F $= 182$, p < 0.0001). The normal value for nGFR is 120 ml/min/m^2; the normal value for a_{13} is therefore 0.016.

There is another problem: the distribution volume (DV) that we found is not the extracellular fluid volume (ECF) predicted by Peters (82) and Bird (83) (ECF $= 0.02154 \times W^{0.6469} \times H^{0.7236}$) ml.[dd] In fact ECF $= 1338 + 1.22 \times DV$. In

---

[dd] Unless stated otherwise, H is height in cm, W is weight in kg.

DV vs BSA

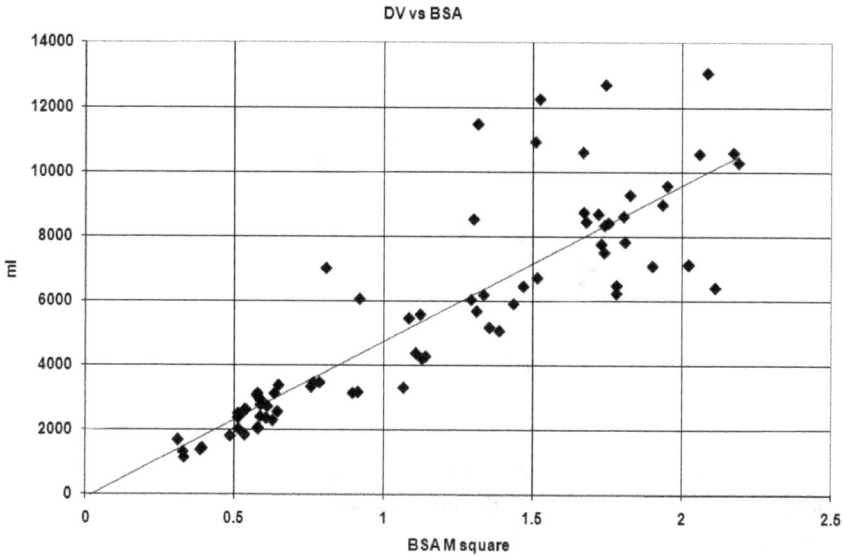

Figure 1.9   The distribution volume of the tracer in compartment 1 is plotted against the BSA computed by the Dubois and Dubois method. The error is very large, but against expectations the relation between a volume (cm^3) and an area (m^2) is linear.

addition, the difference between DV and ECF correlates with age: $(DV - ECF) = -966 - 110 \times ECF$.

Surprisingly, the measured distribution volume DV is related to the BSA (85) by linear regression as DV (ml) $= 4820 \times BSA(m^2)$-65 (Figure 1.10). The SEE is 1550.0 or 28% of the average DV value (Figure 1.9).

There are two crucial data. First, if a_{13} is known, the normalized GFR can be derived from the coefficients of the regression equation $nGFR = 20.4 + 6256 \times a_{13}$.

Second, if a_{13} is known, the GFR normalized to $1.73\,m^2$ is derived by $nGFR = a_{13} \times (4820 \pm 1550 \times 1.73 - 65)$.

The two ways to compute nGFR are in fact equivalent, if the standard error of the estimate is taken into account (Figure 1.10).

Bird and Peters (82, 83), like us, assumed that in children, the BSA would not be a good predictor of the ECF volume, because the BSA of children would be relatively larger (because smaller volumes have a relatively larger surface than larger volumes). Their normalization was therefore based on a predicted volume. The normalized GFR (nGFR) would be, they claimed, more accurate by using the formula $nGFR = GFR*12.9/ECV$, where 12.9 liter was the expected ECV for a standard man (or woman). Our data suggest 8.33 (Figure 1.9). Nevertheless, to

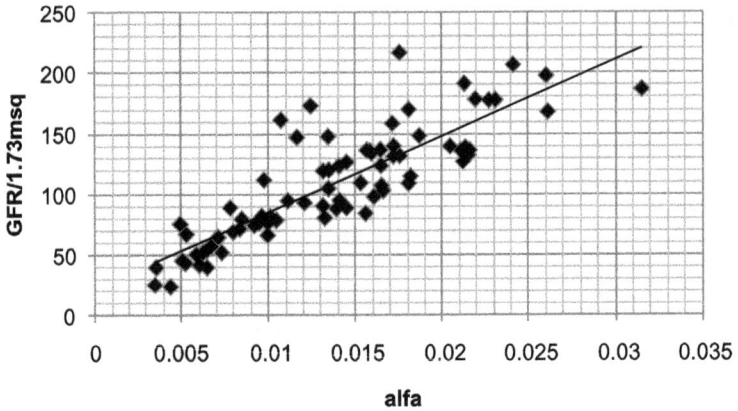

Figure 1.10 The normalized GFR (ml/min/m^2) is plotted against the fractional excretion rate alfa (a_{13} in the text), to illustrate that they correlated but are not identical. The Standard error of the estimate is 28 ml/min/m^2).

eliminate the assumption that BSA and distribution volumes are linearly related is useful. However, in the two-compartmental model, the product $a_{13} \times DV$ may be subject to error propagation, because the measurements of the injected dose (D) requires dilution of a standard and because the intercept value (A + B) by curve peeling may vary greatly for small error in the slopes. In the single-slope model used by Peters, however, there is an assumption that underestimates in the slope are compensated (partially) by overestimates of the distribution volume. It follows that the single exponential method would be more robust than the two-compartmental model with two exponentials and curve peeling (Figure 1.11 and Section 8.2.5).

In the single-slope method, only the late data points are fitted, and to a single exponential (Figure 1.12).

The difference in scale between DV (and PDV) and ECF by Peters is due to the single-slope method. The intercept of the single-slope method would lie between the values of (A + B) and (B), but closer to B, depending on the timing of the sampling and the kinetics of the exchange rates between the compartments. In all cases, the intercept of the single exponential (B) is lower than (A + B), which explains that our DV corresponding to a 1.73 m^2 is smaller than the value given by Peters and Bird (82, 83).

Using a "normal" or average value for the distribution volume as well as for the normalization factor eliminates the discrepancy between the primary metric a_{13} and the normalized GFR, regardless of the patient's status.

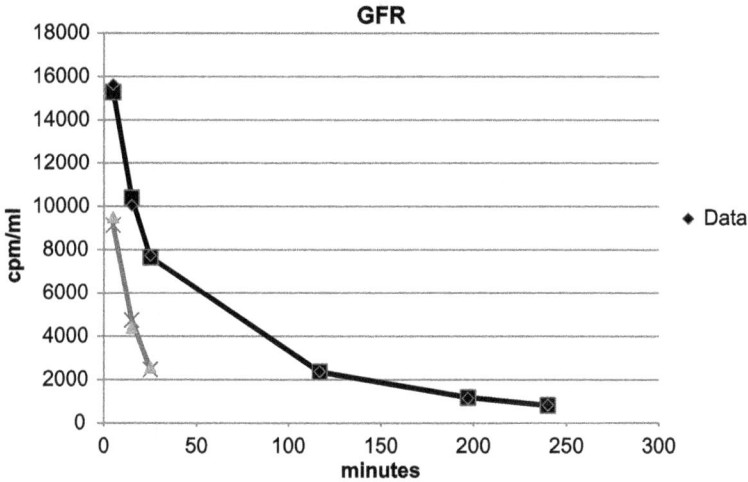

Figure 1.11 The figure illustrates curve peeling in the analysis of GFR plasma sampling data. The last three points are fitted to an exponential ($C_B e^{-\beta t}$), which is extrapolated towards earlier time, and the extrapolated values are subtracted from the early three points. The resulting values are again fitted to an exponential ($C_A e^{-\alpha t}$); what Peters does is equivalent to utilizing the last three points only.

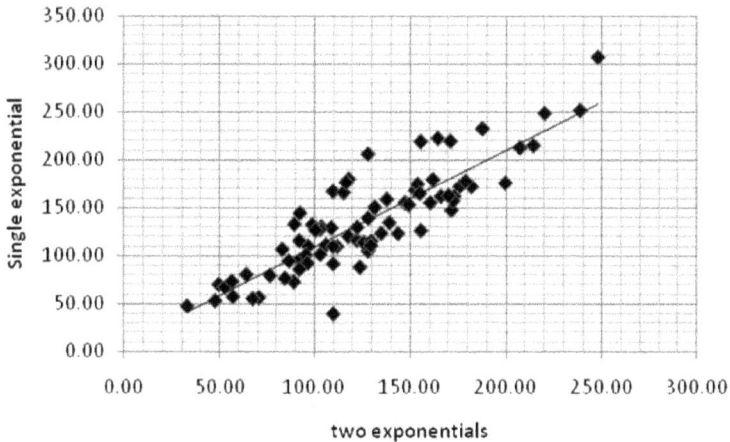

Figure 1.12 Correlation between GFR values obtained for two exponential and single exponential fitting. The regression line is not significantly different from the identity line.

Table 1.5   Patient population.

82 patients, 29 females
Weight: 38.9 ± 27 (6–99) kg
Height: 128 ± 38.9 (51–189) cm
Age: 13.7 ± 14.8 (0.03–69.4) years

Still, the second and more likely error is the discrepancy of predicted (normal) distribution volume values and the actual values in patients in various states of health or states of hydration (89). The goal should be to avoid measuring distribution volumes, and derive the nGFR from a_{13}.

Finally, one should perhaps rethink the possibility of normalizing differently for males and females, as is done for plasma volumes, although the resulting discrepancy is neither large nor statistically significant (Table 1.5).

1.7.3. *Conclusion*

In conclusion, the usual and clinically accepted method to express GFR as $ml/min/1.73\,m^2$ is an effect of historical development, maintained by acculturation and is unlikely to change. The effort to normalize the results introduces errors as the normalization is based on a ratio of a "normal" distribution volume of a standard man and the actual distribution volume in a potentially sick patient. The direct determination of the fractional excretion rate (1/min) vacates the need for normalization, but the cultural need to transform to a normalized GFR remains. We propose that the normalization should be based on the "normal" distribution volume of the patient's height and weight as well as on the "normal" distribution volume of standard man (H = 175 cm and W = 60 kg).

In a prospective study of 108 cases, the value of a_{13} corresponding to a GFR or $120\,ml/min/m^2$ was still $0.016\,min^{-1}$.

REFERENCES

1. Handmaker H. Etude renale fonctionnelle differntielle simple a l'aide du 99m- technetium DMSA. *Compte rendu du II colloque Intl*, Paris 1975; pp. 225–232.
2. Handmaker H, Young BW, Lowenstein JM. Clinical experience with 99m-Tc-DMSA (dimercaptosuccinic acid), a new renal-imaging agent. *J Nucl Med* 1975; 16(1):28–32.
3. Bubeck B, Brandau W, Weber E, Kälble T, Parekh N, Georgi P. Pharmacokinetics of technetium-99m-MAG3 in humans. *J Nucl Med* 1990; 31:1285–1293.

4. duCret RP, Boudreau RJ, Gonzalez R, Carpenter R, Tennison J, Kuni CC. Clinical efficacy of 99m-technetium mercaptoacetylglycine kit formulation in routine renal scintigraphy. *J Urol* 1989; 142:19–22.

5. Muller-Suur R, Bois-Svennsson I, Mesko L. A comparative study of renal scintigraphy and clearance with technetium-99m-MAG3 and iodine-123-hippurate in patients with renal disorders. *J Nucl Med* 1990; 31:1811–1817.

6. Russell CD, Thorstad B, Yester MV, Stutzman M, Baker T, Dubovsky EV. Comparison of technetium-99m-MAG3 with iodine-131 hippuran by a simultaneous dual channel technique. *J Nucl Med* 1988; 29:1189–1193.

7. Taylor A Jr, Eshima D, Christian PE, Milton W. Evaluation of Tc-99m mercaptoacetyltriglycine in patients with impaired renal function. *Radiology* 1987; 162:365–370.

8. Taylor A Jr, Ziffer JA, Steves A, Eshima D, Delaney VB, Welchel JD. Clinical comparison of I-131 orthoiodohippurate and the kit formulation of Tc-99m mercaptoacetyltriglycine. *Radiology* 1989; 170:721–725.

9. Taylor A Jr, Ziffer JA, Eshima D. Comparison of Tc-99m MAG3 and Tc-99m DTPA in renal transplant patients with impaired renal function. *Clin Nucl Med* 1990; 15:371–378.

10. Stoffel M, Jamar F, Van Nerom C, Verbruggen A, Mourad M, Leners N, Squifflet JP, Beckers C. Evaluation of technetium-99m-L,L-EC in renal transplant recipients: a comparative study with technetium-99m-MAG3 and iodine-125-OIH. *J Nucl Med* 1994; 35:1951–1958.

11. Shames DM and Korebkin M. A Simple Technique for Measuring Relative Renal Blood Flow. *J Nucl Med* 1976; 17:876–879.

12. Harris CC, Ford KK, Coleman RE, Dunnick NR. Effect of Region Assignment on Relative Renal Blood Flow Estimates Using Radionuclides. *Radiology* 1984; 151:791–792.

13. Piepsz A, Dobbeleir A, Ham HR. Effect of Background Correction on Separate Technetium-99m-DTPA Renal Clearance. *J Nucl Med* 1990; 31:430–435.

14. Aburano T, Shuke N, Yokoyama K, Matsuda H, Takayama T, Michigishi T, Tonami N, Hisada K. Renal Perfusion with Tc-99m DTPA–Simple Noninvasive Determination of Extraction Fraction and Plasma Flow. *Clin Nucl Med* 1993; 18:573–577.

15. Patlak CS, Blasberg RG, Fenstermacher JD. "Graphical evaluation of blood-to-brain transfer constants from multiple-time uptake data". *J Cereb Blood Flow Metab* 1083; 3:1–7.

16. Patlak CS, Blasberg RG. Graphical evaluation of blood-to-brain transfer constants from multiple-time uptake data. Generalizations. *J Cereb Blood Flow Metab* 1985; 5:584–590.

17. Kontzen FN, Tobin M, Dubovsky EV, Tauxe WN. Comprehensive Renal Function Studies: Technical Aspects. *J Nucl Med Tech* 1977; 5:81–84.

18. Brock M, Feneley RCL, Davies ER. Renography as a prognostic index of urinary tract problems in childhood. *Br J Urol.* 1977; 49:261–267.

19. Bueschen AJ, Lloyd LK, Dubovsky EV, Tauxe WN. Radionuclide kidney evaluation in the management of urolithiasis. *J Urol* 1978; 120:16–20.

20. Peters AM. Quantification of renal haemodynamics with radionuclides. *Eur J Nucl Med* 1991 (b); 18:274–286.

21. DeGrazia JA, Scheibe PO, Jackson PE, Lucas ZJ, Fair WR, Vogel JM, Blumin LJ. Clinical applications of a kinetic model of hippurate distribution and renal clearance. *J Nucl Med* 1974; 15:102–114.

22. Frøkiaer J, Knudsen L, Fl C, Hansen HH, Eika B, Mortensen J, Jensen FT. Reproducibility of iodine-123-hippuran renoscintigraphy in the normal pig at various (urine) flow rates. *Scand J Urol Nephrol Suppl* 1989; 125:87–93.

23. Kempi V, Persson BR. Evaluation of renal function parameters with simultaneously administered 99mTc-DTPA and 131I-hippuran. *Eur J Nucl Med* 1983; 8:65–71.

24. Stamey TA, Nudelman IJ, Good PH, Schwentker FN, Hendricks F. Functional characteristics of renovascular hypertension. *Medicine* 1961; 40:347–392.

25. Stamey TA. Measurement of renal vein renins or differential renal fraction studies in the diagnosis of curable renovascular hypertension. *Urol Res.* Plenum press. 1972; 131–148.

26. Schaefer AJ, Stamey TA. Urethral Catheterization studies. *Urol Clin North Am* 1975; 2:327–335.

27. Nally JV, Black HR. State-of-the-Art Review. Captopril Renography-Pathophysiological considerations and clinical observations. *Semin Nucl Med* 1992; 22:84–97.

28. Wilcox CS, Smith TB, Frederickson ED, Wingo CD, Phillips MI, Williams CM. The captopril glomerular filtration rate renogram in renovascular hypertension. *Clin Nucl Med* 1989; Jan;14(1):1–7.

29. Kopecky RT, Thomas D, McAffee JG. Furosemide augments the effect of captopril on nuclear studies in renovascular stenosis. *Hypertension* 1987; 10:181–188.

30. de Zeeuw D, Jonker GJ, Hovinga TK, Beekhuis H, Piers DA, Huisman RM, de Jong PE. The mechanism and diagnostic value of angiotensin I converting enzyme inhibition renography. *Am J Hypertens* 1991; 4:741S–744S.

31. Lee HB, Blaufox MD. Technetium-99m MAG-3 clearance after captopril in experimental renovascular hypertension. *J Nucl Med* 1988; 30:666–671.

32. McAfee JG, Kopecky RT, Thomas FD Hellwig B, Roskopf M. Comparison of different radioactive agents for the detection of renovascular hypertension with captopril in the rat model. *J Nucl Med* 1988; 29:509–515.

33. Gale B, Zhang C, Lee HB, Heller S, Blaufox MD. The effect of captopril on glucoheptonate uptake in experimental renal artery stenosis. *Nucl Med Commun* 1992; 13(2):110–113.

34. Peters AM, Brown J, Crossman D, Brady AJ. Noninvasive Measurement of Renal Blood Flow with Technetium-99m-DTPA in the Evaluation of Patients with Suspected Renovascular Hypertension. *J Nucl Med* 1990; 31:1980–1985.

35. Nally JV, Clarke HS, Windham JP, s GP, Gross ML, Potvin WJ. Technetium-99m DTPA renal flow studies in Goldblatt hypertension. *J Nucl Med* 1985; 26:917–924.

36. Nally JV, Gupta BK, Clarke HS, Higgins JT Jr, Potvin WJ, Gross ML. Captopril renography for the detection of renovascular hypertension. *Cleve Clin J Med* 1988; 311–318.

37. Fommei E, Ghione S, Palla L, Mosca F, Ferrari M, Palombo C, Giaconi S, Gazzetti P, Donato L. Renal scintigraphic captopril testing the diagnosis of renovascular hypertension. *Hypertension* 1987; 10:212–220.

38. Dondi M, Franchi R, Levorato M, Zuccala A. Evaluation of Hypertensive Patients by Means of Captopril Enhanced Renal Scintigraphy with Technetium-99m DTPA. *J Nucl Med* 1989; 30:615–621.

39. Dondi M, Monetti N, Fanti S, Marchetta F, Corbelli C, Zagni P, De Fabritis A, Losinno F, Levorato M, Zuccalá A. Use of technetium-99m-MAG3 for renal scintigraphy after angiotensin-converting enzyme inhibition. *J Nucl Med* 1991; 32:424–428.

40. Pedersen EB, Jensen FT, Eiskjoer H, Hansen HH. Differentiation between renovascular and essential hypertension by means of changes in single kidney 99mTc-DTPA clearance induced by angiotensin-converting enzyme inhibition. *Am J Hypertens* 1989; 2:323–333.

41. Setaro JF, Chen CC, Hoffer PB, Black HR. Captopril renography in the diagnosis of renal artery stenosis and the prediction of improvement with revascularization: the yale vascular center experience. *Am J Hypertens* 1991; 4:698S–705S.

42. Roccatello D, Picciotto G, Rabbia C, Pozzato M, De Filippi PG, Piccoli G. Prospective study on captopril renography in hypertensive patients. *Am J Nephrol* 1992; 12(6):406–411.

43. Erbslöh-Möller B, Dumas A, Roth D, Sfakianakis GN, Bourgoignie JJ. Furosemide-131I-hippuran renography after angiotensin-converting enzyme inhibition for the diagnosis of renovascular hypertension. *Am J Med* 1991; 90:23–29.

44. Geyskes GG, de Bruyn AJ. Captopril renography and the effect of percutaneous transluminal angioplasty on blood pressure in 94 patients with renal artery stenosis. *Am J Hypertens* 1991; 4:685S–689S.

45. Geyskes 1991 Geyskes GG, Oei HY, Puylaert CB, Mees EJD. Renography with captopril: changes in a patient with hypertension and unilateral renal artery stenosis. *Arch Intern Med* 1986; 146:1705–1708.

46. Svetkey LP, Wilkinson R Jr, Dunnick NR, Smith SR, Dunham CB, Lambert M, Klotman PE. Captopril renography in the diagnosis of renovascular disease. *Am J Hypertens* 1991; 4:711S–715S.

47. Thorstad BL, Russell CD, Dubovsky EV, Keller FS, Luke RG. Abnormal captopril renogram with a technetium-99m-labeled hippuran analog. *J Nucl Med* 1988; 29:1730–1737.

48. Whitaker RH. Methods of assessing obstruction in dilated ureters. *Br J Urology* 1973; 45:15–22.

49. Bretland PM. The single compartment model applied to the large renal pelvis: a preliminary study. *Nucl Med Commun* 1992; 13:106–109.

50. Kletter K, Nürnberger N. Diagnostic potential of diuresis renography: limitations by the severity of hydronephrosis and by impairment of renal function. *Nucl Med Commun* 1989; 10:51–61.

51. Jakobsen H, Nordling J, Munck O, Iversen P, Nielsen SL, Holm HH. Sensitivity of 131I-hippuran diuresis renography and pressure flow study (Whitaker test) in upper urinary tract obstruction. *Urol Int* 1988; 43:89–92.

52. Conway JJ, Maizels M. The "well tempered" diuretic renogram: a standard method to examine the asymptomatic neonate with hydronephrosis or hydroureteronephrosis. A report from combined meetings of The Society for Fetal Urology and members of The Pediatric Nuclear Medicine Council-The Society of Nuclear Medicine. *J Nucl Med* 1992; 33:2047–2751.

53. Conway JJ. "Well-tempered" diuresis renography: its historical development, physiological and technical pitfalls, and standardized technique protocol. *Semin Nucl Med* 1992; 22:74–84.

54. Koff SA, McDowell GC, Byard M. Diuretic radionuclide assessment of obstruction in infants: guidelines for successful interpretation. *J Urol* 1988; 140:1167–1168.

55. Hjortsø E, Fugleberg S, Nielsen L, Gjrup T, Harding O, Munck O. Diuresis renography in patients with reduced renal function. *Dan Med Bull* 1988; 35:294–295.

56. Britton KE, Brown NJG. *Clinical Renography* (1971). London: Lloyd-Luke.

57. Price RR, Touya JJ, Branch R, Goddar J, Brill AB. Validation of renal transit time calculations using compartmental models and direct measurements. *A Review of Information Processing in Medical Imaging* (1978). pp. 536–554. Oak Ridge National Laboratory Press.

58. Whitfield HN, Britton KE, Kelsey Fry Hendry WF, Nimmon CC, Travers P, Wickham JEA. The obstructed kidney: correlation between renal function and urodynamic assessment. *Br J Urol* 1977; 49:615–619.

59. Whitfield HN, Britton KE, Hendry WF, Nimmon CC, Wickham JE. The distinction between obstructive uropathy and nephropathy by radioisotope transit times. *Br J Urol* 1978; 50:433–436.

60. Mesrobian HG, Perry JR. Radionuclide diuresis pyelography. *J Urol* 1991; 146: 601–604.

61. Koff SA, Thrall JH, Keyes JW. Assessment of hydroureteronephrosis in children using diuretic radionuclide urography. *J Urol* 1980; 123:531–534.

62. Zechmann W. An experimental approach to explain some misinterpretations of diuresis renography. *Nucl Med Commun* 1988; 9:283–294.

63. Rossleigh MA, Thomas MY, Moase AL. Determination of the normal range of furosemide half-clearance times when using Tc-99m MAG3. *Clin Nucl Med* 1994; 19:880–882.

64. O'Reilly PH, Testa HJ, Lawson RS, Farrar DJ, Charlton Edwards E. Diuresis renography in equivocal urinary tract obstruction. *Br J Urol* 1978; 50:76–80.

65. Brown SC, Upsdell SM, O'Reilly PH. The importance of renal function in the interpretation of diuresis renography. *Br J Urol* 1992; 69:121–125.

66. Upsdell SM, Leeson SM, Brooman PJ, O'Reilly PH. Diuretic-induced urinary flow rates at varying clearances and their relevance to the performance and interpretation of diuresis renography. *Br J Urol* 1988; 61:14–18.

67. Jamar F, Piret L, Wese FX, Beckers C. Influence of ureteral status on kidney washout during technetium-99m-DTPA diuresis renography in children. *J Nucl Med* 1992; 33:73–78.

68. Lupton EW, Testa HJ, O'Reilly PH, Gosling JA, Dixon JS, Lawson RS, Charlton Edwards E. Diuresis renography and morphology in upper urinary tract obstruction. *Br J Urol* 1979; 51:10–14.

69. Lupton EW, Testa HJ, Lawson RS, Charlton Edwards E, Carrol RNP, Barnard RJ. Diuresis renography and the results of pyeloplasty for idiopathic hydronephrosis. *Br J Urol* 1979; 51:449–453.

70. Lupton EW, Lawson RS, Shields RA, Testa HJ. Diuresis renography and parenchymatic transit times in the assessment of renal pelvic dilatation. *Nucl Med Commun* 1984; 5:451–459.

71. Carlsen O, Kvinesdal B, Nathan E. Quantitative evaluation of iodine-123 hippuran gamma camera renography in normal children. *J Nucl Med* 1986; 27:117–127.

72. Anaise D, Oster ZH, Atkins HL, Arnold AN. Cortex Perfusion Index. A Sensitive Detector of Acute Rejection Crisis in Transplanted Kidneys. *J Nucl Med* 1986; 27:1697–1701.

73. Ash J, DeSouza M, Peters M, Wilmot D, Hausen D, Gilday D. Quantitative Assessment of Blood Flow in Pediatric Recipients of Renal Transplants. *J Nucl Med* 1990; 31:580–585.

74. Hilson AJW, Maisey MN, Brown CB, Ogg CS. Dynamic Renal Transplant Imaging with Tc-99m DTPA (Sn) Supplemented by a Transplant Perfusion Index in the Management of Renal Transplants. *J Nucl Med* 1978; 19:994–1000.

75. Tauxe WN, Dubovsky EV, Kidd T Jr, Diaz F, Smith LR. New formulas for the calculation of effective renal plasma flow. *Eur J Nucl Med* 1982; 7:51–54.

76. Tauxe WN. Tubular function, in Tauxe WN, Dubovsky EV (eds.), *Renal Transit Time* (1985). pp. 78–90. Connecticut: Century-Crofts/Norwalk.

77. Tauxe WN, Dubovsky EV, Kidd T Jr, Smith LR, Lewis R, Rivera R. Prediction of urinary excretion of 131I-orthoiodohippurate. *Eur J Nucl Med* 1982; 7(3):102–103.

78. Yester MV. Tubular Function, in Tauxe WN, Dubovsky EV (eds.), *Renal Transit Time* (1985). pp. 78–90. Connecticut: Century-Crofts/Norwalk.

79. Dubovsky EV. Renal Transplantation, in. Tauxe WN, Dubovsky EV (eds.), *Nuclear Medicine in Nuclear Urology and Nephrology* (1985). pp. 233–278. Norwalk, Connecticut: Appleton-Century-Crofts.

80. Sapirstein LA, Vidt DG, Mandel MJ, Hanusek G. Volume distribution and clearances of intravenously injected creatinine in the dog. *Am J Physiol* 1955; 181:330–336.

81. Blaufox MD, Sanderson DR, Tauxe WN, Wankim KG, Orvis AL, Owen CA Jr. Plasmatic diatriozate-I-131 disappearance and glomerular filtration in the dog. *Am J Physiol* 1963; 204:536–540.

82. Peters AM. The kinetic basis of glomerular filtration rate measurement and new concepts of indexation to body size. *Eur J Nucl Med Mol Imaging* 2004; 31(1):137–149.

83. Bird NJ, Henderson BL, Lui D, Ballinger JR, Peters AM. Indexing glomerular filtration rate to suit children. *J Nucl Med* 2003; 44:1037–1043.

84. DuBois D, DuBois DF. A formula to estimate the approximate surface area if height and weight be known. *Arch Int Med* 1916; 17:863–871.

85. Gehan EA, George SL. Estimation of human body surface area from height and weight. *Cancer Chemother Rep* 1970; 54:225–235.

86. Haycock GB, Schwartz GJ, Wisotsky DH. Geometric method for measuring body surface area: a height weight formula validated in infants, children and adults. *J Pediatr* 1978; 93:62–66.

87. Mosteller RD. Simplified calculation of Body Surface Area. *N Engl J Med* 1987; 317:1098.

88. Boyd E. The Growth of the Surface Area of the Human Body (1935). University of Minnesota Press.

89. Pandey CK, Singh RB. Fluid and electrolyte disorders. *Indian J Anaesth* 2003; 47:380–387.

Chapter 2

Ventilation Perfusion Imaging

2.1. VENTILATION AND PERFUSION COMPARISONS

The purpose is to measure whether the relative regional distribution of pulmonary perfusion and ventilation are proportional.

2.1.1. Basic Paradigm

Primary pulmonary parenchymatic disease, which affects the ventilation of the alveoli, will secondarily affect the pulmonary capillary flow; unventilated regions will not be perfused for a long time.[a] On the other hand, primary vascular pulmonary disease does not generally affect ventilation.[b] In the adult, the most primary vascular pulmonary disease is either thromboembolic disease or pulmonary embolism.

2.1.2. Pulmonary Perfusion Imaging

In perfusion imaging, small particles, large enough to block capillaries, are injected intravenously. During their passage through the large veins, right atrium and (mainly) right ventricle, they are mixed, and are distributed in the various branches of the pulmonary artery in proportion with the fraction of the cardiac output or pulmonary flow to those branches (see Sections 5.2.1 and 9.6). They will however be stopped in the pulmonary capillaries. Their spatial distribution is then the spatial distribution of the pulmonary capillary flow. If an artery branch is partially or totally blocked, the dependent capillary bed is less or not perfused, and less or no

---

[a]Pulmonary perfusion in a non-ventilated area would result in a functional right-to-left shunt.
[b]The lung tissues are fed by the bronchial circulation. A pulmonary artery branch obstruction does not necessarily lead to pulmonary infarction.

tracer will be present. It is important to remember that, in the absence of a right to left shunt, all of the intravenously injected tracer must eventually end in the pulmonary capillary bed. The activity in segment i, A_i, is the fraction of the total flow to the lungs to segment i; the symbol $\dot{Q}$ represents blood flow.[c]

$$A_i = \frac{\dot{Q}_i}{\sum_j \dot{Q}_j}.$$

Well-perfused regions have high activity levels; low perfused regions have low activity levels and appear as defects.

2.1.3. *Pulmonary Ventilation Imaging*

Ventilation, broadly understood, conflates three different functions. First, there is the volume inhaled and exhaled in each ventilator cycle. Multiplied by the number of cycles per unit of time, it defines the ventilation rate $\dot{V}$. The total lung volume V is the volume of gas in the lungs (including trachea and bronchi). The fractional ventilation rate is $\dot{V}/V$. In Section 8.5, $\dot{V} = F$, and $\dot{V}/V = a_{21}$.

2.1.3.1. *Pulmonary ventilation imaging with xenon-133 (^{133}Xe)*

In ventilation imaging, the tracer is a radioactive inert and water-insoluble gas. The prototype is ^{133}Xenon. It has a half-life of 5.4 days. In relation to the ventilation study's time range, decay is insignificant.

In the classical set-up, the tracer is in a spirometer chamber preloaded with ^{133}Xe. The volume in the spirometer is V_s. The patient breathes in and out of the spirometer. In Section 8.5, $\dot{V}/V_s$ is a_{12}.

At the end of the first inspiration, the amount of activity in each lung compartment is the inhaled volume multiplied by the starting concentration in the spirometer; the activity distribution in the lungs is proportional to the distribution of the ventilation rates.

$$A_i = \frac{\dot{V}_i}{\sum_j \dot{V}_j}.$$

The patient has to hold his or her breath, to allow an imaging time for sufficient counts (the technique is called breath-holding), but there is a limit to the capacity of the breath-holding of the patient.

As the patient resumes breathing from the spirometer, equilibrium is eventually reached. At equilibrium, all compartments (the spirometer and the lungs) share

---

[c]The symbol $\dot{X}$ with the dot denotes a first derivative or in this context flow rate.

the same concentration (C_∞) and the activities in different parts of the lungs are proportional to the ventilated volumes in different parts of the lungs.

$$A_i = V_i C_\infty.$$

When equilibrium is reached, the connection between the subject and the spirometer is broken, the patient breathes fresh air, and the activity washes out. The washout is exponential for each region of the lung with a uniform fractional ventilation rate[d] (see Section 8.1). In the region of the lung "i", the fractional ventilation rate $(\dot{V}/V)_i$ acts as the fractional turnover rate and the decrease in activity or washout is (nearly) exponential.

$$A_{wo,i,(t)} = A_{i,(0)} e^{-(\dot{V}/V)_i t}.$$

In reality, the (single-compartment) model is not adequate because the bronchial system lays between the alveoli and the outside, but in practice, the model works well (1).

The importance of xenon kinetics is that they illustrate three very distinct metrics of pulmonary ventilation: the ventilation rate $\dot{V}$, measured by a first breath, the ventilated volume V or total lung volume, measured at equilibrium, and the fractional ventilation rate $(\dot{V}/V)$.

The interesting thing is what happens if two lung regions with equal lung volumes ($V_1 = V_2$) have a different ventilation rate ($\dot{V}_1 > \dot{V}_2$). It follows that $(\dot{V}/V)_1 > (\dot{V}/V)_2$: Early during the inhalation phase, the activity in V_1 will be higher than V_2 ($A_1 > A_2$), but eventually (at equilibrium), the concentration is constant throughout the system and the activity is proportional to the volumes. During washout, the lung region with the larger fractional ventilation rate will empty faster (Figure 2.1).

The usual method to perform ventilation imaging is to start with a posterior view, and have the patient take a deep breath of the concentrated dose. Imaging is performed during breath-holding after this first breath, but the imaging time is obviously limited. In the image collected during breath-holding or very early in the inhalation phase, poorly ventilated regions (with a lower ventilation rate) will contain less activity, and appear as defects (Section 2.1.2).

The patient then resumes breathing, long enough to reach near equilibrium in the poorly ventilated regions. At this time, activity is proportional to volume and does not reflect ventilation rate or fractional ventilation rate.

The patient is then disconnected and washout images are collected. In some laboratories, multiple views are acquired during the washout. If the fractional ventilation rate is low, retention of activity in the lungs remains for a longer time: poorly

---

[d]The dead space of bronchi and trachea are not taken into consideration.

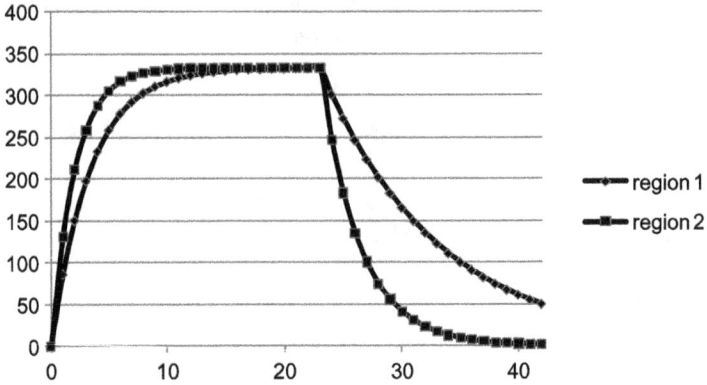

Figure 2.1 Activity in region 1 is slower to rise and reach equilibrium and slower to decrease.

ventilated areas appear as hot spots later during washout. This is easy to detect, but difficult to compare with the perfusion images in which abnormal regions appear as "cold" regions or defects. The deep breath and breath-holding techniques do illustrate the ventilation rate, which is assumed to be proportional to the perfusion rate, but cannot be imaged at leisure, because of the breath-holding. It has the advantage that, like the perfusion (rate) image, an abnormal region appears as "cold". Even so, Alderson (2) did a study in 1980 demonstrating that hot spot imaging in the washout technique was superior to the breath-holding technique. However, in 1976, the same Alderson (3) imaged during tidal breathing, presumably to equilibrium, and then acquired sequential washout images.

The ventilated volume is a purely anatomical metric, and is not expected to correlate with the perfusion rate image.

2.1.3.2. Pulmonary ventilation imaging with krypton-81m

An alternative is found using a very short-lived inert radioactive gas: Krypton-81m (^{81m}Kr) (4–9). In the case of ^{81m}Kr, with decay constant $\lambda = 0.053\,\text{sec}^{-1}$, the situation is different: Krypton is mixed with the inspired air at a constant concentration[e] C_{input}. Equilibrium is reached when the rate of accumulation equals the loss from the alveoli either by decay (λ) or the fractional expiration rate ($\dot{V}/V$).

---

[e]Air is passed over a solid Rubidium generator, with a long half-life. The generator produces gaseous ^{81m}Kr at a constant rate.

The situation is that of the constant infusion model (Section 8.3)

$$\frac{dA}{dt} = k - aA.$$

However, in this case:

$$k = \dot{V}C_{input},$$

$$a = \lambda + \frac{\dot{V}}{V}.$$

The equilibrium activity is therefore defined by:

$$\frac{dA}{dt} = 0,$$

$$k = aA_\infty,$$

$$A_{(\infty)} = \frac{k}{a},$$

$$A_{(\infty)} = \frac{\dot{V}C_{input}}{\lambda + \dot{V}/V},$$

$$C_\infty V = \frac{\dot{V}C_{input}}{\frac{\lambda V + \dot{V}}{V}},$$

$$C_\infty = \frac{\dot{V}}{\lambda V + \dot{V}}C_{input}.$$

If there is no ventilation in a particular region, the concentration remains zero. If the ventilation rate is very high, the concentration in the lung approaches the input concentration. In between we have the following (Table 2.1 and Figure 2.2):

If the lung volume is 5 liters, with the fractional ventilation rate between zero and 60% per respiratory cycle, and the respiration rate is 20/min, the fractional ventilation rate ranges from 0 to 1000 ml/min.

It is generally assumed that in [81m]Kr ventilation imaging, the distribution of activity is proportional to the distribution of the ventilation rates (7), and (presumably) in normal cases to the distribution of perfusion rates (8,9). The great advantage of ventilation perfusion imaging with [81m]Kr is the possibility to carry out both image ventilation and perfusion simultaneously[f] and to have images which are immediately and quantitatively comparable.[g]

---

[f]Simultaneously because the emission energies differ sufficiently for non-overlapping windows.

[g]In both images, decrease in ventilation or perfusion rates results in defects.

Table 2.1 Effect of ventilation rates on the equilibrium values of ^{81m}Kr.

λ/sec	C_{input}	V ml	$\dot{V}/V$	$\frac{\dot{V}}{V}\,sec^{-1}$	$\dot{V}$ ml/sec	$C_{(\infty)}$
0.053308	10	5000	0	0.00	0.00	0.00
0.053308	10	5000	0.1	0.03	166.67	3.85
0.053308	10	5000	0.2	0.07	333.33	5.56
0.053308	10	5000	0.3	0.10	500.00	6.52
0.053308	10	5000	0.4	0.13	666.67	7.14
0.053308	10	5000	0.5	0.17	833.33	7.58
0.053308	10	5000	0.6	0.20	1000.00	7.90

In reality, however, the proportionality is not linear (Figure 2.2). Still the inhalation and perfusion rate images are very similar (Figures 2.3 and 2.4).

2.1.3.3. *Pulmonary ventilation inhalation imaging*

Inhalation imaging is performed after the patient has inhaled an aerosolized tracer. In ideal circumstances, the aerosol is deposited deeply into the bronchial tree.

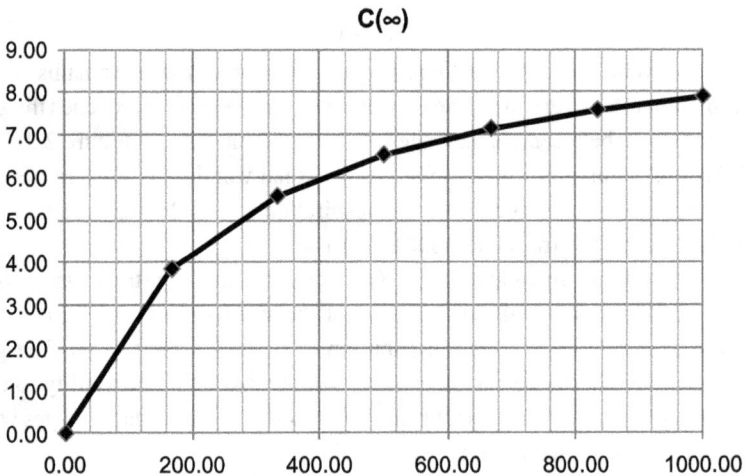

Figure 2.2 The plot shows the relation between the fractional ventilation rate (x-axis) and the activity level obtained with ^{81m}Kr. The relation is not exactly linear and the proportionality decreases at higher ventilation rates.

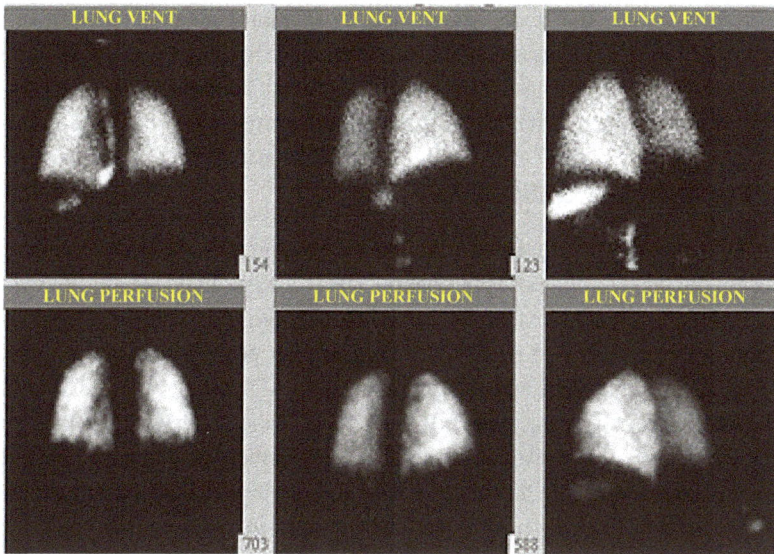

Figure 2.3 Top: The aerosol ventilation image is normal with some activity seen in the esophagus and stomach. Bottom: The perfusion image shows small non-segmental defects.

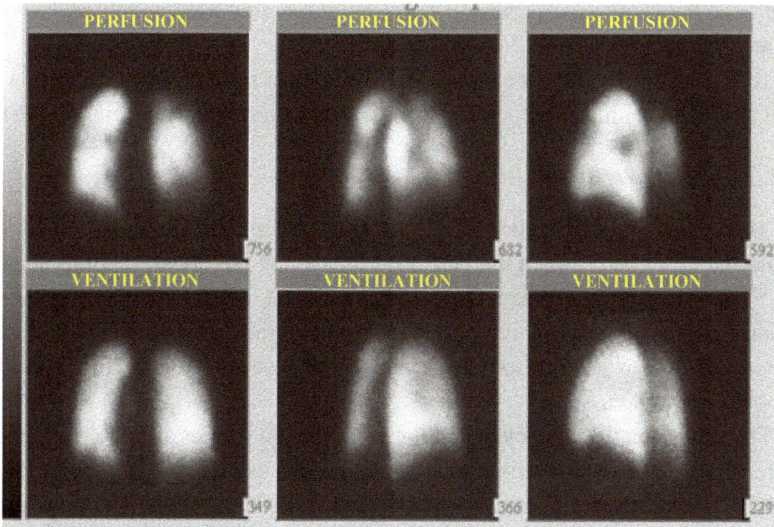

Figure 2.4 Top: Perfusion image. Bottom: ^{81m}Kr ventilation image. The right lung shows an apical unmatched perfusion defect. The left lung shows a middle lobe unmatched defect.

Too often however, the tracer stays partially in major airways, mainly in the presence of bronchial stenosis or partial obstruction, or in patients with chronic obstructive pulmonary disease (10). The distribution of activity, when all goes well, is proportional to the distribution of the ventilation rate (Figures 2.3 and 2.4).

2.2. PULMONARY EMBOLISM

There is controversy (11) around the use of scintigraphic studies (ventilation-perfusion imaging) to diagnose pulmonary emboli. The problem is far from trivial if we accept the fact that more than 50% of pulmonary emboli found on autopsy were undiagnosed at the time of death (12). The defining procedure is the pulmonary arteriogram or angiogram and today probably the CT angiography. The risk of pulmonary angiography is small; in 1111 patients who underwent the procedure during the Prospective Investigation of Pulmonary Embolism Diagonsis (PIOPED) (13) study, there were five deaths (or 0.5%) and major non-fatal complications in nine cases (1%) (14). Most complications occurred in unstable patients (5/122). Surveillance after a negative angiography showed PE in 4 of the 675 cases. However, there is a clinical need for a less invasive and less expensive procedure, either to obtain a diagnosis (negative or positive) or to rationally select the patients in whom an angiogram would be appropriate. The most commonly used procedure used to be the ventilation-perfusion study, but it has now been widely replaced by CT angiography.

Today, it is difficult to remember that at one time only perfusion studies were used (15). The ventilation study has been shown to add mainly specificity (16).

2.2.1. *Interpretation*

We expect that the distribution of $\dot{Q}$ and $\dot{V}$ to be similar. The easy comparison would therefore be between the perfusion image and the breath-holding image,[h] or a ^{81m}Kr or inhalation image. On the other hand, late washout is easily observed, because it presents as an activity in an empty field, rather than a defect within an activity; but, the exact correspondence between the washout and perfusion images is more difficult to assess.

The studies on the efficacy of ventilation perfusion images are much influenced by the method utilized for ventilation imaging, as discussed above. But they are also much influenced by the classification of the scintigraphic outcomes, as we will see. There has, in fact, been a large number of meta-analysis but on a small number of patients of the method and results (17, 18).

---

[h]But that would allow one view only.

2.2.2. *PIOPED*

The investigators in the PIOPED (12) study use three different sets of criteria or attributes of the perfusion abnormality, but in incomplete combinations.[i]

1. Size and shape: Lobar (L), Segmental (S), Subsegmental (SS) and non-segmental (N).
2. Number of defects.
3. Matching of perfusion defects with ventilation abnormalities.
4. Matching with chest X-ray abnormalities.

The investigators then grouped outcomes in what they call high, intermediate, low probability and normal or very low probability (Table 2.2). It is unclear from published reports on what basis. It is certainly true that making normal chest X-rays and normal ventilation studies equivalent is questionable (see Section 2.2.3).

Table 2.2 PIOPED categories.

Large	> 75% of a segment
Moderate	25–75% of a segment
Small	< 25%
Matched	Matching X-ray or V-scan abnormality
Unmatched	No V or CXR abnormality
Category	**Number size and comparison with CXR or V scan**
High probability (HP)	≥ 2 Large segmental; Unmatched
	1 large and ≥ 2 moderate; Unmatched
	≥ 4 moderate; Unmatched
Intermediate (IP)	Not HP or LP
	Borderline HP or LP
	Difficult to categorize
	Matched VQ and pleural effusion
Low probability (LP)	Non-segmental or anatomical explained
	Single moderate mismatched with normal CXR
	Any large defect matched by CXR
	Matched by larger CXR abnormality
	> 3 small with normal CXR
Very low (VL)	≤ 3 small with normal CXR
Normal (NL)	No perfusion defect

---

[i]In the sense that not all perfusion defects are characterized by all attributes. In some cases, the ventilation and/or the chest X-ray findings are omitted.

Table 2.3   Note that the prevalence in the intermediate category is essentially the same as the global prevalence. It is more interesting to compute the operating characteristics. LR is the likelihood ratio (see Section 7.2).[j]

	PE present	PE absent	Prevalence
HP	102	14	0.9
IP	105	217	0.3
LP	39	199	0.2
VL	5	50	0.1
Total	251	480	0.3

The ventilation images were based on early ^{133}Xe (inhalation phase), with first breath-holding and equilibrium for posterior views and washout images for posterior views and 45 degree left and right posterior oblique (45LPO and 45RPO) views (see above: fractional ventilation rate). Therefore, the comparison was $\dot{Q}$ versus $\dot{V}$ for the posterior view only, and $\dot{Q}$ versus $\dot{V}/V$ for posterior and posterior obliques.

The results were tabulated as the two first columns in Table 2.3, where the authors tabulated for each imaging outcome category, the (defining) results of the pulmonary angiogram. What was tabulated was in fact the positive and negative predictive values. In the third column, we tabulated the global prevalence in the population of the verified cases. The operating characteristics are shown in Table 2.4 (Section 7.1).

2.2.3. Worsley

Worsley (19) reviewed and modified the PIOPED categories. First, he defines the perfusion defect attributes (size and corresponding abnormalities in either ventilation image (V) or chest X-ray (CXR). He introduces a separate category for matches in the V/Q scan and a separate matching with a CXR abnormality.

The categories are defined as a post-test probability (independent of prior probability except that in this paper, there is some data about the presence of signs of increased risk). The categories are slightly modified from the original PIOPED categories (Table 2.5).

---

[j]The semantics were badly chosen: The predictive values are not independent of the prior probability (see Section 7.1). Furthermore, what is the probability that a scan was not performed? Finally, an outcome that does not change the prior probability does not yield an intermediate result, but is non-diagnostic.

Table 2.4 The IP category has a sensitivity almost equal to the non-specificity, and a likelihood ratio near 1, therefore a non-diagnostic outcome. Practically speaking, only the categories HP and VL are diagnostic, amounting to 23% of the cases (171/731).

	P(S+|D+)	P(S+|D−)	LR
HP	0.406	0.029	13.93
IP	0.418	0.452	0.93
LP	0.155	0.415	0.37
VL	0.020	0.104	0.19

Table 2.5 Worsley's categories.

Category	Number size and comparison with CXR or V scan
High probability (HP)	< 2 Large segmental unmatched 1 large and ≥ moderate unmatched ≥4 moderate unmatched
Intermediate (IP)	1 moderate to < 2 large unmatched 1 moderate matched normal CXR Matched in lower fields and opacity in CXR Matched VQ and pleural effusion
Low probability (LP)	Multiple matched and normal CXR Matched in upper and middle fields and opacity in CXR Matched and large pleural effusion Matched by larger CXR abnormality Stripe sign >3 small with normal CXR Non-segmental
Very low (VL)	≤3 small with normal CXR
Normal (NL)	No perfusion defect

He starts, like PIOPED to present the results as predictive values (Table 2.6). The overall prevalence of pulmonary embolism in the patients who underwent an arteriogram was 18%. In this population, patients in the intermediate category have a significantly higher prevalence than the population as a whole. However, the LP population has an unchanged prevalence, and should properly have been called non-diagnostic. Indeed, looking at the operating characteristics (Table 2.7), the categories with the LR really different from 1 are HP and (perhaps) IP (>1)

Table 2.6   Predictive values.

Category	PE positive	PE negative	Prevalence
HP	160	24	0.87
IP	169	318	0.35
LP	68	501	0.12
VL	2	78	0.03
Nl	0	960	0.00
Total	399	1881	0.18

Table 2.7   Sensitivities and non-specificities.

Category	P(S+|D+)	P(S+|D−)	LR
HP	0.401	0.013	31.429
IP	0.424	0.169	2.505
LP	0.170	0.266	0.640
VL	0.005	0.041	0.121
Nl	0.000	0.510	0.000

and VL and Normal (<1). Fifty-three percent of the patients fell into the diagnostic category, excluding IP.

2.2.4. *Freitas*

Freitas (20) uses formally, but not substantially different, definitions of the categories as shown in Table 2.8.

Table 2.8   Definitions.

No Q defect	Normal
Q defect < 25% of segment	Low
Q defect > 25% of segment matched X-ray abnormality	Low
Q defect > 25% of segment unmatched X-ray abnormality	Intermediate
Q defect > 25% of segment matched by V abnormalities	Low
> 2 defects > 25% of segments unmatched by X-ray or V scan	High
> 2 segmental equivalent normal X-ray and V scan	High
Defects >50% of lungfield matched by X-ray and V scan	Intermediate

Table 2.9 Predictive values.

	PE positive	PE negative	Prevalence
High	5	1	83.3
Intermediate	29	62	31.9
Low	2	34	5.6
All	36	97	27.1

Table 2.10 Sensitivities and non-specificities.

Category	P(S+|D+)	P(S+|D−)	LR
HP	0.14	0.01	13.47
IP	0.81	0.64	1.26
LP	0.06	0.35	0.16

In his report, the overall prevalence is 27.1%. The intermediate category is non-diagnostic. The low category is a negative result. The diagnostic outcomes cover only 32% of the cases (Tables 2.9 and 2.10).

Noting that the sensitivity for HP is very low, the positive predictive value (PPV) is very high for a population prevalence of 27.1%.

2.2.5. *The Society of Nuclear Medicine*

The Society of Nuclear Medicine has produced some guidelines (21), with some variations of the original PIOPED, specifically doubtful HP and IP categories.

2.2.5.1. *High probability (≥80% probability of PE)*

i. ≥ 2 large mismatched segmental perfusion defects or the arithmetic equivalent in moderate or large and moderate defects.

ii. Two large mismatched segmental perfusion defects, or the arithmetic equivalent,[k] are borderline for "high probability". Individual readers may correctly

---

[k]A large segmental defect, 75% of a segment, equals 1 segmental equivalent; a moderate defect, 25–75% of a segment, equals 0.5 segmental equivalents; a small defect, < 25% of a segment, is not counted. A large segmental defect, 75% of a segment, equals 1 segmental equivalent; a moderate defect, 25–75% of a segment, equals 0.5 segmental equivalents; a small defect, < 25% of a segment, is not counted.

interpret individual images with this pattern as "high probability". In general, it is recommended that more than this degree of mismatch be present for the "high probability" category.

2.2.5.2. Intermediate probability (20%–79%)

i. One moderate to two large mismatched perfusion defects or the arithmetic equivalent in moderate or large and moderate defects.
ii. Single-matched ventilation-perfusion defect with a clear chest radiograph is borderline for "low probability" and thus should be categorized as "intermediate" in most circumstances by readers, although individual readers may correctly interpret individual scintigrams with this pattern as "low probability".
iii. Difficult to categorize as low or high or not described as low or high.

2.2.5.3. Low probability (<19%)

i. Non-segmental perfusion defects (e.g. cardiomegaly, enlarged aorta, enlarged hilar, elevated diaphragm).
ii. Any perfusion defect with a substantially larger chest radiographic abnormality.
iii. Perfusion defects matched by ventilation abnormality provided that there are:

    a. clear chest radiograph; and
    b. some areas of normal perfusion in the lungs.

iv. Any number of small perfusion defects with a normal chest radiograph.

2.2.5.4. Normal

No perfusion defects or perfusion exactly outlines the shape of the lung seen on the chest radiograph (note that hilar and aortic impressions may be seen and the chest radiograph and/or ventilation may be abnormal).

2.2.5.5. Gestalt interpretation

The experienced nuclear medicine physician may be able to provide a more accurate interpretation of the ventilation-perfusion study than is provided by the criteria alone; however, his/her opinion is usually informed by detailed knowledge of the various lung image interpretive criteria.

The major features of PIOPED are that the CXR can be used as a surrogate for ventilation, the number of defects determines the category, but a summed abnormality is introduced. It is amusing that the categories are superseded by gestalt interpretation.

2.2.5.6. *McNeil*

McNeil (22) simplified the categorization of the V/Q results by having small or large perfusion defects, matched or unmatched by ventilation abnormalities. She did, however, eliminate and place in an undetermined category, perfusion defects matched by a CXR abnormality. That group did not get a ventilation scan and is not further characterized. The prevalence of PE in that group was 37% (13/22), somewhat higher than the 26% in the patients with ventilation scans. The ventilation scan was a ^{133}Xe breath-holding scan.

She did also distinguish between single abnormalities and multiple abnormalities. But the number of single perfusion abnormalities was too small for a separate analysis. Her data is tabulated in Table 2.11.

The operating characteristics come out as follows in Table 2.12.

Table 2.11 Predictive values.

Size	Character	PE+	PE−	Prevalence
Large	Unmatched	39	5	0.886
Small	Unmatched	2	6	0.250
All	Unmatched	41	11	0.788
Large	Matched	12	62	0.162
Small	Matched	1	76	0.013
All	Matched	13	138	0.086
Large	All	51	67	0.432
Small	All	3	82	0.035
Total				0.266

Table 2.12 Sensitivities and non-specificities.

		P(S+|D+)	P(S+|D−)	LR
Large	Unmatched	0.722	0.034	21.522
Small	Unmatched	0.037	0.040	0.920
All	Unmatched	0.759	0.074	10.285
Large	Matched	0.222	0.416	0.534
Small	Matched	0.019	0.510	0.036
All	Matched	0.241	0.926	0.260
Large	All	0.944	0.450	2.100
Small	All	0.056	0.550	0.101

Large unmatched defects have a very large LR, large enough to change a prior probability from 0.266 to a post-test probability of 0.886, and with a sensitivity of 0.722, not reached with any other classification. Small matched defects have a LR of 0.013, and moves the prior from 0.266 to 0.036. The convincingly diagnostic outcomes are "Large Unmatched" and "Small Matched" and cover 60% of all outcomes.

2.2.5.7. *Stanford*

Following the criteria suggested by McNeil, we did a study utilizing Krypton-81m for ventilation imaging (7). There were 273 consecutive cases, of which 39 had a normal perfusion image, and on whom no arteriogram was performed. Only 15% of the remaining patients eventually underwent a pulmonary angiogram. The perfusion defect attributes are size, shape and ventilation match or mismatch:

- Segmental (>75%) or lobar defects: SL
- Sub- or non-segmental: SS
- All matched by ventilation abnormalities: MM
- All unmatched by ventilation abnormalities: UU
- Mixed matched and unmatched: MU

For those, the results are shown in Table 2.13.

The problem is the same as the one faced by the PIOPED group: Some outcomes are too rare to contribute statistically by themselves, and the temptation to amalgamate is compelling. However, on what criteria can different outcomes be placed in the same category? The only logical one on a physio-pathological basis (see Section 2.1.1) is the presence of unmatched defects. Unmatched defects may

Table 2.13 Predictive values.

	PE positive	PE negative	Prevalence
SLUU	13	0	1.00
SLMU	2	1	0.67
SLMM	3	9	0.25
SSUU	4	1	0.80
SSMU	1	0	1.00
SSMM	3	17	0.15
Total	26	28	0.48

Table 2.14 Predictive values.

	PE positive	PE negative	Prevalence
Any unmatched	20	2	0.91
All matched	6	26	0.19
Total	26	28	0.48

Table 2.15 Sensitivities and non-specificities.

Category	PE positive	PE negative	LR
Any unmatched	0.77	0.07	10.77
All matched	0.23	0.93	0.25

not have been recognized with ^{133}Xenon studies,[1] but ^{81m}Kr and to some extent aerosol inhalation studies, yield comparable resolution and views as the perfusion study.

In this case, the amalgamation leads to the results in Tables 2.14 and 2.15.

Unlike Sostman (23), we did not find that mostly uncertain scintigraphic outcomes were more likely to be confirmed by pulmonary angiography. At the end of the study, the cases with outcome "large perfusion abnormalities, unmatched", were referred as pulmonary angiography in 34% of the cases, large matched in 13.9% of the cases. One cannot exactly know what additional information was available to the clinician (24), but the data do not support the alleged overuse of pulmonary angiography (there are not too many negative angiograms (11)).

In general, the categories from PIOPED are probably too complex, and not obviously based on the basic paradigm of a primary vascular pulmonary disease. The sensitivities of the HP category is very low, but the specificity is high. With better ventilation imaging and a simple categorization, the operating characteristics improve dramatically, but do not become perfect.

---

[1]The low gamma emission energy results in poor resolution, and often there is only one view.

Interestingly, and unexplained, general gestalt interpretation (by experienced observers) outperforms original and modified PIOPED criteria. Still with all its imperfections, the clinical performance of VQ lung imaging is not bad. As an example, patients without documented thromboembolic disease who have low likelihood results from their lung scintigraphy have little thromboembolic disease in follow-up (25) sessions.

2.2.6. *PIOPED II and PIAPED*

Finally, with the advent of CT angiography and perhaps in the US, a lack of good inhalation agents (26–28), an attempt was made to bypass the ventilation study, and use only the perfusion scan and the CXR (29).

Two schemes are suggested in Table 2.16.

The conclusion here is shown in Table 2.17.

Table 2.16   Categories.

	PIOPED II: Prospective Investigation of Pulmonary Embolism Diagnosis	**PISAPED: Prospective Investigative Study of Pulmonary Embolism Diagnosis**
Positive	$\geq$ 2 segments of CXR mismatched segmental perfusion defects	$\geq$ Wedge-shaped perfusion defect(s)
Negative	Normal perfusion	Normal perfusion
	Non-segmental, prominent hilum, cardiomegaly, elevated diaphragma, linear atelectasis, costophrenic angle effusion, CXR larger than perfusion defect	Near normal
	1–3 small segmental defects	Contour defect anatomical
	1 CXR matched in mid or upper lung	Not wedge shaped perfusion defect
	Stripe sign	
	Pleural effusion 1/3 of pleural cavity	
Non diagnostic	All other findings	Not negative or positive

Table 2.17 Comparisions between PIOPED II and PISAPED.

	PIOPED II	PISAPED
Sensitivity	0.849	0.805
Specificity	0.927	0.996

There were only 21% non-diagnostic studies in the PIOPED II and none in the PISAPED classification scheme.

The remaining question is the nature of uncertainty. Ralph (30) points out that agreement between observers is good in the high probability and normal classes, but not in the intermediate and low probability classes of the PIOPED study. One would expect that the interpretation could (marginally) be improved by complex encoding schemes. Tourassi (31, 32) investigated the use of an artificial neural network as a computer-aided diagnostic tool for predicting pulmonary embolism from ventilation-perfusion lung scans and chest radiographs. The neural network significantly outperformed the physicians involved in the PIOPED study (two-tailed P-value = 0.01). Patil (33) used the artificial neural network on the clinical characteristics of the patients. Characteristics of the history, physical examination, electrocardiograph, chest radiograph, and arterial blood gases of patients with suspected acute PE were presented to a back propagation neural network. Areas under ROC curves for PIOPED clinical assessment combined with ventilation/perfusion (V/Q) scan results were compared with neural network clinical assessment combined with V/Q scan results. The data showed that neural networks were able to predict the clinical likelihood of PE with an accuracy comparable to that of experienced clinicians.

The relative success of neural networks suggest that a prior stratification could be used. However, once we accept that the positive predictive value is a function of the prior probability, we can study the value of additional stratification, rather than exhaust image interpretation refinements. One defining factor is the presence of deep vein thrombosis. Hull (34, 35) found that if deep vein thrombosis is used as a predictor of pulmonary embolism, the sensitivity is 70%, and the specificity is 66% if venography is used. The sensitivity is 43% and the specificity is 81% if impedance plethysmography is used. The efficacy of impedance plethysmography is subject to caution. Ginsberg (36) found that the sensitivity for proximal deep vein thrombosis was 65% (26/40) and for deep calf vein thrombosis 0% (0/7); the specificity was 93% (79/85). Still, according to Stein (37), the inclusion of a test for deep vein thrombosis would reduce the need for an arteriogram significantly. Newer methods for deep vein thrombosis detection may encourage this approach. Using a monoclonal antibody with a high affinity to the DD domain, Bautovitch (38) was able to detect all deep vein thrombosis sites detected by venography (calf 7, popliteal 6, femoral 5), and almost all duplex ultrasound proven ones (calf 15/17, popliteal 14/14, femoral 12/12). Pelvic thrombosis was also detected, but not always verified.

Chest X-ray signs are not helpful in the stratification of patients (39). The most common chest radiographic finding in patients with pulmonary embolism was atelectasis and/or parenchymal areas of increased opacity. However, the prevalence was not significantly different from that in patients without pulmonary embolism. Oligemia (the Westermark sign on the CXR), prominent central pulmonary artery (the Fleischner sign), pleural-based area of increased opacity (the Hampton hump), vascular redistribution, pleural effusion, elevated diaphragm, and enlarged hilum were also poor predictors.

Perrier (40) has suggested that D-dimer measurements of less than $500 \, \mu g/L$ could be reliably used to exclude pulmonary embolism in patients with an abnormal but not high-probability (inconclusive) lung scan. D-dimer measurements of greater than $500 \, \mu/L$ however have no positive predictive value for pulmonary embolism.

Finally, there are other primary vascular disturbances than pulmonary emboli: congenital pulmonary artery abnormalities, mass effects affecting pulmonary vessels (achalasia (41), sarcoidosis (42), bronchogenic cyst (43) and aortic dissection (44)).

2.3. CILIARY FUNCTION AND EPITHELIAL PERMEABILITY

DTPA aerosol clearance has been related to lung epithelial permeability and thickening of alveolar epithelium (45–47).

The study is easy to perform: The patient inhales an aerosol, and is imaged in a dynamic continuous acquisition, usually in a posterior, or a combined anterior and posterior view. Caner (48) found a decrease in clearance rates in complicated diabetes. In normal cases, the clearance was mono-exponentials with half-lives of 91.97 ± 18.21 minutes. In uncomplicated cases, 93.67 ± 21.23 and in complicated cases, 133.05 ± 46.97 minutes.

Fanti (49) found an increased rate in systemic sclerosis: 59.8 ± 19.8 minutes, (normal > 53 minutes) in a mono-exponential analysis.

Mason (50) studied it in pulmonary edema, Susskind (51) in anthracosis; Bradvick (52) looked at smoking. The clearance was bi-exponential (83 ± 19 and

13 ± 4), while in controls, it was monoexponential (67+18 minutes). In sarcoidosis, the half-life was shortened (Stage I: 59 ± 15, Stage II: 54 ± 17, Stage III: 45 ± 15). Mason (53) also studied the effect of smoking.

Wells (54) studied fibrosing alveolitis, Tateno (55) studied scleroderma while Thunberg (56) studied sarcoidosis.

2.4. DETECTING RIGHT TO LEFT SHUNTING

This application is quiet, old and simple (57–60). The patient is intravenously injected with macroaggregates or labeled microspheres that would usually be stopped by the pulmonary capillary bed. If there is an intracardiac shunt with an Eisenmenger syndrome or a pulmonary shunt due to pulmonary arteriovenous malformations (60), significant activity will be found in organs perfused through the aortic system. On a whole body scan, a region of interest is placed to include the whole body (W), one over the lungs (L) and one outside the body but within the imaging field (B). The R > L shunt fraction is computed as:

$$\frac{L - B \times \frac{A_L}{A_B}}{W - B \times \frac{A_W}{A_B}}.$$

In this equation, L are the counts over the lungs, W over the whole body and B outside the body in the imaging field (the background). A_B, A_W, and A_L are the areas or the number of pixels in the three regions. If one uses conjugate views, the geometric means from anterior and posterior views are used, but after the background correction (Figure 2.5).

There are some caveats:

1. Imaging must be performed soon (within 5 minutes of the injection) to prevent elution of the label from the macroaggregate or microspheres.
2. If the intravenous injection has left some activity at the injection site, that site should not be included in the body region.
3. In the case of a positive shunt, the visible organs should include the brain (15% of cardiac output).
4. Visualization of the kidneys and bladder only suggest elution of the label or fragmentation of the tracer.

The singular advantage is the ease by which infrapulmonary shunting can be detected, when a cardiac shunt has been excluded (61).

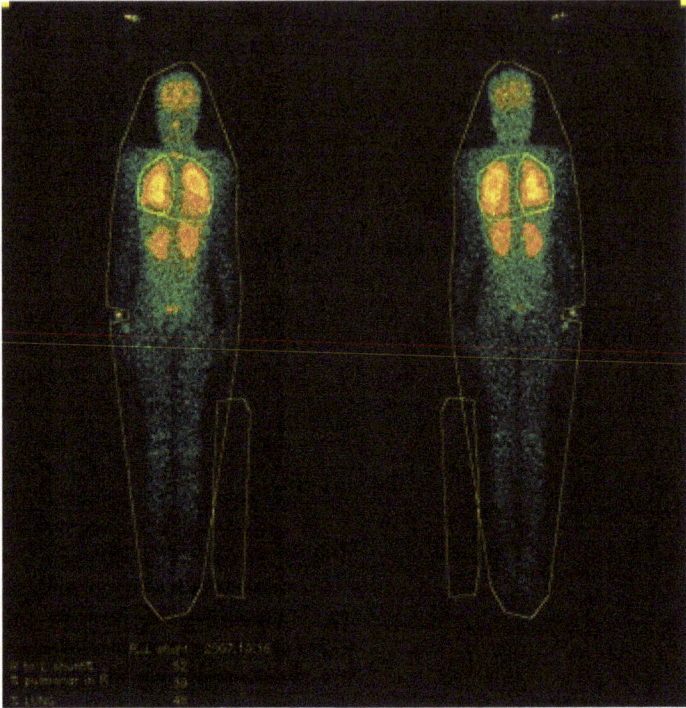

Figure 2.5   The figure illustrates a positive case of R > L shunting. The brain is as visible as the kidneys. The tracer was a macroaggregate of albumin labeled with ^{99m}Tc. Some of the technetium must have come free, because there is activity in the bladder. The computation was performed on data from anterior and posterior conjugate views. An infiltration in the R wrist is not included in the regions (Section 10.5).

Grimon (62) bizarrely eschewed whole body scanning and devised an index using a brain-to-lung activity ratio. The rational is the avoidance of error due to free pertechnetate and the difficulty in avoiding scatter from the lungs.

2.5. MONITORING PULMONARY BLOOD FLOW DISTRIBUTION

In certain circumstances, it is useful to know how pulmonary flow is distributed between the lungs and lung regions. One application is the evaluation of pulmonary atresia and tetralogies (63, 64, 65). While relative lung perfusion distributions are cited in clinical decision-making for congenital and acquired pulmonary vascular diseases, normal values and ranges have not been published for a large population of normally perfused lungs. Common wisdom accepts that the split should be between 55% and 45%.

In actuality, a study in more than 200 patients, who had no ventilation abnormality nor perfusion abnormalities, the average R:L ratio was in the range of 52.5%:47.5% with a population standard deviation of 2.1% (66). The clinical relevance is not clear for such small differences (55 vs. 52.5) but the fact that the natural range was not defined until relatively late, speaks volumes about evidence-based medicine.

An application that used to be common was the evaluation of the fraction of pulmonary function that would be lost in a lobectomy or pneumonectomy in patients with marginal pulmonary function (67).

The simple approach is to use the perfusion study only. Complications arise when a ventilation and perfusion study is requested and both use a ^{99m}Tc-labeled agent.[m] In the case of perfusion imaging only, the usual dose is 1 mCi. Anterior and posterior views are acquired with a dual-headed camera so that they are registered "in line". One of the images is flipped around the y-axis, and a geometric mean is computed. The geometric mean image is usually displayed as a posterior view (left lung to the left of the viewer). In well-registered images, the geometric mean can be computed on a pixel by pixel basis, but with the danger that in one of the views a pixel has zero value and not in the other.

The regions of interest (ROI) should include regions of non-perfused lung, which requires some set strategy. One way is to place the base of the lungs for both lungs on the basis of the lung with the lowest base, and to do the same for the apex. Judgment needs to be used for that approach. The contours of the lungs are drawn,

Table 2.18 Perfusion distribution net.

Percentage of lung		
	Left lung	**Right lung**
Apical	13.3	31.4
Middle	44.6	49.7
Basal	42.1	18.9
Percentage of total Q	31.9	68.1

[m]The influence of the first set of images on the second set needs to be corrected, but this does not amount to cross-talk, but to shine through.

Chapter 2

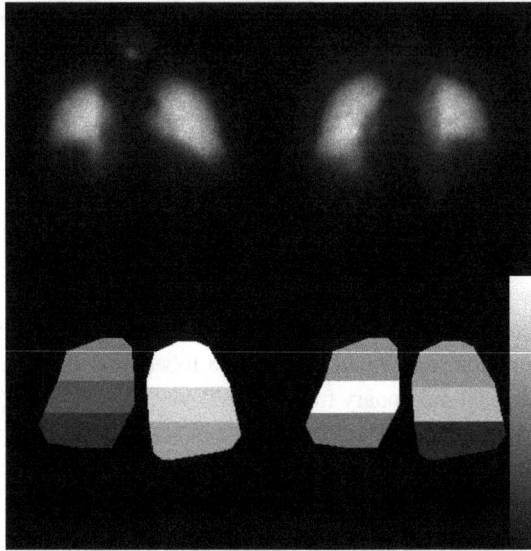

Figure 2.6 In the top row, the anterior (on the left) and posterior planar perfusion images are shown. On the bottom left, the regions, and on the right, the average count rate per segment or region are shown.

and three regions per lung are defined. Quantitative results are shown in Table 2.8 and the illustration is in Figure 2.6.

REFERENCES

1. De Roo MJK, Goris M, Van Der Schueren, Cosemans J, Billiet L, Gyselen A. Computerized dynamic scintigraphy of the lungs. *Respiration* 1969; 26:408–424.
2. Alderson PO, Biello DR, Khan AR, Barth KH, McKnight RC, Siegel BA. Comparison of 133-Xe single-breath and washout imaging in the scintigraphic diagnosis of pulmonary embolism. *Radiology* 1980; 137:481–486.
3. Alderson PO, Rujanevech N, Secker-Walker RH, McKnight RC. The role of 133-Xe ventilation studies in the scintigraphic detection of pulmonary embolism. *Radiology* 1976; 120:633–640.
4. Fazio F, Jones T. Assessment of regional lung ventilation by continuous inhalation of radioactive Krypton-81m. *Br Med J* 1975; 3:673–676.
5. Goris ML, Daspit SG, Walter JP, McRae J, Lamb J. Applications of ventilation lung scanning with 8lm-Krypton. *Radiology* 1977; 122:399–403.
6. Goris ML, Daspit SG. Lung ventilation studies with Kr-8lm, in Guter M (ed.), *Progress in Nuclear Medicine: New Radiogases in Practice* (1978). pp. 69–92. S. Karger, Basel, Munich, London, New York, Sydney.

7. Goris ML, Daspit SG. Krypton-81m ventilation scintigraphy for the diagnosis of pulmonary embolism. *Clin Nucl Med* 1981; 6:207–212.

8. Nosil J, Bajzer Z, Spaventi S. The use of 81m-Kr gas for the measurement of absolute regional lung ventilation. *Nuklearmedizin* 1977; 16:13–17.

9. Nosil J, Spaventi S, Slaus I. 81m-Kr: production, application, and use of computer for ventilation studies. *Eur J Nucl Med* 1977; 2:1–8.

10. Laube BL. Homogeneity of bronchopulmonary distribution of 99m-Tc aerosol in normal subjects and in cystic fibrosis patients. *Chest* 1989; 95:822–830.

11. Robin ED. Overdiagnosis and overtreatment of pulmonary embolism: the emperor has no clothes. *Ann Intern Med* 1972; 87:775–781.

12. Goldhaber SZ, Hennekens CH, Evans DA, Newton EC, Godleski JJ. Factors associated with correct antemortem diagnosis of major pulmonary embolism. *Am J Med* 1982; 73:822–826.

13. PIOPED investigators: Value of the ventilation/perfusion scan in acute pulmonary embolism. Results of the prospective investigation of pulmonary embolism diagnosis. (PIOPED). *JAMA* 1990; 263:2753–2759.

14. Stein PD, Athanasoulis C, Alavi A, Greenspan RH, Hales CA, Saltzman HA, Vreim CE, Terrin ML, Weg JG. Complications and validity of pulmonary angiography in acute pulmonary embolism. *Circulation* 1992; 85:462–468.

15. Anderson TM, Mall JC, Hoffer PB, Tetalman MR, Hendrix RW. Efficacy of emergency radionuclide perfusion lung studies. *Radiology* 1976; 120:125–130.

16. McNeil BJ. A diagnostic strategy using ventilation-perfusion studies in patients suspect for pulmonary embolism. *J Nucl Med* 1976; 17:613–616.

17. McCartney WH. Ventilation-perfusion lung scanning in pulmonary embolus. *Clin Nucl Med* 1981; 6:P27–P36.

18. Webber MM, Gomes AS, Roe D, La Fontaine RL, Hawkins RA. Comparison of Biello, McNeil and PIOPED Criteria for the diagnosis of pulmonary emboli on lung scans. *AJR* 1990; 154:975–981.

19. Worsley DF, Alavi A. Comprehensive Analysis of the Results of the PIOPED Study. *J Nucl Med* 1995; 36:2380–2387.

20. Freitas JE, Sarosi MG, Nagle CC, Yeomans ME, Freitas AE, Juni JE. Modified PIOPED criteria used in clinical practice. *J Nucl Med* 1995; 36:1573–1578.

21. Society of Nuclear Medicine. Procedure guidelines.

22. McNeil BJ. Ventilation-perfusion studies and the diagnosis of pulmonary embolism (concise communication). *J Nucl Med* 1980; 21:319–323.

23. H. Sostman HD, Coleman RE, DeLong DM, Newman GE, Pain S. Evaluation of revised criteria for ventilation perfusion scintigraphy in patients with suspected pulmonary embolism. *Radiology* 1994; 193:103–107.

24. Stein PD, Willis II PW, Dalen JE. The importance of clinical assessment in selecting patients for pulmonary angiography. *Am J Cardiol* 1979; 43:669–671.

25. Kahn D, Bushnell DL, Dean R, Perlman SB. Clinical outcome of patients with a "low probability" of pulmonary embolism on ventilation-perfusion lung scan. *Arch Intern Med* 1989; 149:377–379.

26. Ashburn WL, Belezzuoli EV, Dillon WA, Mensh BD, Hoogland D, Yeung DW, Coade GE. Technetium-99m labeled micro aerosol "Pertechnegas". A new agent for ventilation imaging in suspected pulmonary emboli, *Clin Nucl Med* 1993; 18:1045–1052.

27. Ballinger JR, Andrey TW, Boxen I, Zhang ZM. Formulation of technetium-99maerosol colloid with improved delivery efficiency for lung ventilation imaging. *J Nucl Med* 1993; 34:268–271.
28. Peltier P, Bardies M, Chetamieau A, Chatal JF. Comparison of technetium-99mC and phytate aerosol in ventilation studies. *Eur J Nucl Med* 1992; 19:349–354.
29. Sotman HD, Miniati M, Gottschalk A, Matta F, Stein PD, Pistolesi M. Sensitivity and specificity of perfusion scintigraphy combined with chest radiography for acute pulmonary embolism in PIOPED II. *J Nucl Med* 2008; 49:1741–1748.
30. Ralph DD. Pulmonary embolism, The implications of prospective investigation of pulmonary embolism diagnosis. *Radiol Clin North Am* 1994; 32:679–687.
31. Tourassi GD, Floyd CE, Sostman HD, Coleman RE. Acute pulmonary embolism: artificial neural network approach for diagnosis. *Radiology* 1993; 189:555–558.
32. Tourassi GD, Floyd CE, Sostman HD, Coleman RE. Artificial neural network for diagnosis of acute pulmonary embolism: effect of case and observer selection. *Radiology* 1995; 194:889–893.
33. Patil S, Hemy JAN, Rubenfire M, Stein PD. Neural network in the clinical diagnosis of acute pulmonary embolism. *Chest* 1993; 104:1685–1689.
34. Hull RD, Hirsh J, Carter CJ, Jay RM, Dodd PE, Ockelford PA, Coates G, Gill GJ, Turpie AG, Doyle DJ, Buller HR, Raskob GE. Pulmonary angiography, ventilation lung scanning, and venography for clinically suspected pulmonary embolism with abnormal perfusion lung scan. *Ann Intern Med* 1983; 98:891–899.
35. Hull RD, Hirsh J, Carter CJ, Raskob GE, Gill GJ, Jay RM, Leclerc JR, David M, Coates G. Diagnostic value of ventilation-perfusion lung scanning in patients with suspected pulmonary embolism. *Chest* 1985; 88:819–828.
36. Ginsberg JS: Impedance plethysmography: reevaluating its sensitivity for deep vein thrombosis. *Cardiology review* 1995; 12:20–22.
37. Stein PD, Hull RD, Saltzman HA, Pineo G. Strategy for diagnosis of patients with suspected acute pulmonary embolism. *Chest* 1993; 103:1553–1559.
38. Bautovich G, Angelides S, Lee FT, Greenough R, Bundesen P, Murray P, Schmidt P, Waugh R, Harris J, Cameron J. Detection of deep venous thrombi and pulmonary embolus with technetium-99m-DD-3B6/22 anti-fibrin monoclonal antibody Fab' fragment. *J Nucl Med* 1994; 35:195–202.
39. Worsley DF, Alavi A, Aronchick JM, Chen JT, Greenspan RH, Ravin CE. Chest radiographic findings in patients with acute pulmonary embolism: observations from the PIOPED study. *Radiology* 1993; 189:133–136.
40. Perrier A, Desmarais S, Goehring C, de Moerloos P, Morabia A, Unger PF, Slosman D, Junod A, Bounameaux H. D-dimer testing for suspected pulmonary embolism in outpatients. *Am J Respir Crit Care Med* 1997; 156:492–496.
41. Butler RR Jr, Wilf LH. Mismatch on Tc-99m DTPA aerosol ventilation-perfusion lung scan caused by achalasia. *Clin Nucl Med* 1994; 19:1028–1030.
42. Finestone H, Colp C, Rackson M, Shames J, Gallagher R. Ventilation-perfusion imaging in sarcoidosis: potential for nonembolic segmental mismatch. *J Nucl Med* 1994; 35: 476–478.
43. Worsley DF, Johnson RDA, Kwong JS. Bronchogenic cyst causing unilateral ventilation-perfusion mismatch. *Clin Nucl Med* 1996; 21:249–250.

44. Slonim SM, Molgaard CP, Khawaja IT, Seldin DW. Unilateral absence of right lung perfusion with normal ventilation on radionuclide scan as a sign of aortic dissection. *J Nucl Med* 1994; 35:1044–1047.

45. Oberdorster G, Utell MJ, Morrow PE, Hyde RW, Weber DA. Bronchial and alveolar absorption of inhaled 99mTc-DTPA. *Am Rev Respir Dis* 1986; 134:944–950.

46. Schmekel B, Bos JAH, Kahn AR, Wohlfart B, Lachmann B, Wollmer P. Integrity of the alveolar-capillary barrier and alveolar surfactant system in smokers. *Thorax* 1992; 47:603–608.

47. Coates G, O'Brodovich H. Measurement of pulmonary epithelial permeability with 99mTc-DTPA aerosol. *Semin Nucl Med* 1986; 16:275–284.

48. Caner B, Ugur O, Bayraktar M, Ulutuncel N, Mentes T, Telatar F, Bekdik C. Impaired lung epithelial permeability in diabetics detected by technetium-99m-DTPA aerosol scintigraphy. *J Nucl Med* 1994; 35:204–206.

49. Fanti S, De Fabritis A, Aloisi D, Dondi M, Marengo M, Compagnone G, Fallani F, Cavalli A, Monetti N. Early pulmonary involvement in systemic sclerosis assessed by Technetium-99m-DTPA clearance rate. *J Nucl Med* 1994; 35:1933–1936.

50. Mason GR, Effros RM, Uszler 3M, Mena I. Small solute clearance from the lungs in patients with cardiogenic and noncardiogenic pulmonary edema. *Chest* 1985; 88: 327–334.

51. Susskind H, Rom WN. Lung inflammation in coal miners assessed by uptake of 67-Ga-citrate and clearance of inhaled 99mTc-labeled DTPA. *Am Rev Respir Dis* 1992; 146: 47–52.

52. Bradvick I, Wollmer P, Evander E, Lárusdóttir H, Blom-Bülow B, Jonson B. Different kinetics of lung clearance of Technetium-99m labeled diethylene triamine penta-acetic acid in patients with sarcoidosis and smokers, *Eur J Nucl Med* 1994; 21: 1218–1222.

53. Mason GR, Uszler JM, Effros RM, Reid E. Rapidly reversible alternations of pulmonary epithelial permeability induced by smoking. *Chest* 1983, 83:6–11.

54. Wells AU, Hansell DM, Harrison NK, Lawrence R, Black CM, du Bois RM. Clearance of inhaled 99mTc-DTPA predicts the clinical course of fibrosing alveolitis. *Eur Respir J* 1993; 6:797–802.

55. Tateno M, Nakano A, Hasegawa A, Watanabe N, Oriuchi N, Inoue T, Endo K, Sasaki Y. Pulmonary clearance of 99mTc-DTPA aerosol in patients with progressive systemic scleroderma. *Kaku Igaku* 1992; 29:585–590.

56. Thunberg S, Larsson K, Eklund A, Blaschke E. 99mTc-DTPA clearance measured by a dual head gamma camera in healthy subjects and patients with sarcoidosis. Studies of reproducibility and relation to bronchoalveolar lavage findings. *Eur J Nucl Med* 1989; 15:71–77.

57. Gates GF, Goris ML. Suitability of radiopharmaceuticals for determining cardiac shunting. *J Nucl Med* 1975; 16:528.

58. Gates GF, Goris ML. Suitability of radiopharmaceuticals for determining right to left shunting. *J Nucl Med* 1977; 18:255–257.

59. Gates GF, Goris ML. Hypoxemia unassociated with anatomic shunting in pulmonary disease. *Clin Nucl Med* 1977; 2:227–231.

60. Robin ED, Laman PD, Goris ML, Theodore J, A shunt is (not) a shunt is (not) a shunt. *Ann Rev Resp Dis* 1077; 115:553–557.

61. Lu G, Shill W-J, Chou C, Xu J-Y. Tc-99m MAA total body imaging to detect intrapulmonary right-to-left shunts and to evaluate the therapeutic effect in pulmonary arteriovenous shunts. *Clin Nucl Med* 1996; 21:197–202.
62. Grimon G, Andre L, Bernard O, Raffestin B, Desgrez A. Early radionuclide detection of intrapulmonary shunts in children with liver disease. *J Nucl Med* 1994; 35:1328–1332.
63. Dowdle SC, Human DG, Mann MD. Pulmonary ventilation and perfusion abnormalities and ventilation perfusion imbalance in children with pulmonary atresia or extreme tetralogy of Fallot. *J Nucl Med* 1990; 31:1276–1279.
64. Houzard C, Andre M, Guilhen S, Thivolle P, Berger M. Perfusion lung scan in patients operated for transposition of the great arteries. *Clin Nucl Med* 1989; 14:268–270.
65. Matsushita T, Matsuda H, Ogawa M, Ohno K, Sano T, Nakano S, Shimazaki Y, Nakahari K, Arisawa J, Kozuka T, Kawashima Y, Yabuuchi H. Assessment of the intrapulmonary ventilation-perfusion distribution after the Fontan procedure for complex cardiac anomalies: Relation to pulmonary hemodynamics. *J Am Coll Cardiol* 1990; 15:842–848.
66. Cheng CP, Taur AS, Lee GS, Goris ML, Feinstein JA. Relative lung perfusion distribution in normal lung scans: observations and clinical implications. *Congenit Heart Dis* 2006; 5:210–216.
67. Corris PA. Use of Radionuclide scanning in the preoperative estimation of pulmonary function after pneumonectomy. *Thorax* 1987; 42:285–291.

Chapter 3

Renal Imaging with DMSA and the Generation of 3D Regions of Interest in Volume Images

3.1. CLINICAL CONTEXT

Dimercaptosuccinic acid (DMSA) usually labeled with ^{99m}Tc is one of the tubular tracers without excretion [1, 2]. If imaged properly, it allows for the evaluation of kidney size, their relative tubular function and the homogeneity of the tubular function (e.g. the presence or absence of "defects", often but not always, associated with renal scarring or acute pyelonephritis).

There are two aspects of the use of DMSA that at first appear confusing. First, the imaging modality is always scintigraphic, but could be planar (imaged with a parallel hole collimator PHC), planar (imaged with a pinhole collimator or PH), or single photon emission tomography (SPECT).

Second, the diagnostic context is not necessarily a question about the kidneys directly. In some cases, the DMSA image is used as a surrogate for vesicoureteral reflux (VUR), in the sense that in the case of a first (upper) urinary tract infection (UTI), a normal DMSA makes the diagnosis with a voiding cystourethrogram (VCUG) unnecessary. Sometimes, in an acute phase, abnormal "early" DMSA images define, confirm or illustrate the diagnosis of acute pyelonephritis (APN). Finally, early DMSA is used to predict later scarring after an UTI, APN or reflux (VUR), as defined by "late" DMSA imaging.

However, serious efforts at quantification are all based on the analysis of PHC planar imaging (for relative function) or SPECT imaging for defect quantification and not PH.

There are some experimental or empiric data about the sensitivity of DMSA imaging for "defects" in the acute phase or late phase. The sensitivity to detect histologically verified APN in piglets with DMSA was 92% for SPECT and 83% for pinhole scintigraphy. But the specificity was lower for SPECT (82% vs. 95%) (3). In an experimental model of UTI and VUR in piglets, Risdon (4) finds that DMSA imaging has a specificity of 100% with APN lesions, but smaller lesions are not detected, with the sensitivity being 80%. In a similar experimental setup but in the chronic phase, Arnold (5) finds a sensitivity of 85% for macroscopic scarring and a specificity of 97%. Again, the sensitivity decreases with minor lesions. The importance of those numbers will be underscored when the operating characteristics of ultrasound (US) is evaluated against DMSA as a "gold standard" (see also Section 7.1).

Rossleigh (6) also used pig models and histology as a standard to compare different methods of imaging; in this case, late DMSA PHC, PH, SPECT and US. He found that PHC had the best operating characteristics. The operating characteristics (sensitivity and specificity) were: for PHC 62% and 100% respectively, for PH 74% and 99%, for SPECT 59% and 98%, and for US 29 and 92%. The size of pigs, when used for late studies, becomes a handicap, specifically for US. The near equivalence of PH and planar may also be explained by the subject's size. Strangely enough, the authors reject SPECT, because no quantification is available (see Section 3.2.2).

In patients, Itoh (7) found SPECT to be more sensitive than planar imaging by a factor of 1.5 in detecting abnormalities and loss of function, at least in grades III and IV reflux, and the abnormalities correlated with the degree of reflux. This introduces DMSA as a surrogate of VUR. Simiou (8) defines the controversy: 72 neonates (144 renal units) with a first (symptomatic) UTI are included in the study. DMSA imaging was performed within 72 hours and a VCUG within 2 months. DMSA imaging was repeated after 6 months.[a] APN was detected by DMSA in 19% of the renal units, VUR in 22%. However, 71% of the grade III or higher cases of VUR had normal DMSA imaging. The sensitivity of DMSA imaging for grade III or higher RUV was only 29%, with a specificity of 82%. However, all the units (N = 75) with scarring had an early abnormal DMSA scan. At this time, we would conclude that a normal early DMSA scan does not exclude significant RUV, but does exclude late scarring.[b] In addition, Chiou (9) used DMSA SPECT

---

[a]This sets the stage for early and late DMSA imaging, where abnormalities in the former connote APN and in the latter, scarring.
[b]As defined by DMSA imaging.

to measure a defect volume and radioactivity ratio in the acute phase and again at the late phase. Larger volumes in the acute phase were more likely to predict scarring in the late study with a sensitivity and specificity of 96% and 92%.

Does a normal DMSA scan voids the need for a VCUG? In infants (< 2 years, N = 220) with a febrile UTI, Lee (10), looking separately at high and low grade VUR, and in combination of US and DMSA, did not find a high diagnostic yield. VUR was detected in 67 cases (30.4%). If a distinction is made between low and high grade VUR, the results are that of the Table 3.1 (sensitivity only).

The authors speculate, however, that negative US and DMSA scans (in a logical AND[c]) have a high predictive value for improvement after either high or low grade reflux.

The prevalence of VUR in children with a first UTI was 14.3% (139/974) in a large Chinese study (11), and more frequent in toddlers (< 2 years). In that case, with a sensitivity and specificity of 24.8% and 94.3% respectively for US, the positive predictive value is not high (see Table 3.2 and Section 7.1).

The contrary opinion is given by Lin (12). The patients are infants with a first UTI (N = 114). Lin does not see the value of a VCUG in infants with a UTI with a negative DMSA, mainly because late scarring was not correlated to VUR as demonstrated by VCUG, and was absent with a negative early DMSA. Again, the

Table 3.1   Sensitivities (10).

	US	DMSA	Either one
Low grade	41.7	37.5	62.5
High grade	86%	88.4	95.3

Table 3.2   Derived from Ref. 11.

$P(S+|D+)$	0.248
$P(S+|D-)$	0.057
$P(D+)$	0.143
$P(D+)P(S+|D+)$	0.035
$1 - P(D+)$	0.857
$(1 - P(D+))P(S+|D-)$	0.049
$P(D+|S+)$	0.421

---

[c]See Section 7.7.

prevalence of VUR was 14.9. In support of that thesis, Tseng (13) reported a small number of patients (toddlers ≤ 2 years, N $= 142$) with their first UTI. The VCUG was positive in 42 toddlers while early DMSA was positive in 99 patients, but only two had renal scarring. The operating characteristics of the DMSA scan for the detection of VUR were as follows:

Sensitivity   88% (95% confidence: 73–100%)
Specificity   36% (95% confidence 26–46%)
PPV   37% (95% confidence 27–46%)
NPV   0.33% (95% confidence 0–0.88%)

A negative DMSA in those circumstances practically excludes the possibility of a VUR; Moorthy (14) agrees. The value of the observation is that the dose for a radiological VCUG is much higher than for a DMSA scan; this may also be true for a scintigraphic VCUG. But could an US not do as well? In this case the question is: If a defect is detected by DMSA, what is the chance that it be detected by some form of US? In effect, DMSA becomes a gold standard. But is that reasonable?

The data[d] suggest that in the first UTI, the prevalence of VUR is $\pm 15\%$. The sensitivity of DMSA may be as high as 0.9, in which case, out of 100 renal units, 13.5 would come out positive. The specificity is high (0.94), in which case 81.4 out of the 100 units would be negative. If US were perfect, there would have been 15 positive and 85 negative cases. At best, the discrepancy would have been an apparent 1.5 false positive and an apparent 3.6 false negative cases. Therefore, in the best case, the US would have had a sensitivity of 73% and a specificity of 98% (Table 3.3).

In actuality, all the forms of US do not perform at that level, but the results are not as bad as they seem, considering that the gold standard is not pure gold.

Narshi (15) found that in infants with UTI, early Doppler US detected only 33% of late DMSA scarring. Stogianni (16) used DMSA as a standard for the number

Table 3.3   Deriving US operating characteristics.

	DMSA	Perfect	False	Specificity	Sensitivity
Positive	13.50	15.00	1.50	0.98	—
Negative	81.40	85.00	3.60	—	0.73

[d]Taken from the patient studies for the prevalence and from the piglet and pig studies for the sensitivity and specificity for defect or scarring.

of scars, and power Doppler ultrasound (PDUS). The PDUS sensitivity was 73.8, while the specificity was 85.7. Basiratnia (17) compared power Doppler US in the acute phase to early DMSA and the sensitivity and specificity were found to be 89% and 53% respectively. Wang (18) compared US with SPECT DMSA in the acute phase, and found US sensitivities and specificities for the detection of APN to be 49.2% and 88% respectively. Biggy (19) looked at US abnormalities in APN, also documented by DMSA and find the sensitivity and specificity of US to be 27% and 89% respectively.

In general, the specificity of US is close to what the ideal specificity would be if DMSA is the gold standard; the sensitivity is significantly lower than expected. The lowest values for the sensitivity were recorded by Moorthy (20) who found the sensitivity for US (vs. late DMSA) to be 5.2% with a specificity of 98.3%. However, for diffuse scarring, the sensitivity of US was 47.2%. One expects that unilateral diffuse scarring would also be detected by a quantitative DMSA study, in which asymmetry in DMSA renal uptake would show.

Some authors (21, 22) compared DMSA to intravenous urography (IVU). Ozen (22) found the two methods equivalent for the number of scars, but DMSA superior in the evaluation of the scar (scoring). Shanon (21) found that the sensitivity and specificity of DMSA, IVU and US were 94% and 100%, 76% and 100% and 65% and 96% respectively.

Acosta (23) presented some evidence that segmental abnormalities can be detected with DMSA after captopril, and thus help in the diagnosis of renovascular hypertension (RVH), even though the effect of captopril on tubular agents is believed to be minimal. In fact, since the glomerular fraction would decrease under captopril, tubular uptake should increase or remain unchanged (24, 25).

Estorch (26) considers the problem of the difference between a small kidney with less uptake and a large kidney with less uptake and proposes a size correction. Indeed, a small kidney, perfused in proportion to its size would not be ischemic. A small kidney, less perfused than proportionally with size, would be ischemic and could explain hypertension. Rossleigh (6) uses renal length as a measure of size, but that is difficult to accept unless one assumes that the kidney's long axis is always parallel to the imaging plane. A 3D image would allow a direct measure of renal volume. In fact, other quantitative measures also require a volumetric image: Hitzel (27) in one paper describes three methods to quantificate abnormalities in planar DMSA images, with the goal to define the predictive value of DMSA in the acute phase (of APN) for the late phase renal scarring. One of the methods is successful: it is essentially the ratio of counts at a given threshold (70%) comparing to the counts at a 20% threshold. If this ratio is less than 0.45, late scarring is more likely. But he also compares the volumes at different thresholds, even though projection images do not yield volumes directly. In what follows, we will explore the contribution of volume or 3D images to the quantification and characterization of DMSA images.

3.2. ANALYZING IMAGES AS TRULY THREE-DIMENSIONAL

Three-dimensional or volumetric imaging dominates radiology, MRI and to a certain extent, nuclear medicine. And while tools for the quantitative analysis of planar images (regions of interest and time-activity curves) do exist in nuclear medicine, it is worthy to note that few exist for volumetric images. The direct application of planar methods to multiple slices in a volume is tedious, work intensive and imprecise at the cranial and caudal ends in transverse slices. Groshar (28) partially overcomes it by selecting thick slices in the three orthogonal displays, and settling on a best (inclusive) slice.

The interesting aspect of most approaches is that the SPECT image is not really recognized as a volume image (29). But there is a method to delineate an organ in 3D in a volumetric image, and to extract the activity and volume in the next step. To evaluate and demonstrate the method, we have applied the method to renal imaging with DMSA although the original application was splenic imaging in children treated for hypersplenism.

In planar renal imaging, in addition to the visual evaluation of cortical irregularities due to scarring, the relative uptake in each kidney is also measured. This is mostly done with conjugate views (simultaneously acquired anterior and posterior projections). If the counts in the anterior image in a kidney are A, and in the posterior B, the "true" count in the kidney is assumed to be $\sqrt{AB}$, the geometric mean (see Section 10.5). But, as pointed out by Estorch (26), renal activity and volume are not identical metrics. Even so, anatomical imaging does not have an easy metric for function, and tends to use volume as surrogates.

Traditionally, renal size has been expressed as renal length (6). There should be a correlation between renal length and volume, but not in planar imaging. The renal length cannot be truly evaluated, because the kidneys do not, in general, have their long axis parallel to the detector plane. That does not necessarily deter people from using that approach. Lin (31) uses DMSA SPECT for renal length, but strangely enough in the summation image of coronal slices, which reduces the method to the limitation of planar imaging. In a volumetric image, if the upper pole is in location $[x_1, y_1, z_1]$ and the lower pole in $[x_2, y_2, z_2]$, the renal length would be $L = \sqrt{(x_2 - x_1)^2 + (y_2 - y_1)^2 + (z_2 - z_1)^2}$ and not $y_2 - y_1$.

Ultrasound imaging does not have that limitation, because the imaging plane can be selected to include the long axis (30). Using CT, Morrisroe (32) finds that function (by DMSA) generally correlates with volume by CT, but not at lower function. The metric is not an absolute volume, but a percentage volume and DMSA on the right or left.

Song (33) found a correlation between the surgical reduction of renal volume and GFR (by DTPA). His volumes are absolute (millimetric), but the volume is defined by analyzing the image slice by slice. Kim (34) finds with 3D US a good correlation with renal volumes defined by CT. Again, the method is very artisanal. Fowler (35) uses contrast CT (portal venous phase) with DMSA as the gold standard, again on a slice basis (thick slices), but sophisticated in the sense that fatty and non-contrast enhanced tissue is eliminated. The correlation is good, but the comparison is fraction of volume to L and R, not actual volume.

In general, little effort was expanded on using a volumetric approach (36). Marcuzzo (37) uses planar imaging (PHC), but a rather sophisticated segmentation; however the comparison is with visual interpretation.

In volumetric images, if an organ can de-delineated, since the size of the voxels is known, the volume of the organ can be determined. If the volumes can be determined from DMSA SPECT images, what can one learn?

The answer lies in the nature of SPECT imaging:

- The organs occupy space exclusively. There is no overlap, therefore no background subtraction is required.
- While in anatomical imaging, size is used as a surrogate for function, in planar DMSA imaging, activity is used as a surrogate for size; the two are conflated.
- In SPECT, size (volume) and function (activity) can be evaluated separately.

There are a number of questions that can be answered using SPECT. First, is there an advantage in the use of conjugate views even in small subjects? Second, is the activity distribution between both kidneys different if derived from conjugate planar imaging or from volumetric imaging (SPECT)? Third, are the volumes derived from volumetric images in concordance with the expected value (30)? Fourth and last, is there a fixed relation between relative DMSA uptake and relative volume (26)?

In what follows, we describe a study devised to answer those questions.

3.2.1. *Material and Methods*

With Hongyun June Zhu and Paolo Castaneda.

3.2.1.1. *Patient population*

The patient population consists of 41 patients who underwent a renal study with DMSA, and from whom planar and SPECT images were obtained. All identifying information (name, medical record number, accession number, date of study and date of birth) were removed from the data except the millimetric values of the voxels and the age at the time of the study. In 10 of the cases, mainly very small and young subjects, the planar acquisition consisted only of a posterior projection. In nine cases, only one kidney was detected by either method. The average age was 56 months, the median was 18 months, with a minimum of 2.9 months and a maximum of 21 years.

3.2.1.2. SPECT data

The SPECT data were reconstructed by filter back-projection, with a Butterworth filter and with a cut-off frequency and order adapted to the noise of the images and the size of the kidneys.

3.2.1.3. 3D regions of interest

Three-dimensional (3D) regions of interest were produced as follows: coronal, sagital and transverse maximum intensity projection (MIP) images were produced. On each, the organ was delineated by a ROI, as would be done on a projection image. In the volume, a voxel with coordinates (K, L, M) is considered part of a preliminary 3D ROI, if and only if, the coordinates (K, L) define a point within the ROI of the transverse MIP, the coordinates (K, M) define a point within the ROI of the coronal MIP and the coordinates (L, M) define a point within the sagital MIP. Then, within this preliminary 3D ROI, a maximum count value "max" is determined, and all voxels with values below max/10 are set at zero.[e] What remains is a perfectly contoured 3D ROI around the organ (Figure 3.1).

All voxel values within this refined region are added to define the organ counts (A) in the final ROI. The number of voxels in this 3D ROI multiplied by the x, y and z dimensions (in cm) of the voxels define the organ volume (ml). The relative uptake (A%) in one kidney or volume (V%), is computed as $100X/(X+Y)$ where X and Y are the counts or volumes in the respective kidneys (Figure 3.2).

3.2.2. Results

In general, the relation between age and volume is identical for the expected and the observed volumes. For the expected, $\ln(E) = 0.45*\ln(age) + 4.2$ and $\ln(O) = 0.43*\ln(age) + 4.11$.

---

[e]This value can be changed either interactively or according to the application.

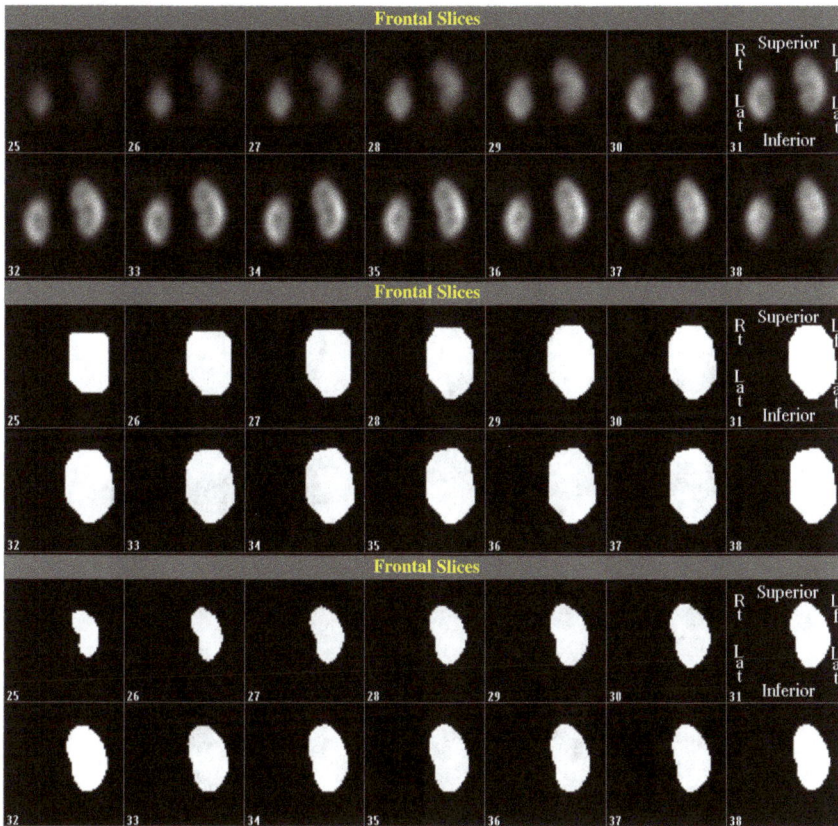

Figure 3.1 The top two rows show coronal slices through the two kidneys in the reconstructed SPECT volume. The next two rows are the coronal slices through the intersection of the three orthogonal planar ROIs for the left kidney. The third set of two rows are the coronal slices through the final left renal ROI.

First, the obvious: If taken directly, the length of the kidney (cm) is not equivalent to the volume (cm^3 or ml). In fact, the length cubed yield a better correspondence (Figure 3.3).

The results for the activity split from conjugate views correspond closely with those from SPECT data. Converging values from two different approaches are reassuring but not proof. One should indeed remember that the mathematics underlying the conjugate views and geometrical means approach, does in fact only apply to point sources (Section 10.5), however, if the renal function is good, tissue crosstalk is minimal, and the subjects are generally small (Figure 3.4).

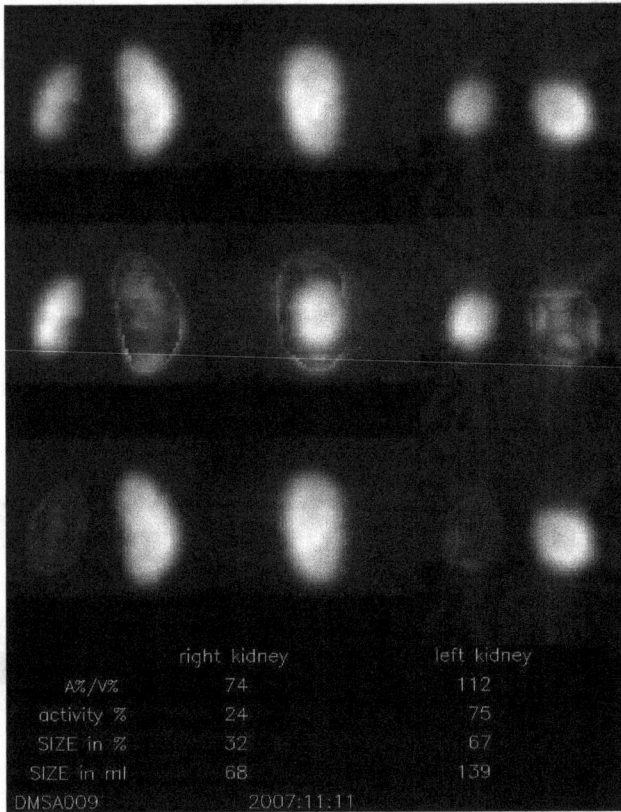

Figure 3.2   The top row shows the MIP[f] images of the reconstructed volume image. The next rows show the MIPs images after the removal of the left and right kidneys respectively. The results are the sizes in ml, the size in percentage of the sum of R and L kidneys, the percentage activity in each kidney, and the ratios of activity percentage/volume percentage.

Organ volumes (ml) derived with 3D ROI from volumetric data, in this case the kidneys, seem to agree with volumes acquired from other modalities. Also, in general, relative function (A%) correlates closely with relative volume (V%) but this is not always true (26). This is due to the patient population, in whom the decrease in perfusion is secondary to scarring, in contradistinction to the

---

[f]Maximum Intensity Projection images.

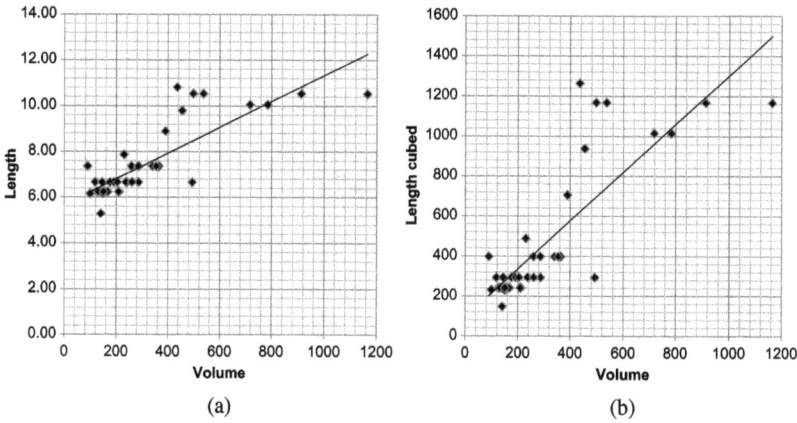

(a)   (b)

Figure 3.3   (a) Relationship between renal volume (ml) and renal length (cm). The regression is L(cm) = 5.7 + 0.006 × V(ml). (b) Relationship between renal volume (ml) and renal length (cm^3). The regression is $L(\text{cm}^3) = 95 + 1.2 \times V(\text{ml})$.

case in renovascular hypertension, where the flow is less than the anatomy would predict (Figure 3.4).

Finally, A% and V% are closely related. For each case, if we were to take the smallest kidney, the relation is V% = 1.04 * A% − 2.49 ± 7.54 (Paired t-test p = 0.638). The aberrant values are due to a large polycystic kidney in one case. The smallest kidney accumulated 50% of the activity, and was the only normal size; however V% was 35%. The other case, with a near normal volume (V% = 44%) and a very low uptake (Figure 3.4) may represent a failure of the set 10% thresholding. With those two cases eliminated, it appears that for smaller kidneys the volume is overestimated or the activity underestimated (A/V = 0.0107 * V% + 0.50), but the relation is a weak one (Figure 3.4 and Table 3.4).

3.3. DISCUSSION AND CONCLUSION

In other applications, 3D ROI analysis for volumetric data may be more useful, as in comparing the size of the spleen and the relative uptake in the spleen, versus size and uptake in the liver (38, 39). Another application is the determination of the mass and total SUV in lesions on PET (40, 41) volumes. The major point is that the analysis of SPECT data a true 3D analysis is possible, not difficult nor particularly work intensive, in comparison with methods based on organ delineation slice by slice.

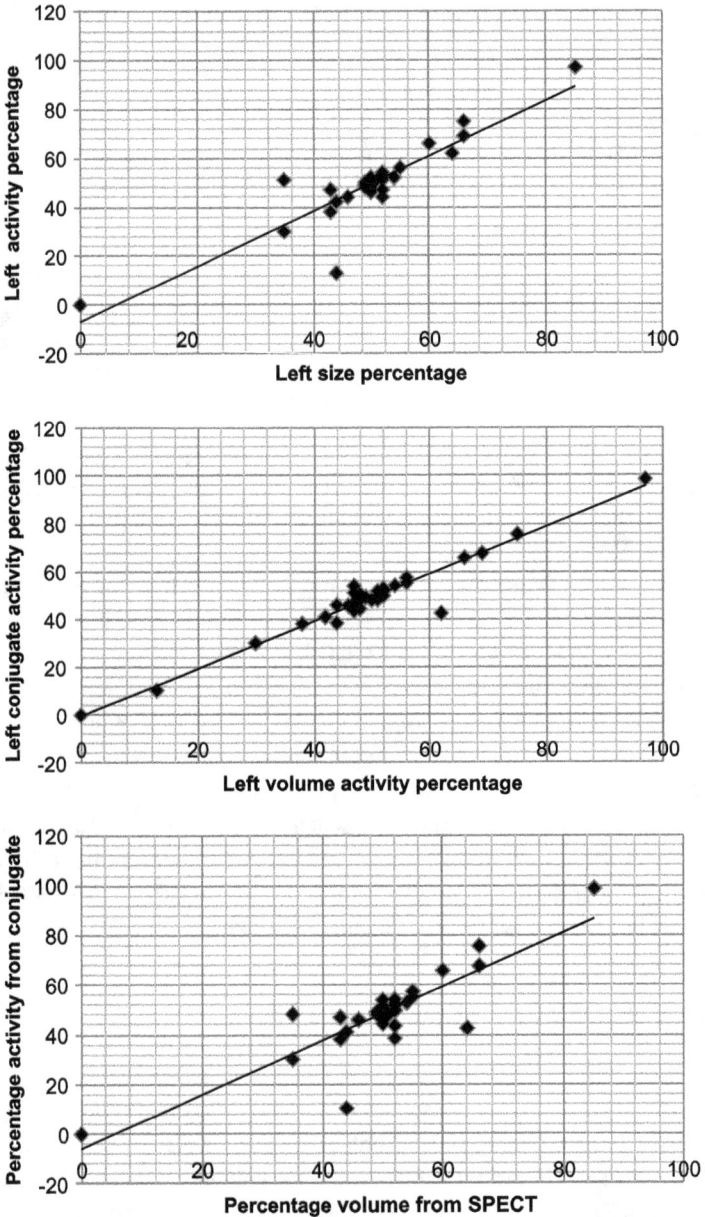

Figure 3.4 Comparison of three relations between a 3D volume, 3D counts and conjugate counts. The counts are expressed as a percentage of left activity, the volumes a percentage of total volume. Quantitative comparison is given in Table 3.4.

Table 3.4   Results of linear regression between the variables are illustrated in Figure 3.4. The "best" regression is between counts (%) from 3D and conjugate images. The worse was between 3D volume and planar counts.

	Parameter	Value	Std error	P	P	F
3D volume vs. 3D counts	**Intercept**	−7.0812	5.1476	0.1788	NS	128
3D volume vs. 3D counts	**Slope**	1.1277	0.0994	0.0000	S	
3D counts vs. planar counts	**Intercept**	−0.3244	2.3533	0.8912	NS	476
3D counts vs. planar counts	**Slope**	0.9878	0.0452	0.0000	S	
3D volume vs. planar counts	**Intercept**	−6.1268	6.2481	0.3344	NS	81
3D volume vs. planar counts	**Slope**	1.0902	0.1207	0.0000	S	

REFERENCES

1. Handmaker H. Etude renale fonctionnelle differntielle simple a l'aide du 99m-technetium DMSA. *Compte rendu du II colloque Intl*, Paris 1975; pp. 225–232.

2. Handmaker H, Young BW, Lowenstein JM. Clinical experience with 99mTc-DMSA (dimercaptosuccinic acid), a new renal-imaging agent. *J Nucl Med* 1975; 16(1): 28–32.

3. Majd M, Rushton HG, Chandra R, Andrich MP, Tardif CP, Rashti F. Technetium-99m-DMSA renal cortical scintigraphy to detect experimental acute pyelonephritis in piglets: comparison of planar (pinhole) and SPECT imaging. *J Nucl Med* 1996; 37(10):1731–1734.

4. Risdon RA, Godley ML, Parkhouse HF, Gordon I, Ransley PG. Renal pathology and the 99mTc-DMSA image during the evolution of the early pyelonephritic scar: an experimental study. *J Urol* 1994; 151(3):767–773.

5. Arnold AJ, Brownless SM, Carty HM, Rickwood AM. Detection of renal scarring by DMSA scanning — an experimental study. *J Pediatr Surg* 1990; 25(4):391–393.

6. Rossleigh MA, Farnsworth RH, Leighton DM, Yong JL, Rose M, Christian CL. Technetium-99m dimercaptosuccinic acid scintigraphy studies of renal cortical scarring and renal length. *J Nucl Med* 1998; 39(7):1280–1285.

7. Itoh K, Yamashita T, Tsukamoto E, Nonomura K, Furudate M, Koyanagi T. Qualitative and quantitative evaluation of renal parenchymal damage by 99mTc-DMSA planar and SPECT scintigraphy. *Ann Nucl Med* 1995; 9(1):23–28.

8. Siomou E, Giapros V, Fotopoulos A, Aasioti M, Papadopoulou F, Serbis A, Siamopoulou A, Andronikou S. Implications of 99mTc-DMSA Scintigraphy Performed During Urinary Tract Infection in Neonates. *Pediatrics* 2009.

9. Chiou YY, Wang ST, Tang MJ, Lee BF, Chiu NT. Renal fibrosis: prediction from acute pyelonephritis focus volume measured at 99mTc dimercaptosuccinic acid SPECT. *Radiology* 2001; 221(2):366–370.

10. Lee HY, Hyun Soh B, Hee Hong C, Joon Kim M, Won Han S. The efficacy of ultrasound and dimercaptosuccinic acid scan in predicting vesicoureteral reflux in children below the age of 2 years with their first febrile urinary tract infection. *Pediatr Nephrol* 2009; 24(10):2009–2013.

11. Wang Z, Xu H, Liu HM, Rao J, Shen Q, Cao Q. Clinical analysis of 139 cases of primary vesicoureteric reflux in children. *Zhonghua Er Ke Za Zhi* 2008; 46(7): 518–521.

12. Lin CH, Yang LY, Wamg HH, Chang JW, Shen MC, Tang RB. Evaluation of imaging studies for vesicoureteral reflux in infants with first urinary tract infection. *Acta Paediatr Taiwan* 2007; 48(2):68–72.

13. Tseng MH, Lin WJ, Lo WT, Wang SR, Chu ML, Wang CC. Does a normal DMSA obviate the performance of voiding cystourethrography in evaluation of young children after their first urinary tract infection? *J Pediatr* 2007; 150(1):96–99.

14. Moorthy I, Easty M, McHugh K, Ridout D, Biassoni L, Gordon I. The presence of vesicoureteric reflux does not identify a population at risk for renal scarring following a first urinary tract infection. *Arch Dis Child* 2005; 90(7):733–736.

15. Narchi H, Donovan R. Renal power Doppler ultrasound does not predict renal scarring after urinary tract infection. *Scott Med J* 2008; 53(4):7–10.

16. Stogianni A, Nikolopoulos P, Oikonomou I, Gatzola M, Balaris V, Farmakiotis D, Dimitriadis A. Childhood acute pyelonephritis: comparison of power Doppler sonography and Tc-DMSA scintigraphy. *Pediatr Radiol* 2007; 37(7):685–690.

17. Basiratnia M, Noohi AH, Lotfi M, Alavi MS. Power Doppler sonographic evaluation of acute childhood pyelonephritis. *Pediatr Nephrol* 2006; 21(12):1854–1857.

18. Wang YT, Chiu NT, Chen MJ, Huang JJ, Chou HH, Chiou YY. Correlation of renal ultrasonographic findings with inflammatory volume from dimercaptosuccinic acid renal scans in children with acute pyelonephritis. *J Urol* 2005; 173:190–194.

19. Biggi A, Dardanelli L, Pomero G, Cussino P, Noello C, Sernia O, Spada A, Camuzzini G. Acute renal cortical scintigraphy in children with a first urinary tract infection. *Pediatr Nephrol* 2001; 16(9):733–738.

20. Moorthy I, Wheat D, Gordon I. Ultrasonography in the evaluation of renal scarring using DMSA as the gold standard. *Pediatr Nephrol* 2004; 19:153–156.

21. Shanon A, Feldman W, McDonald P, Martin DJ, Matzinger MA, Shillinger JF, McLaine PN, Wolfish N. Evaluation of renal scars by technetium-labeled dimercaptosuccinic acid scan, intravenous urography, and ultrasonography: a comparative study. *J Pediatr* 1992; 120(3):399–403.

22. Ozen HA, Basa I, Erbas B, Ozen S, Ergen A, Balkanci F, Bakkaloglu A. DMSA renal scanning versus urography for detecting renal scars in vesicoureteral reflux. *Eur Urol* 1990; 17:47–50.

23. Acosta Gómez MJ, Llamas Elvira JM, Rodríguez Fernández A, Gómez Río M, López Ruiz JM, Muros De Fuentes MA, Moral Ruiz A, Ramírez Navarro A. Diagnosis of renovascular hypertension by pre- and post-captopril renal scintigraphy with 99mTc-DMSA. *Rev Esp Med Nucl* 2001; 20(7):537–543.

24. Lee HB, Blaufox MD. Technetium-99m MAG-3 clearance after captopril in experimental renovascular hypertension. *J Nucl Med* 1988; 30:666–671.

25. McAfee JG, Kopecky RT, Thomas FD, Hellwig B, Roskopf M. Comparison of different radioactive agents for the detection of renovascular hypertension with captopril in the rat model. *J Nucl Med* 1988; 29:509–515.

26. Estorch M, Torres G, Camacho V, Tembl A, Prat L, Mena E, Flotats A, Carrió I. Individual renal function based on 99mTc dimercaptosuccinic acid uptake corrected for renal size. *Nucl Med Commun* 2004; 25(2):167–170.

27. Hitzel A, Liard A, Dacher JN, Gardin I, Ménard JF, Manrique A, Véra P. Quantitative analysis of 99mTc-DMSA during acute pyelonephritis for prediction of long-term renal scarring. *J Nucl Med* 2004; 45(2):285–289.

28. Groshar D, Frankel A, Iosilevsky G, Israel O, Moskovitz B, Levin DR, Front D. Quantitation of renal uptake of Technetium-99m DMSA using SPECT. *J Nucl Med* 1989; 30: 246–250.

29. Goris ML, Boudier S, Briandet PA. Interrogation and display of single photon emission tomography data as inherently volume data. *Am J Physiol Imaging* 1986; 4: 168–180.

30. Rosenbaum DM, Korngold E, Teel RL. Sonographic assessment of renal length in normal children. *AJR Am J Roentgenol* 1984; 142:467–469.

31. Lin E, Connolly LP, Zurakowski D, DiCanzio J, Drubach L, MichellK, Tetrault T, Laffin SP, Treves ST. Reproducibility od renal length measurements with ^{99m}Tc-DMSA SPECT. *J Nucl Med* 2000; 41:1632–1635.

32. Morrisroe SN, Su RR, Bae KT, Eisner BH, Hong C, Lahey S, Catalano OA, Sahani DV, Jackman SV. Differential renal function estimation using computerized tomography based renal parenchymal volume measurement. *J Urol* 2010; 183:2289–2293.

33. Song C, Bang JK, Park HK, Ahn H. Factors influencing renal function reduction after partial nephrectomy. *J Urol* 2009; 182:395–396.

34. Kim HC, Yang DM, Lee SH, Cho YD. Usefulness of renal volume measurements obtained by 3-dimensional sonographic transducer with matrix electronic arrays. *J Ultrasound Med* 2008; 27:1673–1681.

35. Fowler JC, Breadsmoore C, Gaskart MTG, Cheow HK, Bernal R, Hegarty P, Bullock KM, Taylor H, Dixon AK, Peters AM. A simple processing method allowing comparison of renal enhancing volumes derived from standard portal venous contrast-enhanced. *Br J Radiol* 2006; 79:935–942.

36. Kistler AD, Poster D, Krauer F, Weishaupt D, Raina A, Senn O, Binet I, Spanous K, Wütrich RP, Serra AL. Increases in kidney volume in autosomal dominant plycystic kidney disease can be detected within 6 months. *Kidney Int* 2009; 75:235–242.

37. Marcuzzo M, Masiero PR, Scharcanski J. Quantitative parameters for the assessment of renal scintigraphic images. *Proc IEEE Engl Med Biol Soc* 2007; 3431–3441.

38. Héry G, Becmeur F, Méfat L, Kalfa D, Lutz P, Lutz L, Guys JM, de Lagausie P. Laparoscopic partial splenectomy: indications and results of a multicenter retrospective study. *Surg Endosc* 2007; Oct 18.

39. Choi YS, Han HS, Yoon YS, Jang JY, Kim SW, Park YH. Laparoscopic splenectomy plus cholecystectomy for treating hereditary spherocytosis combined with cholelithiasis in siblings. *Minim Invasive Ther Allied Technol* 2007; 16(5):317–318.

40. Goris ML, Mari C, Zhu H, Wapnir IL. Volumetric regions of interest (3D-ROI) in small animal's SPECT studies: the definition of the appropriate metric at the limit of spatial resolution. Presented at the Annual Congress of the European Association of Nuclear Medicine, Vienna, Austria, August 31, September 4, 2002. *Eur J Nucl Med* 2002; 29:S139.
41. Zhu HJ, Vasanawala M, Wang Y, Mari C, Goris ML. In FDG PET, SUVs are dependent on a competitive system and hence dependent of uptake in other tissues, and excretion. SNM 2006. *J Nucl Med* 2006; 47:361.

Chapter 4

Therapy with Radionuclides

4.1. INTRODUCTION

Therapy with radionuclides is a form of radiation therapy characterized by three factors:

- The radiation source is inside the patient, thus in that sense it is similar to brachytherapy.[a] Brachytherapy is performed using solid radioactive sources that are placed (surgically) next to the target, and can be removed when the planned dose of radiation has been delivered. With soluble sources, the "placement" depends on the biodistribution of the substrate to which the radioisotope is attached.
- The radiation rate and total dose are connected by the physical characteristics of the radionuclide and the biological behavior of the substrate. The dose cannot be removed as in brachytherapy.
- To the extent that the biodistribution is not perfect (in the sense that only the target would accumulate the substance), other organs will be affected by the radiation originating from the substrate's label. Also, unlike external beam radiotherapy, the radiation originating in the substance cannot be focused towards the target. Activity in one organ will affect the radiation absorbed dose in surrounding organs.

---

[a]From Wikipedia, the free encyclopedia: Brachytherapy (from the Greek word *brachys*, meaning "short-distance"), also known as internal radiotherapy, sealed source radiotherapy, curietherapy or endocurietherapy, is a form of radiotherapy where a radiation source is placed inside or next to the area requiring treatment. Brachytherapy is commonly used as an effective treatment for cervical [1], prostate [2], breast [3], and skin cancer [4] and can also be used to treat tumors in many other body sites [5]. Brachytherapy can be used alone or in combination with other therapies such as surgery, external beam radiotherapy (EBRT) and chemotherapy.

First, we will review the basis of dosimetry with (soluble) radioactive substances. Second, we will review some treatment applications, and third, we will discuss the radiation protection aspect of releasing a radioactive patient.

4.2. DOSIMETRY: INTERNAL RADIATION DOSIMETRY

In this chapter, we review dosimetry resulting from radioactivity in organs and tissues. The formalism for those computations is usually referred to as MIRD formalism, where MIRD stands for Medical Internal Radiation Dosimetry.

4.2.1. Radiation Depends on the Amount of Radioactivity and the Length of the Exposure: Cumulative Activity

If the activity is expressed as A mCi and does not leave the organ (no biological excretion), then the cumulative activity is the integral of the exponential function $Ae^{-\lambda t}$, where λ is the decay constant. The conventional expression is the activity multiplying the average residency time. In the hypothesis of no excretion, the average residency time is the initial activity times 1.44 the physical half life (T_p). But the hypothesis is unrealistic in most cases. All the activity is not in its final location from time zero, nor is the physical decay the only way by which the activity decreases.

$$\bar{A} = \int_0^\infty A_{(0)}e^{-\lambda t}dt,$$

$$\bar{A} = \frac{A_{(0)}}{\lambda},$$

$$\bar{A} = 1.44\, T_p A_{(0)}. \quad \text{(see Equation 8.9)}$$

In general, the cumulative activity is expressed as mCi.hr (millicurie.hour).[b] In the simple case that only the physical decay is in play, if the physical half-life is given as 8.6 days, it becomes 8.6 days $\times 24\frac{\text{hrs}}{\text{day}} = 206.4$ and the corresponding decay constant $\lambda = 0.080581^{-\text{day}}$, becomes $\frac{0.080581}{day} = \frac{0.080581}{day} \times \frac{day}{24}hr = \frac{0.003358}{hr}$.

However, the functional description of the kinetics of a tracer in a particular organ is not often well described by a single exponential. Often, the sampling

---

[b]If the physical half-life is 8.6 days, in hours it becomes 8.6 days $\times$ 24 (hrs/day).

density is lower than a full description of the kinetics would require. In what follows, we give an example:

The kinetics of a particular tracer in an organ is exactly described by the equation:

$$A(t) = A_0 \frac{a_{12}}{a_{12} - a_{21}} (e^{-a_{21}t} - e^{-a_{12}t}) \quad \text{(see Equation 8.41)}$$

In this example, the activity is expressed as μCi/injected dose in μCi, and $A_0 = 0.4$. The exponents are $a_{12} = 0.5\,\text{hr}^{-1}$ and $a_{21} = 0.01\,\text{hr}^{-1}$. As we have seen, the area under the curve is average time × activity. In this case,

$$\int_0^\infty A(t)dt = \frac{A_0 a_{12}}{(a_{12} - a_{21})} \left[\frac{1}{a_{21}} - \frac{1}{a_{12}} \right] = \frac{A_0}{a_{21}} = 40\,\mu Ci \cdot hr.$$

However (see Figure 4.1), there is some undersampling.

The solution is a numerical integration. In this case, we use the trapezoidal method. The method is explained in Table 4.1.

4.2.2. *Radiation Depends on the Energy Emitted Over the Cumulative Time: Equilibrium Absorbed Dose Constant*

What we want to determine first is the amount of energy that will be emitted to be potentially deposited in the tissues (see why in Section 4.2.3). The ultimate goal is to measure RAD, whose units are 100 erg/g.

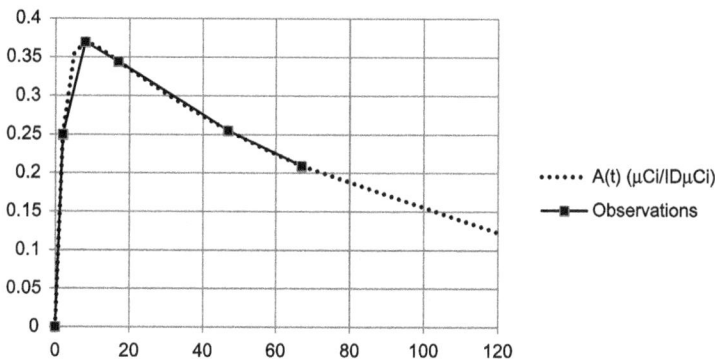

Figure 4.1 The functional expression of the kinetics are shown as a stippled line and are μCi/injection dose in μCi. The observations are the black squares. The lines connecting them (full thin line) deviate from the true functional form.

Table 4.1   The table shows the time (in hours) and the activity measured in an organ at those times. The integration is done by averaging the values of two subsequent data points and multiplying them by the time between those data points. Hence, the integration between the 2-hour and 8-hour samples is computed as $[(0.37+0.25)/2] \times (8-2) = 1.86$. For the last data point this cannot be done, but in that case one can conservatively (if radiation toxicity is a concern) extrapolate the last value with the physical decay (in this case $\lambda = 0.008(0.21/0.008) = 26.11$. The result is not bad since the total (45.06) is not very different from the theoretical 40 (μCi.hr).

Observation times (Hr)	Observations (μCi/ID μCi)	Trapezoidal integration
0.00	0.00	0.25
2.00	0.25	1.86
8.00	0.37	3.21
17.00	0.34	8.99
47.00	0.26	4.64
67.00	0.21	26.11
	Total	45.06

The definition of "activity" is the number of disintegrations. One microcurie is defined as 3.7×10^4 disintegration per seconds. How much energy is actually emitted per disintegration or per hour? The total number of disintegrations over one hour is easily computed:

$$3.7 \times 10^4 \frac{dis}{\mu Ci \cdot sec} \times 3.6 \times 10^3 \frac{sec}{hr} = 1.332 \times 10^8 \frac{dis}{\mu Ci \cdot hr}.$$

As an example, let us consider a β-emitter with three γ emissions of which two are in series (Figure 4.2). The β-emitter has energy 0.07 MeV with an abundance (N_β) of 1, and the gammas have energies respectively of 0.300, 0.200 and 0.100 MeV with abundance of $N_1 = 0.4$, $N_2 = 0.6$ and $N_3 = 0.6$ respectively.

The equilibrium absorbed dose constant (Δ) can be calculated for each of the emissions, but the units have to be changed from MeV to erg and then to Rad (100 erg/g). In what follows, N is the abundance and E the energy in MeV:

$$\Delta = \frac{N \times E\, MeV}{dis} \times \frac{1.332 \times 10^8 dis}{\mu Ci \cdot hr} \times \frac{1.602 \times 10^{-6}\, erg}{1\, Mev} \times \frac{Rad \times g}{100\, erg}$$

$$= 2.13NE \frac{Rad \times g^c}{\mu Ci \cdot hr}.$$

---

[c] $1.33 \times 1.00\,E+08 \times 1.602 \times 1.00\,E-06 \times 0.010 = 2.133864.$

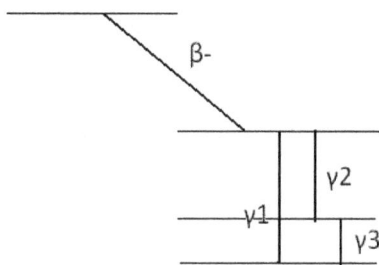

Figure 4.2 Decay scheme of the example used in the computation of the equilibrium absorbed dose constant Δ.

For the three emissions in the example, we have:

$$\Delta_\beta = 2.13 \times N_\beta \times 0.07 \, \text{Rad} \cdot \text{g}/\mu\text{Ci} \cdot \text{hr}$$

$$\Delta_{\gamma 1} = 2.13 \times N_1 \times 0.300 \, \text{Rad} \cdot \text{g}/\mu\text{Ci} \cdot \text{hr}$$

$$\Delta_{\gamma 2} = 2.13 \times N_2 \times 0.200 \, \text{Rad} \cdot \text{g}/\mu\text{Ci} \cdot \text{hr}$$

$$\Delta_{\gamma 3} = 2.13 \times N_3 \times 0.100 \, \text{Rad} \cdot \text{g}/\mu\text{Ci} \cdot \text{hr}$$

4.2.3. *Emitted Dose and Absorbed Dose* (Φ)[d]

If, in our example the $\mu Ci \cdot hr$ was 40, and the isotope was concentrated in one organ, the radiation burden to the organ would not necessarily be the sum of the Δ values defined above, because not all the radiation would be absorbed in the organ. The absorbed dose fraction Φ needs to be defined.

The amount absorbed depends on the type and energy of the emission. Beta emission does not penetrate far into the tissues, while low-energy gamma rays penetrate less than high-energy gamma rays. In the MIRD system, an average man electronic image has been created, in which the relative position, size and density of organs is represented. For all emission "i", and each organ "j", one computes the absorption in all other organs and in the organ itself.

$$\text{Total energy absorbed in organ } k = \sum_i N_i \Delta_i \sum_j \bar{A}_{ij} \varphi_{ij}(r_k \leftarrow r_j). \quad (4.1)$$

In this formulation, $\bar{A}$ is the cumulative activity and is different for all the organs "j", Φ_{ij} is the emission "i" and organ-specific radiation from organ "j" into organ r,

---

[d] Φ is the Greek capital letter Phi.

where r can be equal to j (the organ is irradiated by its contents) or not equal (the organ is irradiated by the contents of other organs).

The units are now Rad · g since $\bar{A}$ has unit $\mu Ci \cdot hr$. If the weight of the organ is W g, then $\sum_i N_i \Delta_i \sum_j \bar{A}_{ij}\varphi_{ij}(r_k \leftarrow r_j)/W$ represents the dose in RAD.

4.2.4. *Actual Application*

- In animal studies, if the animals can be sacrificed, the actual data tend to be percentage injected dose/g, which is not entirely rational for animals weighing a few grams altogether. But with care, $\bar{A}$ can be computed if the organ size or total organ activity is included. What would be missing is a reasonable estimate of Φ for all organs. In principle, one could concentrate on the β emissions only, since their range is not very large, but still, for a small animal, a range of 0.1 cm is not insignificant (1). However, if the activity is expressed as A per organ, the biodistribution can be applied to estimate what the radiation burden would be with a comparable biodistribution in man.

- Estimations of organ cumulative activity has been performed using planar whole body imaging, but the overlap of multiple tissues makes the estimates uncertain.[e] Even so, planar whole body imaging has been used. Sometimes, conjugate views are obtained, but more often the ROI's are applied to anterior and posterior and the counts are combined in a geometric average (Figure 4.3 and Table 4.2). The administered dose (in μCi) is derived from the first whole body images, before any excretion has occurred.

- In general, if the isotope (label) is the same for dosimetry and therapy, decay correction is not applied since the absorbed dose is delivered while the isotope decays. If the labels are different, a double correction is applied for each data point. If A are the actual counts at time t with the dosimetric tracer that has a decay constant a, and the therapy tracer has a decay constant b, the corrected count at time t is computed as follows:

$$A_{corrected} = Ae^{(a-b)t}.$$

- If the images are volumetric images with attenuation correction (as in PET/CT), the observations are more secure. Most PET imaging systems are calibrated for dose. The advantage is that the images are volumes, but the manufacturers do

---

[e]Delineation of adjacent "background" is reassuring but not well founded.

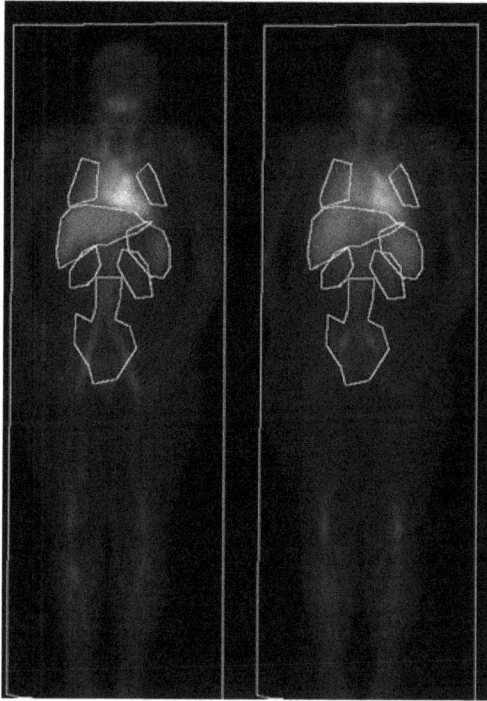

Figure 4.3 Representation of a planar whole body scan with ROIs over the liver, spleen, kidneys, lumbar sacral spine and lungs. The values obtained from anterior and posterior views are combined as geometric means ($\sqrt{Ant \times Post}$) or the equivalent of conjugate views (see Section 10.5).

not provide many truly volume tools. What is needed is true 3D ROIs, as the one described in Section 3.2.1.3 (Figure 4.4).

- The dosimetric methods discussed here are best described as macroscopic for two reasons. First, at the microscopic level, the distribution of the tracer is not homogeneous and second, while the range of the emission may be of a scale in mm, the deposition of the energy tends to concentrate close to the origin, because the volume is proportional to the cube of the radius and the range is the maximum of ranges with higher frequencies for shorter ranges (2, 3). Efforts have been made (4) to refine dosimetry to the microscopic level, but have not penetrated clinical practice.

Table 4.2   The table is the final tabulation prior to the computation of the cumulative activity. The time is in hours, while the counts are transformed in mCi by using the injected dose measured by the dose calibrator and the geometric average of the whole body counts in the first acquisition.

Hours	WB counts	WB milliCi	Kidney counts	Kidney milliCi
0.32	2802425	5.019	92819	0.166
4.08	2684519	4.808	104072	0.186
16.65	2360731	4.228	116411	0.208
64.45	1295777	2.321	49533	0.089
164.25	325905	0.584	10119	0.018

Hours	Liver counts	Liver milliCi	Lungs counts	Lungs milliCi
0.32	343012	0.614	128543	0.230
4.08	319086	0.571	110884	0.199
16.65	324182	0.581	95006	0.170
64.45	185805	0.333	55386	0.099
164.25	56051	0.100	7784	0.014

Hours	Marrow counts	Marrow milliCi	Spleen counts	Spleen milliCi
0.32	165274	0.296	116806	0.209
4.08	137448	0.246	90391	0.162
16.65	145662	0.261	88781	0.159
64.45	72685	0.130	39473	0.071
164.25	19197	0.034	9466	0.017

4.3. THERAPY

4.3.1. *Introduction and Survey*

It seems to be a small conceptual step to deduce that if a labeled substance can be shown to concentrate in a malignant lesion, with an appropriate change of radioactive label, the substance could be used to treat the lesion (with internal

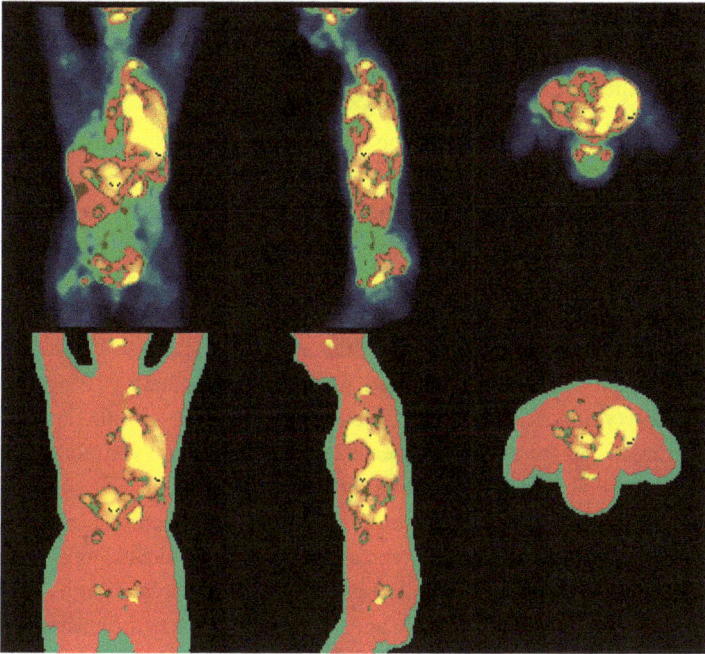

Figure 4.4 The top row shows the original MIP of PET image of a patient with lymphoma. The bottom row shows orthogonal MIP's of the 3D regions for the whole body, the lean body mass and the lesions.

radiotherapy). Tumor imaging agents, with relatively long residency times, do not exactly abound, but they exist. Consider the list of agents that have been used to image tumors:

- Aspecific agents
  - Gallium (macrophages-ferritin)
  - Bone tracers (Strontium, Fluor, Phosphanates, Samarium)
- Cellularity agents
  - 201-Thallium
  - ^{99m}Tc-Sestamibi/Tetrofosmin
- Metabolic agents
  - Fluorodeoxyglucose
  - Iodine (^{123}I, ^{131}I, ^{125}I)
  - MIBG

- Receptor-specific agents
  - Octreotide (Somatostatin)
  - Antibodies

There is, however, a fundamental question: Is the fact that tumors are sufficiently targeted for imaging sufficient to assume that they will be effective for therapy? As we have seen above, unlike imaging where a time interval is needed when the contrast is favorable, for therapy we need a longer residency time. In addition, not all labels have the physical characteristic (non-penetrating radiation emission).

As examples for bone metastases, one can use EHDP labeled with ^{99m}Tc, or labeled with Samarium-153[f] as Quadramet,[g] or Strontium-89.[h] Thallium-201 and ^{99m}Tc agents have not been used for therapy, nor have ^{18}F agents, as in ^{18}F-fluorodeoxyglucose. But iodine isotopes have been used for therapy, both ^{125}I and ^{131}I, directly to treat thyroid disease (in which case, they are both label and tracer), and as labels for metaiodobenzylguanidine (MIBG).

MIBG works as a norepinephrine (NE) analogue, and accumulates in cytoplasmic vesicles by the NE re-uptake mechanism. This re-uptake exists in adrenergic nerves, adrenal medulla and neural crest tissues. The application as diagnostic agent (with ^{123}I) (5) and therapeutic agent (with ^{131}I) are neuroblastoma (6) and potentially pheochromocytoma (7).

Octreotide is a somatostatin analog (8, 9, 10) and has been used both for imaging and therapy labeled with indium-111, and for therapy with 90-yttrium and 177-lutesium (11).

4.3.2. *Radioimmunotherapy in Lymphomas*

If radioimmunotherapy had to be tried, lymphomas would have been the malignancies of choice. This is because, generally speaking, lymphomas are radiosensitive. However, before reviewing radioimmunotherapy of (low-grade) lymphomas, a more general review of radioimmunotherapy will be useful.

A first useful distinction is between the medical and surgical models in medicine. In medical models, the therapeutic agent has an effect only if it meets

---

[f]Samarium-153 emits both medium-energy beta particles and a gamma photon, and has a physical half-life of 46.3 hours (1.93 days). Samarium-153 has average and maximum beta particle ranges in water of 0.5 mm and 3.0 mm, respectively.

[g]Quadramet® is a therapeutic agent consisting of radioactive samarium and a tetraphosphonate chelator, ethylenediaminetetramethylenephosphonic acid (EDTMP).

[h]Strontium-85 used to be utilized as an imaging agent for bones.

the target. The examples are antibiotics having effects on the bacteria they meet but not (one hopes) on other tissues. Immunotherapy is another good example, since in the absence of a receptor, the antibody would have no effect. In the medical model, specificity resides in the mechanism (a specific interaction between agent and target).

In the surgical model, the effect of the treatment is not specific to the target. The specificity originates in the precision of the anatomical aim towards the target. In radiation therapy, the goal of therapy planning is to concentrate the dose of radiation over the target. The knife and radiation are indifferent in their effect and work against the target only if well directed. In the surgical model, specificity resides in the location.

Second, if we consider radioimmunotherapy as a step beyond immunotherapy of cancer, the step was prompted by the (relative) failure of the latter. The conventional way to explain the failure is a lack of intrinsic killing effect and a lack of penetration into poorly vascularized tumor masses. The addition of a radioactive label (usually a β-emitter) to the antibody would improve both. Radiation is lethal and the type of radiation used (β rays) has a sufficient range to overcome the lack of penetration.

The introduction of radioimmunotherapy involves a transition from the medical to surgical model; even those antibodies that have not reached their target (yet) are irradiating the tissues in which they are in. A quick and complete delivery of the antibody to the target(s) therefore becomes crucial. Additionally, if the goal of radioimmunotherapy is to increase the reach and killing effect, what should the range (and the energy) of the β ray be? A higher energy and longer range would seem advantageous in larger masses, but in submicroscopic diseases, most of the energy would be dispensed to surrounding normal tissues. Finally, the fact that the specificity lies in the location, combined with the fact that the target is not rapidly reached, suggests that the half-life of the label should be longer than the average time needed for an optimal accumulation in the tumor.

All available data, for all forms of disease, suggest that tumor doses are not high enough to have a curative effect and that measured tumor doses do not predict response (12). Yet there is, at least in lymphomas, a curative effect. This discrepancy has preoccupied researchers (13). Some of the magnified effect of what is effectively a relatively small radiation dose can be assigned to the continuous nature of the irradiation by radiolabeled antibodies (14, 15). In addition, in external beam irradiation, the dose is distributed in a relatively homogeneous distribution within the tumor, while in radioimmunotherapy at a microscopic level, the dose is very heterogeneous (16). This heterogeneity may in fact increase the dose at a microscopic level to vital tumor elements. In a phase II study, the calculated (average) tumor dose did not predict response (17). In fact, even tumor visualization does not predict the effect of therapy (18) to the probable dismay of Britton (19) who claims non-imaged lesions should not be treated. The apparent paradox is at least partially explained by the known fact that tumor volume or burden is a negative predictor of therapeutic success and that larger volumes are more easily visualized.

Low-grade lymphomas are refractory to most treatments, and each subsequent treatment is less effective (20). Radioimmunotherapy seemed a possibility to improve treatment options.

At present, the most successful (and FDA approved) radioimmunotherapy agents for lymphomas are anti-CD20 monoclonal antibodies. Rituximab (Rituxan^{TM}) is a chimeric antibody, used as a non-radioactive antibody and to pre-load the patient when Zevalin^{TM} is used. Zevalin^{TM} is yttrium-90 (^{90}Y) or the indium-111 (^{111}In) labeled form of Ibritumomab tiuxetan. Bexxar^{TM} is iodine-131 (^{131}I) labeled form of tositumomab. Ibritumomab tiuxetan and tositumomab are mouse anti-CD20 monoclonal antibodies.

The treatments with both tracers are very similar. In both cases, the injection of the labeled antibody is preceded by the injection of a large amount of unlabeled antibodies (Rituximab before Zevalin^{TM} and tositumomab before Bexxar^{TM}) (21). This "pre-loading" occupies easily reachable sites (bone marrow and spleen), and "forces" the labeled antibody to circulate for a longer period of time, thus increasing its probability of reaching the lymphoma sites (Figure 4.5).

In the case of Zevalin^{TM}, a biodistribution study, with ^{111}In-Zevalin^{TM}, precedes the therapeutic dose with the ^{90}Y-labeled Zevalin^{TM}. With Bexxar^{TM}, the dosimetric and therapeutic phases of the study are performed with ^{131}I-Bexxar^{TM} (but with different doses). However, because of the large inter-patient variability in whole body retention of ^{131}I, in the case of Bexxar^{TM}, an estimation of the amount that will deliver a dose of 75 cGy to the whole body is calculated.

This estimation of the whole body dose is based on measuring the whole body retention time, from whole body imaging (scanning) over a week period. Surprisingly, the data are well fitted by a single exponential, but that is because most of the activity remains in the vascular system, and what transfers to the tissues releases the iodine, which is quickly excreted in the urine.[i] The system works approximately as a catenary system with two compartments, of which the second compartment has a faster transfer rate.

---

[i]The thyroid is blocked.

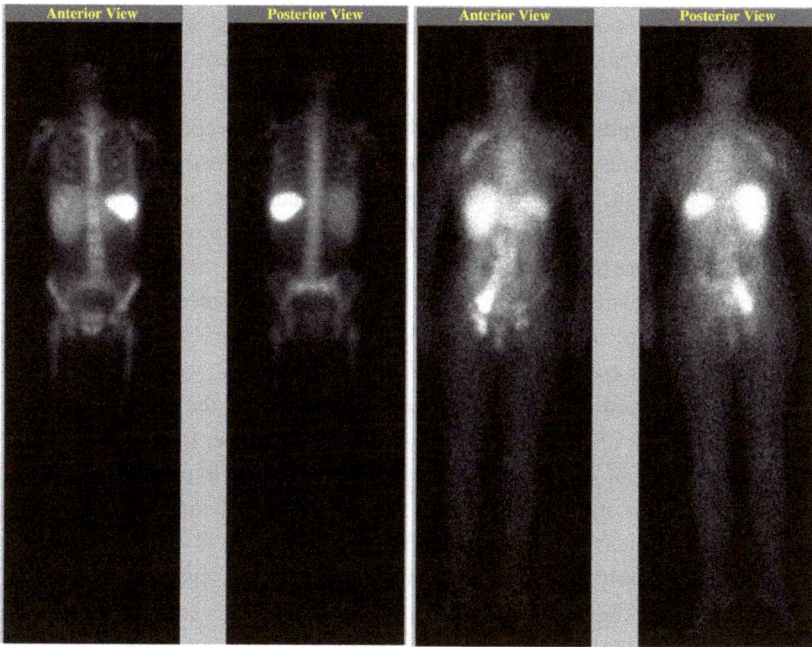

Figure 4.5 Effect of the pre-infusion of cold antibodies on the biodistribution of the radiolabeled antibody. In this case, the image was recorded on day 6 after the infusion of ^{111}Indium labeled anti-CD20. On the left, the radioactive infusion was given without a pre-infusion; on the right, the radioactive infusion was given within 2 hours after a pre-infusion of cold anti-CD20 (1mg/kg).

If the whole body retention is well described by a single exponential[j] $A(t) = A_0 e^{-\lambda t}$, with λ having dimensions hr^{-1}, the dose is not difficult to compute. In one example, the patient is a male, of 92 kg and 178 cm. Because the platelets are low (102 000), the prescribed dose should yield 65 cGy whole body. Since the residency time is 53 hours, the dose to prescribe is 160 mCi.

In neither case is the dose to the tumor calculated, because current *in vivo* imaging methods only allow the calculation of a macroscopic and average tumor dose, probably irrelevant in view of the microscopic heterogeneity. The administered quantity is limited by considerations of toxicity.

---

[j]In general it would not be. In the case of complete antibodies, the fractional transfer rate from plasma to extra-plasma space (α_{12}) would be small (see Figure 8.9).

Horning (22) reported on a series of 40 patients treated with Bexxar^{TM}. The median number of prior treatments was four. Most patients were low grade lymphomas (70%). Some were transformed low grade (25%), a few intermediate grade. Thirty-five (88%) patients were rituximab refractory. The overall response rate was 68% with a median response duration of 16 months (1+ to 38+ months). A complete response was seen in 33% of the patients. The median duration was not reached.

Similar results were reported by Kaminski (23) about a series of 60 patients. Again, the group was handicapped by a median of four prior treatments. Low grade, transformed low grade and intermediate grade were distributed as 56%, 38% and 2% respectively. The overall response and complete response were 47% and 20%, with median duration of 12 and 47 months respectively.

When the method was used as the first treatment (24), the complete response rate was higher than 72% and the 5-year survival rate higher than 55%.

In the context of other treatments and outcomes for low grade b-cell lymphomas, the results are remarkable. Toxicity is primarily hematological, but rare and reversible with actual clinical protocols.

Interestingly, only one paper reports on a prospective and randomized study on the additional effect of the radioactive label (25). In this study, with the same amount of antibody in identical regiments, but with the addition of radioactivity, the complete response rate was 33% in the radioactive group, and 8% in the unlabeled group. The overall response rate was 55% and 19% respectively.

The same (positive) results should not be expected for all tumors (26, 27). However, improvement will come by making the delivery more efficient by labeling the antibody, already joint to the target (28).

4.3.3. *Predicting Outcome*

With Hongyun Zhu and Daniel Y Sze.

In some cases, external dosimetry can be used to predict response because the microscopic distribution seems to be more homogeneous. Such a case occurs in SIR therapy for intrahepatic tumors. SIR-Spheres® are biocompatible radioactive microspheres that contain yttrium-90 and emit β radiation. SIR-Spheres® are implanted by intra-arterial infusion in the hepatic artery, since intrahepatic tumors are preferentially perfused by the hepatic arterial system, while the normal liver gets most of its blood flow from the portal system. The SIR-Spheres® are trapped in the tumor's capillary. This approach is more akin to brachytherapy than therapy with soluble radioactive substances, but can be used as a model for prediction of toxicity and response.

The treatment protocol has a particular aspect: The dose is calculated on the basis of a body surface area (BSA),[k] the fraction of the liver dependent to the hepatic artery branch to be infused (H%), and the tumor volume as a percentage of liver (T%). The infused dose is modulated by the degree of shunting to the lungs (P), to avoid toxicity. In reality, the calculation of the infused dose is odd, since the absorbed dose is a function of the activity per gram tumor. The formula is (if the pulmonary shunt is less than 10%):

$$GB_q = (BSA - 0.2) + \frac{H\% \times T\%}{100 \times 100}.$$

This approach seems inconsistent. If we assume a patient with a BSA of $1.75 \, m^2$ and a liver volume of 1500 ml, as the tumor volume progressively increases, the administered dose per ml decreases (Table 4.3).

This apparent inconsistency prompted us to look for the factors predicting success or failure, with failure being either no response or toxicity.

4.3.3.1. *Background: Fusion*

Fusion is the simultaneous and combined analysis of two images mapping identically in the same object space, but recording a different attribute of the object. Most fusion has been performed as a visual representation in which the attributes are represented (independently) into overlapping but different color scales. In this work we explore fusion, in which the attributes are combined in a mathematical or logical manner, to address a specific goal.

Table 4.3   The calculated dose is derived from the formula given in the text. As the tumor volume doubles, the activity per ml almost halves.

Liver volume (ml)	H%	T%	Calculated infused dose	Tumor volume (ml)	GBq/ml tumor
1500	0.6	0.1	1.61	150	0.0107
1500	0.6	0.2	1.67	300	0.0056
1500	0.6	0.3	1.73	450	0.0038
1500	0.6	0.4	1.79	600	0.0030
1500	0.6	0.5	1.85	750	0.0025
1500	0.6	0.6	1.91	900	0.0021

[k]One assumes that this is a predictor of normal liver mass.

In preparation for a treatment of liver metastases with intra-arterially infused radioactive ^{90}Y-labeled microspheres, the liver is infused intra-arterially with ^{99m}Tc-labeled macroaggregates, imaged, and reinjected with ^{99m}Tc colloid and re-imaged without changing position. Before reconstruction, the projection images are corrected for crosstalk (because both the MAA and the colloid are labeled with ^{99m}Tc) then the images are reconstructed. The result is a set of two in-line registered image volumes, defining MAA perfused tumor and liver, and functional liver (colloid) with or without MAA (Figure 4.6).

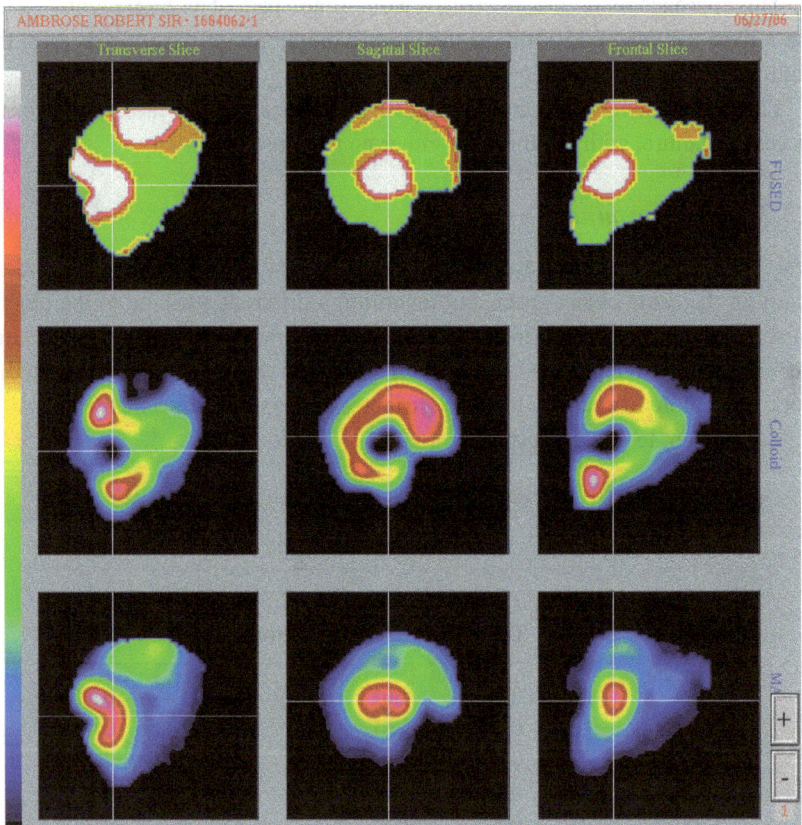

Figure 4.6 The figure shows three orthogonal slices, centered on the center of the liver. In the top row, the three categories are shown (white = pure tumor or MAA only, green = pure liver or colloid only and brown = a mixture (affected liver)). The second row shows the colloid distribution and the third, the MAA distribution.

Table 4.4 Regression between survival time and the doses and volumes. T/L is the dose ratio between tumor and liver.

Survival	Single regression		
	Coefficients	t Stat	P-value
Tumor RAD	0.037	3.50	0.0008
Affected liver RAD	0.050	2.76	0.0075
Affected liver ml	−0.096	−2.59	0.0118
T/L	122	2.44	0.0175
Unaffected liver ml	0.068	1.19	0.2377
Tumor ml	−0.057	−1.14	0.2571

The analysis of the fusion allows the computation of relative and absolute volumes, and relative doses to liver and tumor. The logic defines pure liver (image volume with colloid only), pure tumor (MAA only) and affected liver (MAA mixed with colloid). The total liver is the combination of class 1 and 3, the total tumor class 2 and 3. The analysis was performed on 40 patients who had reasonable follow-ups.

4.3.3.2. Results

Survivors had a lower average total liver volume (p = 0.02) and affected liver volume (p = 0.01). They also had a higher relative dose to the tumor. We found that the relative volume of normal liver perfused by MAA is the best predictor of post-therapy toxicity as measured by survival. Other significant predictors of survival length were (positively) the tumor dose and the ratio of tumor dose to liver dose (Table 4.4).

4.4. RELEASING PATIENTS TREATED WITH RADIOACTIVE AGENTS

4.4.1. Background

The Nuclear Regulatory Commission has changed the rules for the release of patients treated with radioactive products. It used to be that a patient treated with more than 30 mCi of iodine-131 (^{131}I) for thyroid disease or who as a source measured more than 7 milliroentgen at 1 m (7 mR@1m) could not be released.

The rule was changed to one where an explicit computation and instructions to the patient would not allow the exposure to the patient's family and those living with the patient, to exceed 500 millirem (500 mrem).[1]

The instructions to the patient were subsumed under the heading of occupancy, generally a 25% occupancy. This would mean that the patient would, on average, be at a distance of 1 m away from the relevant others for 25% of the time, if behavior was not changed. For the rest of the time, the relevant others would not be irradiated at all. The NRC instructions read in part:

> For radionuclides with a physical half-life greater than 1 day and no consideration of biological elimination, it is assumed that the individual likely to receive the highest dose from exposure to the patient would receive a dose of 25% of the dose to total decay (0.25 in Equation U.2), at a distance of 1 meter. Selection of 25% of the dose to total decay at 1 meter for estimating the dose is based on measurements discussed in the supporting regulatory analysis that indicate the dose calculated using an occupancy factor, E, of 25% at 1 meter is conservative in most normal situations.

> For radionuclides with a physical half-life less than or equal to 1 day, it is difficult to justify an occupancy factor of 0.25, because relatively long-term averaging of behavior cannot be assumed. Under this situation, occupancy factors from 0.75 to 1.0 may be more appropriate.

In what follows, we will discuss the instruction that would change the occupancy, but first the kinetics.

4.4.2. *Basis for Occupancy Control: Kinetics*

In the case of radioimmunotherapy, a preliminary low-dose kinetic study has been determined. At the time of treatment, the whole body average retention time is known. As an example, consider a case of a patient eventually treated with 160 mCi of ^{131}I-Bexxar. In the preliminary kinetic study with 5 mCi, the analysis yielded a average retention time of 2 days, or $\lambda = 1/2$ day^{-1} or 0.021 hr^{-1}. Before releasing the patient, the exposure rate is 18 mR[m] at 1 m. Let us first consider exposure in concrete terms. If the patient lives with another person, one can divide the day in three parts of 8 hours: At night, they sleep in the same room, or bed at ≤1 m. During the day, one person leaves the house, and is eventually at an infinite distance or a

---

[1]Assumption follows assumption, but if the exposure is 7 mR/h at 1 m, the dose to the subject is supposed to be 5 mrem/h at 1 m.

[m]mR is milli-Roentgen, an exposure rate.

Table 4.5 The table illustrates occupancy by dividing the day in three equal parts. At an average distance of 1 m for 24 hours, at an exposure rate of 18 mR/hr at 1 m, the daily exposure would be 432 mR. But when the day is divided into the three parts, it becomes 34% of that total. The 34% value is more conservative than the stipulated 25%. The modification easily brings the value down to 2%.

Distance (m)	Time (hr)	Fraction (1/msqr)	Rate (mR/hr @1m)	Exposure
Normal exposure				
1	8	1	18	144.00
3	8	0.11	18	0.89
10	8	0.01	18	0.08
Total				144.97
Exposure (fraction of 432)				**0.34**
Modified exposure				
5	8	0.04	18	5.76
3	8	0.11	18	0.89
10	8	0.01	18	0.08
Total				6.73
Exposure (fraction of 432)				**0.02**

distance ≥ 10 m, and finally, mornings and evenings, they are in the same room at an average of 3 m. If this is not modified, the exposure times would be that as shown in Table 4.5 and would correspond to 33% occupancy (because 100% occupancy would correspond to an exposure of $24 \times 18 = 432$).

A modified exposure would begin by eliminating the nights spent in the same room (or bed). In that case, we assume that the distance is now 5 m and the occupancy to now be 2% (Table 4.5).

Now, consider the following: If the exposure is not modified, the person living with the patient would be exposed to[n]

$$0.33 \times 432 \int_0^\infty e^{-0.5t} dt = \frac{432}{0.5} = 864 \, mR.$$

---

[n]In what follows, the unit for time will be days.

Table 4.6 Computation of occupancy control days. The table is organized with the last equation as a template. The time unit is day. The fractional rate λ is day^{-1}. If the occupancy is not controlled, the total exposure rate would be 864 mR. The table shows the number of days to control the occupancy as a function of the λ value.

mR/day @ 1m	432	432	432
λ	0.25	0.25	0.5
Controlled occupancy	0.02	0.02	0.02
Normal occupancy	0.33	0.33	0.33
T time for controlled	**1**	**2**	**1**
$\exp(-0.5 * T)$	0.778801	0.606531	0.606531
$1 - \exp(-0.5 * T)$	0.221199	0.393469	0.393469
First term	0.017696	0.031478	0.015739
Second term	1.028017	0.80062	0.40031
Total	451.748	359.4663	179.7332

This would be more than the allowed exposure. We need to compute the solution to the equation:

$$0.02 \times 432\,mR \int_0^{T_1} e^{-0.5t}\,dt + 0.33 \times 432 \int_{T_1}^{\infty} e^{-0.5t}\,dt = 500\,mR.$$

What we need to find is the time T that would satisfy the equation. This equation simplifies to the following (and can be solved numerically) (Table 4.6):

$$432 \times \left[\frac{0.02}{0.5}(1 - e^{-0.5T}) + \frac{0.33}{0.5}e^{-0.5T} = 500 \right].$$

4.4.3. *The Case of Thyroid Treatment without Measured Kinetics*

The kinetics are assumed to be dominated by iodine in thyroidal tissue (organified) and iodine in other tissues (ions). The organified iodine has a presumed retention time of 8 days° (a = 0.005 hr^{-1}). The ionic iodine is assumed to have a residency time of 24 hours (b = 0.04 hr^{-1}).

°This is a conservative maximum. In the treatment of hyperthyroidism, it is probably much less. In the case of thyroid cancer treatment, the patient is put back on thyroid medication (and suppression), and the kinetics are slowed.

If occupancy is not controlled, and the initial exposure rate R mR/hr at 1 m the cumulative exposure would be defined by the sum of two exponentials,[P] weighted by the thyroid uptake. If the thyroid uptake measured during the diagnostic study was P% at 24 hours and p = P/100, the thyroid component of the exposure would be well approximated by Rp and the whole body (ionic iodine) by R(1 − p). Without modification, the occupancy is 0.33 and the cumulative exposure rate is

$$\left[0.33Rp \int_0^\infty e^{-at} dt + 0.33R(1-p) \int_0^\infty e^{-bt} dt \right]$$

$$= \left[\frac{0.33Rp}{a} + \frac{0.33R(1-p)}{b} \right] = 837mR.$$

Table 4.7 Releasing thyroid patients. Illustration of the numerical computation of the factors influencing the exposure of the patient's familiars. For the first three columns the thyroid uptake is 35%, but the control of occupancy varies from none to 48 hours. In the fourth column, the thyroid uptake is smaller, and at equal value of T, the cumulative exposure is less.

R (mR/hr at 1 m)	35	35	35	35
a	0.005	0.005	0.005	0.005
b	0.02	0.02	0.02	0.02
RIU% at 24 hours	15	15	15	8
0.33Rp	1.7325	1.7325	1.7325	0.924
0.02Rp	0.105	0.105	0.105	0.056
0.33R(1−p)	9.8175	9.8175	9.8175	10.626
0.02R(1−p)	0.595	0.595	0.595	0.644
T	0	24	48	24
exp(−aT)	1.00	0.89	0.79	0.89
exp(−bT)	1.00	0.62	0.38	0.62
1−exp(−aT)	0.00	0.11	0.21	0.11
1−exp(−bT)	0.00	0.38	0.62	0.38
Thyroid component	347	310	277	165
Ionic component	491	315	206	341
Total exposure (mR)	837	625	483	506

[P]We will use hours as units.

If the occupancy control reduces occupancy to 0.02 and if T is the number of days with occupancy control, we have:

1. Thyroid component: cumulative exposure $= \left(\frac{0.02Rp}{a}(1 - e^{-aT}) + \frac{0.33Rp}{a}e^{-aT} \right)$ mR.

2. Ionic component: cumulative exposure $\left(\frac{0.02R(1-p)}{b}(1 - e^{-bT}) + \frac{0.33R(1-p)}{b}e^{-bT} \right)$ mR.

Again, T is not easily defined analytically, but it is numerically. We start by defining the constants: the decay rates a and b are constants, as are the occupancy fractions 0.33 and 0.22. The variables are R and p and the variable to define is T (in hours). The computation is illustrated in Table 4.7.

REFERENCES

1. Akabani G, Poston JW, Bolch WE. Estimates of beta absorbed fractions in small tissue volumes for selected radionuclides. *J Nucl Med* 1991; 32:835–839.
2. Gillepspie FC, Orr JS. Microscopic dose distribution from 125; I in the toxic thyroid gland and its relation to therapy. *Br J Radiol* 1970; 43:40–47.
3. Makrigiorgos GM. Limitations of conventional internal dosimetry at the cellular level. *J Nucl Med* 1989; 30:1856–1864.
4. Wessels BW. Miniature thermoluminescent dosimeter absorbed dose measurements in tumor phantom models. *J Nucl Med* 1986; 27:1308–1314.
5. Mozley PD, Kim CK, Mohsin J, Jatlow A, Gosfield E 3rd, Alavi A. The efficacy of Iodine-123-MIBG as a screening test for pheochromocytoma. *J Nucl Med* 1994; 35:1138–1143.
6. Vik TA, Pfluger T, Kadota R, Castel V, Tulchinsky M, Farto JCA, Heiba S, Serafini A, Tumeh S, Khutoryansky N, Jacobson AF. 123-I MIBG scintigraphy in patients with known or suspected neuroblastoma: results from a prospective multicenter trial. *Pediatr Blood Cancer* 2009; 2:784–790.
7. Ansari AN, Siegel ME, DeQuattro V, Gazarian LH. Imaging of medullary thyroid carcinoma and hyperfunctioning adrenal medulla using Iodine-131 Metaiodobenzylguanidine. *J Nucl Med* 1986; 27:1858–1860.
8. O'Dorisio MS, Chen F, O'Dorisio TM, Wray D, Qualman SJ. Characterization of somatostatin receptors on human neuroblastoma tumors. *Cell Growth Differ* 1994; 5:1–8.
9. O'Dorisio MS, Hauger M, Cacalupo AJ. Somatostatin receptor in neuroblastoma: diagnostic and therapeutic implications. *Semin Oncol* 1994; 21:33–37.
10. Bong SB, VanderLaan JG, Louwes H, Schuurman JJ. Clinical experience with somatostatin receptor imaging in lymphoma. *Semin Oncol* 1994; 21:48–50.
11. Kwekkeboom DJ, Teunissen JJ, Bakker WH, Kooij PP, de Herder WW, Feelders RA, van Eijck CH, Esser J-P, Kam BL, Krenning EP. Radiolabeled somatostatin analog

[177Lu-DOTA0,Tyr3] octreotate in patients with endocrine gastroenteropancreatic tumors. *J Clin Oncol* 2005; 23:12.

12. Knox SJ, Goris ML, Trisler K, *et al.* 90-Y-labeled anti-CD20 monoclonal antibody therapy of recurrent B cell lymphoma. *Clin Cancer Res* 1996; 2:457–470.

13. Knox SJ, Goris ML, Wessels BW. Overview of animal studies comparing radioimmunotherapy with dose equivalent external beam irradiation. *Radiot Oncol* 1992; 23:111–117.

14. Knox S, Levy R, Miller RA, Uhland W, Schiele J, Ruehl W, Finston R, Day P, Goris ML. Determinants of the anti-tumor effect of radiolabeled monoclonal antibodies. *Cancer Res* 1990; 50:4935–4940.

15. Knox SJ, Sutherland W, Goris ML. Correlation of tumor sensitivity to low dose rate irradiation with G2/M-phase block and other radiobiological parameters. *Radiat Res* 1993; 135:24–31.

16. Langmuir VK, Fowler JF, Knox SJ, Wessels BW, Sutherland RM, Wong JY. Radiobiology of radiolabeled antibody therapy as applied to tumor dosimetry. *Med Phys* 1993; 20: 601–610.

17. Knox SJ, Goris ML, Tempero M, Weiden PL, Gentner L, Breitz H, Adams GP, Axworthy D, Gaffinan S, Bryan K, Fisher DR, Colcher D, Horak ID, Weiner LM. Phase II trial of yttrium-90-Dota-Biotin pretargeted by NR-LU-10 antibody/Streptavidin in patients with metastatic colon cancer. *Clin Cancer Res* 2000; 6:406–414.

18. Iagaru A, Gambhir SS, Goris ML. 90Y-Ibritumomab (Zevalin®) Therapy in Refractory Non-Hodgkin's Lymphoma: Observations from 111In-Ibritumomab Pre-Treatment Imaging. *J Nucl Med* 2008; 49:1809–1812.

19. Britton KE. Radioimmunotherapy of Non-Hodgkin's Lymphoma. *J Nucl Med* 2004; 45:924–925.

20. Johnson PW, Rohatiner AZ, Whelan JS, Price CG, Love S, Lim J, Matthews J, Norton AJ, Amess JA, Lister TA. Patterns of survival in patients with recurrent follicular lymphoma: a 20-year study from a single center. *J Clin Oncol* 1995; Jan;13:140–147.

21. Schiele J, Knox SJ, Goris ML, Ruehl W, Goris ML. The effect of unlabelled monoclonal antibody (MAB) on the biodistribution of 131I-anti-idiotype MAB in murine B cell lymphoma, *Radiot Oncol* 1992; 24:169–176.

22. Horning SJ, Younes A, Kroll S, Jain V, Lucas J, Podoloff D, Goris M. Efficacy and Safety of Tositumomab and Iodine-131 Tositumomab (Bexxar) in B-cell Lymphoma Progressive after Rituximab. *J Clin Oncol* 2005; Feb 1;23(4):712–719.

23. Kaminski MS, Zelenetz AD, Press OW, Saleh M, Leonard J, Fehrenbacher L, Lister TA, Stagg RJ, Tidmarsh GF, Kroll S, Wahl RL, Knox SJ, Vose JM. Pivotal study of iodine I 131 tositumomab for chemotherapy-refractory low-grade or transformed low-grade B-cell non-Hodgkin's lymphomas. *J Clin Oncol* 2001; 19:3918–3928.

24. Kaminski MS, Tuck M, Estes J, Kolstad A, Ross CW, Zasadny K, Regan D, Kison P, Fisher S, Kroll S, Wahl RL. 131I-tositumomab therapy as initial treatment for follicular lymphoma. *N Engl J Med* 2005; Feb 3;352(5):441–449.

25. Davis TA, Kaminsky MS, Leonard J, Gregory SA, Wahl R, Hsu F, Wilkinson M, Frankel S, Cohen P, Serafini A, Zelenetz A, Kroll S, Goris M, Levi R, Know S. The radioisotope contributes significantly to the activity of radioimmunotherapy. *Clin Cancer Res* 2004; 10(23):7792–7798.

26. Deb N, Goris M, Trisler K, *et al.* Treatment of hormone refractory prostate cancer with 90Y-CYT-356 monoclonal antibody. *Clin Cancer Res* 1996; 2:1289–1297.

27. Knox SJ, Goris ML, Tempero M, Weiden PL, Gentner L, Breitz H, Adams GP, Axworthy D, Gaffinan S, Bryan K, Fisher DR, Colcher D, Horak ID and Weiner LM. Phase II trial of yttrium-90-Dota-Biotin pretargeted by NR-LU-10 antibody/Streptavidin in patients with metastatic colon cancer. *Clin Cancer Res* 2000; 6:406–414.

28. Andres Forero, Paul L. Weiden, Julie M. Vose, Susan J. Knox, Albert F. LoBuglio, Jordan Hankins, Michael L. Goris, Vincent J. Picozzi, Don B. Axworthy, Hazel B. Breitz, Robert B. Sims, Richard G. Ghalie, Sui Shen, Ruby F. Meredith. Phase I trial of a novel anti-CD20 fusion protein in pretargeted radioimmunotherapy for B-cell non-Hodgkin's lymphoma. *Blood* 2004; Jul 1;104(1):227–236.

Chapter 5

Myocardial Imaging Studies

In myocardial perfusion studies, a diffusible tracer is injected and the relative distribution of the tracer in the myocardium is evaluated. In the normal case, the distribution in the myocardium of the left ventricle is homogeneous, and does not differ between the distribution after a stress injection from the distribution after a resting injection.

5.1. INDICATIONS

There are four principal clinical indications and two secondary ones:

a. Confirm coronary artery disease (CAD) in patients who are not known to have CAD, but have suggestive symptoms or circumstances.
b. Determine if a known coronary lesion perturbs coronary flow (during stress); determine significance of coronary lesion.
c. Determine if and how much myocardium remains at risk (ischemic) following a myocardial infarction (risk stratification).
d. Determine if myocardium will benefit from a vascular intervention (viability).

The two secondary indications are:

e. Diagnosis of acute myocardial infarction.
f. Surveillance following therapy, e.g. angioplasty.

Indications "a" and "b" can be conflated as an attempt to answer whether the patient is at risk for a cardiac event.[a]

---

[a]And it should be obvious that if a is confirmed by comparing myocardial perfusion studies to coronary arteriograms, then b cannot be considered valid, unless it can be shown that the prognostic value of the myocardial perfusion study supersedes that of the coronary arteriogram.

5.2. TRACERS

There are two types of flow tracers, and a number of metabolic tracers. In addition, there are some tracers which specifically bind to or accumulate in damaged myocardial tissues.

5.2.1. *Flow Tracers*

A flow tracer is a diffusible compound, whose uptake by the tissues is flow limited (rather than diffusion limited), and whose retention by the tissues is prolonged, either because the compound is diluted in the intracellular space, or is bound to cell structures. The prototype of the former is potassium-43 (1). Radioactive potassium has been used for this application (^{43}K) (2, 3) but the physical properties of that isotope were not well suited for scintigraphic imaging.

Potassium-43 was soon replaced by rubidium-81 (4), and later by thallium-201 (^{201}Tl). Finally, two technetium-labeled flow tracers were added to the list.

5.2.1.1. *Potassium analogues*

The first type of flow tracers are tracers that mimic potassium; They diffuse freely, so that their distribution immediately after injection is flow limited. Being intracellular, their initial distribution is maintained for some time, but they eventually redistribute to equilibrate with the native potassium distribution.

The modern prototype is ^{201}Tl. The emission characteristics of ^{201}Tl are suitable for scintigraphic imaging, and this tracer was, at some time, the standard in modern literature. In the same class we find rubidium, of which the isotope ^{82}Rb is a positron emitter that can be obtained from a generator system. With a half-life of 76 seconds, ^{82}Rb can be used for sequential measurements in one session. At higher flow rates, the uptake of rubidium becomes diffusion limited.

An interesting alternative is nitrogen-13 ammonia. Nitrogen-13 ammonia (^{13}NH$_3$) is cyclotron produced. Imaging the distribution of this tracer, however, requires positron imaging capabilities (5, 6). The half-life of ^{13}N is 10 minutes. The distribution of ^{13}NH$_3$ is flow limited in the same range as ^{201}Tl; water labeled with oxygen-15 has also been used.

The advantage of position emission tomography (PET) studies is that they allow absolute blood flow determinations. As an example, Zhao (7) was thus able to demonstrate decrease in absolute blood flow in transplanted hearts, in which the diffuse nature of the disease makes the detection of focal perfusion defects ineffective.

5.2.1.2. *Membrane affinity*

The second type of tracer also has an early flow-limited distribution, and attaches to cell membranes, and does not significantly redistribute except in re-perfused canine myocardium (8). The prototype is Cardiolite labeled with [99m]Technetium (MIBI or hexakis 2-methoxy isobutyl isonitrile)[b] or tetrofosmin, also labeled with [99m]Tc (9–11). In general, at higher flow rates, diffusion limitation becomes a factor, and the relation between early distribution and regional flow is distorted (12).

Teboroxime is a boronic acid (BATO)[c] compound. The radiolabeled compound is neutral and highly lipophilic. The extraction of teboroxime at higher flow rates is reported to be higher than for thallium-201 or ^{99m}Tc-sestamibi. The uptake of the tracer seems unaffected by the metabolic state of the myocardial cell. The fast component of the plasma disappearance function has a half-life of 5 to 6 minutes at rest and 2.5 to 3 minutes during stress. The clearance rate from the myocardium seems to be affected by blood flow (13–17). The myocardial clearance is fast, and early studies were performed with planar imaging (for speed), but Nakajima (18) performed SPECT studies using a three-headed camera with some success. Henzlova (19) compared images taken between 11 and 20 minutes following a stress injection,[d] with images obtained between 1.5 and 4.5 minutes following a resting injection, and found those images to be statistically equivalent in relation to the number of abnormal segments. In dogs, Blumhart (20) found that the post-stenotic washout of teboroxime was slower after adenosine or dipyridamole, but, unlike the classic measurement of thallium washout, which is performed over 4 hours, the measurement here is made at 5 and 10 minutes, when the pharmacological effect may still be present (Sections 5.3 and 5.4).

5.2.2. *Metabolic Tracers*

Metabolic tracers are organic molecules which either accumulate in the myocardium as a function of some specific metabolic activity, or whose myocardial kinetics can be shown to be associated with a specific metabolic activity.

---

[b]Myocardial accumulation and retention is dependent on intact mitochondria and plasma membrane potentials. Indeed the steady state (evidence from cellular pharmacological and biophysical analysis) suggests that ^{99m}Tc-sestamibi is localized within mitochondria.

[c][99]Tc-SQ30217 is a boronic acid adduct of technetium oxide (BATO) and is a neutral lipophilic flow agent.

[d]Which he called washout images.

Free fatty acids carried by serum albumin from adipose tissues are normally the dominating source of energy of the myocardium. With ischemia, the balance is shifted towards glucose. The demonstration of this shift is therefore a demonstration of ischemia, but in live myocardial cells. A number of tracers have been used to demonstrate the shift.

The most, frequently used is a sugar analog, labeled with the positron emitter F-18-fluorodeoxyglucose. This tracer enters the glucose oxidation pathway, but remains blocked before metabolization is complete. Regions where myocardial metabolism favors glucose show relative higher uptake (21). In the fasting state, the distribution of FDG in the myocardium is heterogeneous, to become homogeneous with glucose loading (22). Most studies in which 18-FDG is used are based on PET imaging, but regular scintigraphy either planar (23, 24) or SPECT (25) has been used.[e]

C-11-Palmitate is a fatty acid. The rapid early clearance of palmitate from the myocardium reflects mitochondrial metabolization to $^{11}CO_2$, and correlates with levels of myocardial work. During hypoxia or ischemia, this rate is decreased. Ebert (26) proposed the tracer 14(R,S)-fluorine-^{18}fluoro-6-thia-heptadecanoic acid to evaluate myocardial energy metabolism. Since thia-fatty acids do not undergo complete beta-oxidation, their kinetics are more easily derived.

Beta-methyl iodophenyl pentadecanoic acid (BMIPP) has also been used as 123-I-BMIPP ([123I]15-(p-iodophenyl)-3-R,S-methylpentadecanoic acid). With this tracer, Taki (27) showed that after vascular restoration, there was slow recovery of the fatty acid metabolism, and that this recovery correlated better with function recovery than the reduction of stress or resting perfusion defects measured with ^{201}Tl.

5.2.3. *Cell Damage Tracers: Antimyosin*

Myocytes degeneration is observed during the active phase of myocardial damage. ^{111}Indium antimyosin antibody (AM) is a specific marker of the damaged myocyte. Narula (28) found that the sensitivity and specificity of antimyosin imaging with planar and SPECT imaging varied between 91% and 100%, with a specificity of 28% to 42%. However, spurious or aspecific uptake of ^{111}In-antimyosin in the lungs make a lung ratio quantitative analysis problematic (29). We will not discuss antimyosin.

---

[e]The images would lack spatial resolution because of the very high energy collimator. This loss of resolution ended up as unacceptable and this approach did not catch on.

5.3. THE CENTRAL PARADIGM OF MYOCARDIAL PERFUSION STUDIES

Normal & Equal. In the normal case, regional myocardial perfusion is fairly homogeneous, and the regional myocardial distribution of a flow tracer injected during exercise (or stress), would be close to the regional distribution in all normal patients on average, but even closer to the regional distribution of a tracer injected in the same patient but at rest.

In the presence of a stenosis, the higher blood flow recruited during a higher workload (stress, exercise or dobutamine), or an arteriolar vasodilatation (dipyridamole, adenosine), cannot be accommodated by the stenosed vessel, and the myocardium distal to the stenosis accumulates relatively less tracer than the rest.

Abnormal & Unequal. In that case the "stress" image differs from the "normal" average and from the reference rest image. The abnormality is said to be transient[f] and corresponds to stress ischemia.

Abnormal & Equal. In the presence of scarring or myocardial infarction,[g] there is no or little flow, either at rest or during stress (or vasodilatation). The stress image differs from the normal, but not from the reference rest image. The abnormality is said to be fixed. The finding connotes myocardial infarction or scarring.

It is worth noting that the ideal way to perform a rest and stress perfusion study, is to perform a 2-day study, to avoid interference from the first injection on the second.

On the basis of a paper by Pohost in 1980 (30), a redistribution image, recorded 4 hours following the stress injection, was substituted for the resting injection image. The rationale does not seem outlandish, but the author himself points out that a number of factors play a role to in the redistribution.

In short,

a. if equilibrium is reached by redistribution, the distribution of thallium should be the same as that of potassium, and (see Section 5.10) indicate viability or more precisely cellularity,

---

[f]Stress induced, but also induced by a vasodilation in the normal vascular beds, not distal to a stenosis.

[g]Because one of the characteristic of (functional) scintigraphic imaging is that a lack of target organ (in this case myocardial cells) and lack of function (in this case flow) cannot be distinguished.

b. but the reaching of equilibrium may take longer than expected since tissues starting with a lower concentration, may depend on the availability of the plasma level of circulating tracer.

c. However, the basis to replace a resting injection for resting flow by redistribution for resting flow assumes that resting flow will be proportional to cellularity and intracellular potassium concentration.

It has been generally, (but not universally) accepted, that a transient abnormality could be equally characterized either by the combination of stress and rest imaging, or by the combination of stress and redistribution imaging, and that the match transient-ischemia and fixed-scar remained unmodified. A transient perfusion defect measured with the delayed imaging technique became a synecdoche for myocardial stress ischemia. Normal resting perfusion, however, is underestimated when redistribution or delayed images are substituted to resting injection, as we will see in what follows.

Indeed, it has been shown that many apparently fixed defects on the 4 hour delayed images are transient if imaging is delayed for 24 hours (31) and Nelson (32) demonstrated that the degree of redistribution depends on the amount of circulating thallium during the interval (as noted by Pohost). In addition, it can be shown that there are cases where a true resting flow shows that the abnormality is transient, when the redistribution suggest a fixed lesion. Naruse (33) and Iskandrian (34) in a paper about viability (Section 5.10) had 35 patients with a fixed defect after a stress injection who had a normal resting study.

None of this changed the basic paradigm which remained at:

- Normal/normal: normal physiological response, no significant coronary obstruction
- Abnormal/normal (transient): represents stress (exercise of pharmacological) induced ischemia
- Abnormal/abnormal (fixed): represents scar

5.3.1. *Paradigm Shift*

The paradigm, however, needs to be modified. With high-grade stenosis, a stable state can exist when resting regional flow is also decreased. The myocardium is hibernating but viable, e.g. it would recover if the vascular lesion was corrected. Hibernating myocardium is chronically ischemic, and favors sugar metabolism. Hence, after FDG injection (at rest or during exercise), an excess FDG uptake would be present in living but ischemic myocardium. Hibernating myocardium is also dyskinetic or hypokinetic, and wall motion abnormalities are present. In fact, the definition of viability was originally that in an underperfused myocardial segment at rest with resting wall motion abnormality, the wall motion abnormality reverses to normal when the vascular flow is restored (by CABG or angioplasty) (35).

The interpretation of ^{201}Tl myocardial perfusion studies has been further refined by the observation that increased lung uptake is associated with more advanced diseases (36, 37). We should point out, however, that the mechanism may well be due to congestive heart failure (CHF) during exercise, and that the sign has not been shown to be independent of other clinical characteristics. In one publication, abnormal lung to myocardial uptake was present in 1 out of 6 of single vessel, 6 out of 14 of two vessel and 6 out of 12 of three vessel disease. In normal or negative subjects, the ratio correlated inversely to the peak exercise rate. However, no data are presented making the ratio independent of other clinical or scintigraphic signs.

Finally, in some cases of ^{201}Tl imaging and delayed imaging, the observation made was that new defects appeared in the delayed images. The significance of this phenomenon is unclear. In a recent review, Maddahi (38) attempts to resume the possibilities, which include imaging artifacts, normal washout heterogeneity and the presence of an admixture of viable and necrotic tissue.

5.4. PROCEDURES AND TECHNIQUES

5.4.1. *Imaging*

With ^{201}Tl, the procedure consists, in principle, of two separate imaging sessions. In one session, the patient is injected during peak exercise, and exercise is extended for one or two minutes beyond that time. The patient is then imaged, starting within 10 minutes of the injection. In a separate session, the patient is injected at rest, and imaged. We have mentioned the substitution of a 3- to 4-hour delayed image following the stress injection (39). This approach would be acceptable only for tracers that redistribute, which is not the case for MIBI and tetrofosmin, where two separate injections are required.

Originally, stress and resting injections tended to be separated by a few days however, with technetium agents, 1-day protocols have been proposed. In the second imaging session, the dose is usually tripled. The interpretation does not seem to be affected (40, 41). In an effort to further reduce total procedure time, imaging with ^{201}TI should immediately follow a resting or stress injection; subsequently, a stress or resting ^{99m}Tc-Sestamibi injection (42, 43) and imaging can be used.

There are multiple protocols, of which a number were reviewed by Berman (44). A 90-minute protocol was described by Mahmood (11) for thallium and tetrofosmin.

Recently, there has been interest in shortening the total procedure time even more by combining stress and rest imaging into one imaging session; this requires the use of two tracers. The combination of ^{201}Tl and ^{99m}Tc-sestamibi has been proposed, but the crosstalk from the technetium-scattered photons in the thallium window is a serious drawback (45).

Originally, most imaging was planar (projection imaging) in three views or projections for stress and rest: 45 LAO, anterior and left lateral. Tomographic imaging (Single Photon Emission Computed Tomography[h] (SPECT)) eventually replaced planar imaging, with some gain in the detection of circumflex disease.

SPECT imaging has been proposed (46) to image the patient prone, and to decrease diaphragmatic attenuation of the inferior wall.

5.4.2. *Stress Testing*

In actual stress testing, the actual stress consists of increasing the oxygen requirement of the myocardium. The normal response is the increase of coronary flow. If there is a (significant) coronary obstruction,[i] flow cannot increase beyond the obstruction. In the dependent myocardial domain, the uptake of the flow tracer does not increase in proportion to the flow in the other domains, and in the image that domain appears less active.[j] The usual stress method is graded exercise, in America usually on a treadmill, while in Europe, mainly on an immobile bicycle.

5.4.3. *Pharmacological Challenge*

5.4.3.1. *Dipyridamole*

As an alternative to exercise testing, a pharmacological intervention has been used, with dipyridamole. The usual dose is a 4-minute intravenous infusion of dipyridamole intravenously at dose rate of 0.14 mg/kg/min for 4 minutes (total dose = 0.56 mg/kg, not to exceed a total of 60 mg of dipyridamole), followed by the tracer

---

[h]Generally named SPET in Europe, eliminating the somewhat redundant "computed".

[i]The concept of obstruction is discussed in the chapter on renography. In short, an obstruction is a resistance to increased flow.

[j]The demotic expression is "less perfused", but in fact the "defect" in the stress study may be more perfused than in the rest study, but the expected increase in stress perfusion is either absent or less than in the normal myocardium.

injection. Dipyridamole is a coronary vasodilator causing coronary vasodilatation by inhibiting the reuptake and metabolism of adenosine. It typically increases heart rate from 20% to 40% and decreases systolic blood pressure by 10%. The action of dipyridamole is reversed by aminophylline.

The normal increase in cardiac blood flow is less than the total coronary reserve but sufficient to provoke a contrast between regions supplied by normal coronaries, and regions supplied by stenosed vessels which are unable to accommodate the increased flow.

Contraindications: unstable angina; myocardial infarction within 5 days; history of asthma and COPD; wheezing at the time of study; systolic blood pressure < 90; Class 3 or 4 NYHA;[k] 2 or 3 degree heart block without pacemaker; allergy to medications used for the study and xantines within 24 hours.

During infusion, the patient can be in supine position (and as an option can be asked to perform low-level, hand-grip exercises). Alternatively, infusion or dipyridamole can be performed with the patient upright and walking in place. The radiopharmaceutical is injected 2 to 4 minutes after the end of the dipyridamole infusion.

Reversal of dipyridamole action with slow injection of 100 mg of aminophylline, optimally 5 minutes after the injection of radiopharmaceutical.

Adverse reactions include chest pain, headache, dizziness, hypotension, nausea, EKG changes, and bronchospasm.

Stop infusion of dipyridamole and reverse action with aminophylline if severe adverse reaction occurs. If aminophylline does not alleviate symptom(s), NTG-SL can be administered as BP permits.

5.4.3.2. *Adenosine*

The patient preparation consists of nothing except clear liquids for 6 hours, or caffeine (coffee, tea or coke) for 24 hours. There are absolute and relative contraindications:

- Absolute: Second or third degree block without a pacemaker, ongoing wheezing, hypotension (SBP < 90 mmHg), recent (< 24 hours. Use of dipyridamole or xanthines (aminophylline, caffeine).
- Relative: Remote history of active airway disease (asthma, COPD), sick sinus syndrome, severe sinus (< 40) bradychardia.

---

[k]New-York Heart Association.

The infusion of adenosine must connect close to the distal end of the catheter, to avoid a bolus when the radioactive tracer is injected.

The adenosine (Adenocard™) comes in 6 mg/2 ml. Aim for a 6-minute injection at a rate of 140 μg/kg/min. Inject the tracer (cardiolite or thallium) at 3 minutes.

Terminate the infusion (i) if the patient experiences severe chest, tooth or jaw pain (7/10 or greater), (ii) if there is development of persistent second-degree or complete heart block, (iii) if there are significant ECG ischemic changes (> 2 mm ST segment depression), (iv) if there is severe hypotension (< 90 mm Hg) or severe wheezing.[1]

For mild chest pain, the patient may be given O_2 via nasal cannula.

5.4.3.3. Regadenoson (Lexiscan™)

Administration: 5 ml (0.4 mg) in a rapid (10-second) injection, IV followed by a 5-ml saline flush. The radiotracer is injected 10–20 seconds after the flush. The indications are the same as adenosine, but the procedure is somewhat simplified (inability to exercise on treadmill, pre-operative risk evaluation). For preparation, anti-ischemic medication can be discontinued only on the order of the referring physician. Xanthines should be avoided for at least 12 hours, dipyridamole for 48 hours, aminophylline for 24 hours.

The contraindications are the same as for adenosine: second or third degree AV block, asthma patients with wheezing and a systolic blood pressure less than 90 mm Hg. The antagonist is aminophylline, 50 to 250 mg in a slow IV (50–100 mg/30 to 60 seconds) and a systolic blood pressure of lower than 80 mm Hg, the development of second degree AV block, wheezing, severe chest pain or >2 mm ST segment depression, poor perfusion signs (pallor, cyanosis, cold skin). The patient can request to stop the pharmacological test, but that may invalidate the results of the myocardial perfusion study.

5.4.3.4. Dobutamine

Dobutamine has been used in lieu of exercise, mostly in conjunction with echocardiography. When performed with proper precautions, dobutamine testing is safe, but side effects are common (47). The usual method is to infuse dobutamine in increasing doses of 10, 20, 30, and 40 μg/kg/min at 3-minute intervals. In 729 out of 1012 patients, the maximum dose was reached. The heart rate

---

[1]**Source**: Imaging guidelines: Myocardial Stress Protocols. *J Nucl Cardiol*, Vol. 3, Nr 3; G1–G46 May/June 1996.

increased from 76 ± 14 to 127 ± 20 beats/min and the systolic blood pressure from 141 ± 20 mm Hg to 168 ± 36 mm Hg. The most common side effects were chest pain (31%), headache (14%), dyspnea (12%) palpitations (10%) and flushing (10%). There were no death, myocardial infarction, pulmonary edema, ventricular fibrillation, sustained ventricular tachycardia or cerebral vascular accidents. Non-sustained ventricular tachycardia occurred in 43 patients (4.2%) but did not cause any hemodynamic instability. Chest pain, with characteristics of angina pectoris, was treated with sublingual nitroglycerin in 24 out of 98 patients. Two patients were treated with intravenous digitalis and one with a fast-acting β-adrenergic blocker for control of heart rate (47). Those results are consistent with those of Mertes (48).

5.5. DATA ANALYSIS

5.5.1. *Visual Interpretation*

The interpretation of myocardial perfusion studies does consist, as suggested above, of two comparisons: The case is compared to a virtual image of what the normal should be, and the stress image is compared to the rest image. The defect is characterized as either fixed or transient.

Earlier studies reported mainly results based on the visual interpretation of "unprocessed" data. Unprocessed meant read directly from the photographic medium, assuming that the film characteristics, CRT settings and developing techniques resulted in a universal rendering of the data. If not universal, the photographic display was assumed to be constant within the institution.

Early processing consisted mainly of contrast recovery, whose main goal was to render the stress and rest images more comparable, even though their contrast tended to vary, because higher non-specific activities (tissue crosstalk) were present in the resting images. The best known method became the interpolative background subtraction (49), but multiple modifications have been spawned (50).

5.5.2. *Polar Transformation (Circumferential Profile)*

The next step was an attempt to quantify the distribution of myocardial activity (Vogel 1980, Burow 1979). The methods vary in details, but are essentially based of a polar transformation of the images, or on radial sampling. With an origin at the center of the myocardial cavity, in the original image, n radii, equally spaced over 360 degrees are extended towards the periphery. A pixel located at (x, y) in the original image, is located at (X_p, Y_p) in the transformed or polar image. The relation between x and X_p and between y and Y_p is define by:

$$X_p = \sqrt{(x - x_0)^2 + (y - y_0)^2},$$

$$Y_p = \tan^{-1} \frac{(y - y_0)}{x - x_0} + \alpha_0,$$

where x_0 and y_0 are the coordinates of the center point and α_0 is the angle of the origin. Regardless of the size of the object in the original image, in the y_p dimension of the transformed image, the object will extend of "n" pixels. In the X dimension, the size will remain different (Figure 5.1). But in most applications,

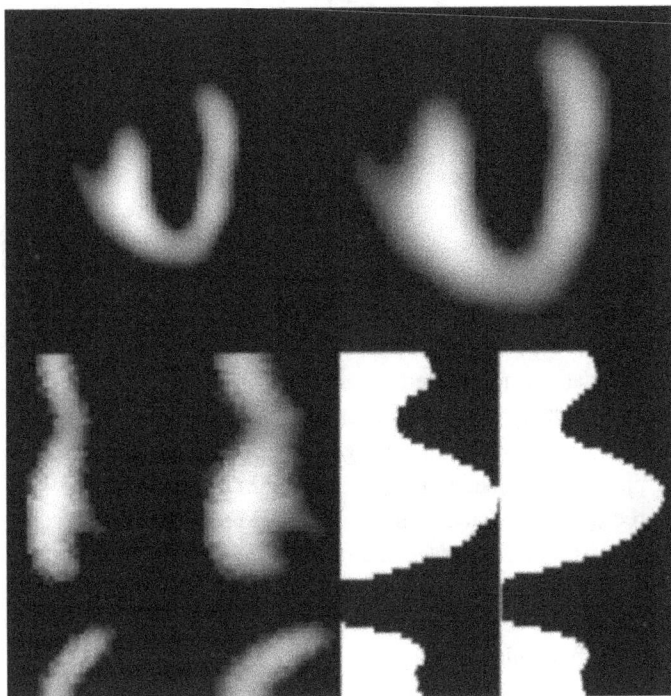

Figure 5.1 The figur is an illustration of a polar transform; in this case of a set of two two-dimensional cartesian images. The images are in fact identical, except for size. The two objects cannot be made to overlap precisely (except by zooming). A polar transform makes the two images of equal length (vertical dimension) and matching in the y_p-axis. On the thickness (x_p) aspect, the images have not become identical, but if one samples along the x_p-axis line by line and records the maximum value for each line, the data are reduced to a one-dimensional vector, were y_p is the x-axis and the maximum value is the x value: It is a circumferential profile The two circumferential profile are identical.

the object is sampled for an attribute which does not include a size dimension, i.e. the highest count rate density along x_p.

This second step reduces the data in the two-dimensional image to a one-dimensional vector (a "circumferential" profile), which except for density differences is comparable, regardless of the shape and size of the myocardium in the image. The advantage is that shape and size differences between patients are eliminated, and the vectors or profiles can be averaged and compared between multiple patients. In planar images, normal population average profiles are produced for each of the three or four standard views and in addition, normal population differences between the stress and rest profiles.

In the case of separate stress and rest imaging, and in inter-patient comparisons (before averaging or comparing) the images are normalized prior to the generation of the profiles, or the profiles are normalized to their maximum value. In the case of stress and redistribution imaging, the profile comparison is expressed as a percentage difference, without count normalization (53). This set of values is generally referred to as the wash-out.

In planar images, the validity of the comparison requires identical projection orientations and equivalent placing of the origin. The acquisition angle or projection angle is calibrated on a first perfect left anterior oblique image.

5.5.3. *3D Polar Transformation (Bull's Eye)*

In the case of tomographic images in most methods, the image volume between the apex and the base is divided in an equal number of thick slices perpendicular to the long axis of the heart. For each slice, an individual circumferential profile is generated. Rather than represent the profiles as many curves, the sampled values are plotted as densities in a two-dimensional image, in which the density of point "i" in the profile of the slice Z is plotted at x and y, and are defined as follows:

If there are S thick slices and the total number of points in the profile is N, and the profile values are mapped in an image of dimension 64×64, the ratio $360\,i/N$ represents an angle in degrees, and

$$x = 32.5 + \frac{Z \cdot S}{32} \cdot cosine\left(\frac{i \cdot 360}{N}\right),$$

$$y = 32.5 + \frac{Z \cdot S}{32} \cdot sine\left(\frac{i \cdot 360}{N}\right).$$

The resulting image has the aspect of a bull's eye. Central values are generally apical, peripheral values are basal.

There is a special problem at the apex, where in a plane perpendicular to the long axis, the origin would be in the myocardial wall. Various methods have been proposed to circumvent that problem. In reality, the approach lacks consistency, since instead of sampling radially in space, sampling is performed in Cartesian coordinates from the base to the apex, and in polar coordinates within the thick slices. A total polar sampling method has been described (54).

There are a number of important features associated to polar sampling:

1. Structures closer to the origin are oversampled relative to structures farther from the origin. The placing of the origin could therefore make a defect appear larger or smaller. Nevertheless, Caldwell (55) found good correlation between defects area in the circumferential analysis and the perfusion defect in the anatomical slices.
2. Misalignment of the zero angle results in a shift in the polar transformed image, and hence a misalignment of the regions of the myocardium.
3. The attribute or sample value is not necessarily representative of the whole distribution across the myocardial wall. This statement needs *a proviso*: in low resolution imaging, the total counts across the myocardial wall tend to correlate with the maximum across the myocardial wall. However, this correlation weakens as the resolution of the imaging system increases.
4. The polar transformation methods have the advantage that they provide a simple and ready-made method to make comparisons between cases and populations. Naruse (33) did compare planar and SPECT normal data files for thallium-201, ^{99m}Tc-sestamibi, ^{99m}Tc-tetrofosmin and ^{99m}Tc-furifosmin. Significant differences were found in the planar image normal profiles, but the differences in SPECT normal profiles were not significant. One explanation is that in projection (planar) imaging, a single rotation correction is not sufficient. The rotation corrects for misalignment in terms of the patient's long axis (cranio-caudal), but not for rotation around that axis.

5.5.4. *Non-Rigid Registration*

An alternative should be considered, and that is a 3-dimensional non-rigid or elastic registration of all cases to a population template (Figure 5.2). There are various methods. The non-rigid registration allows global but independent changes in the x, y and z coordinates and in the xy, yz and xz angles between the coordinates (global affine), and local changes (local splines). One of the advantages is that the results

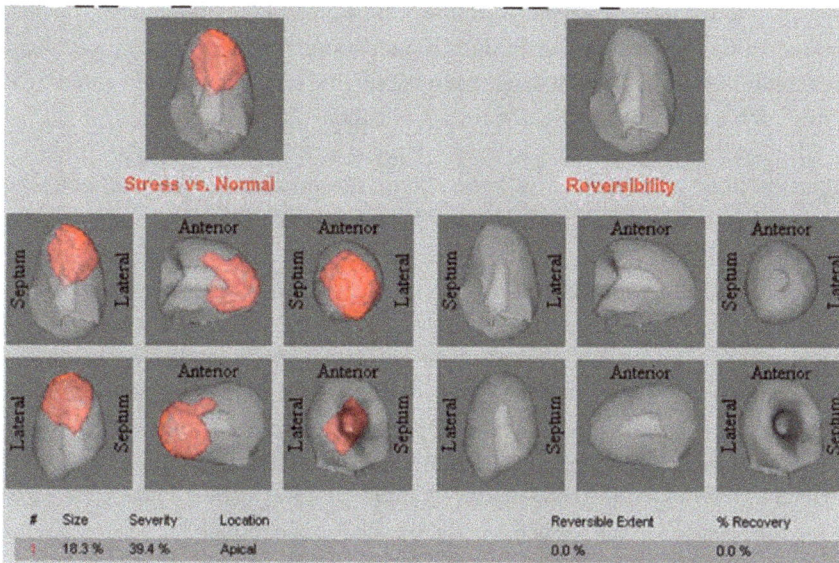

Figure 5.2 Representation of the results of normalizing shapes not by a polar transform, but by a 3-D elastic registration to a population template. The whole of the wall activity is maintained and measured, as opposed to the polar transform method (bull's eye) in which the metric is reduced to the maximum across the myocardial wall. In this example, the (morphologically) transformed myocardium maintained the internal distribution of densities. Shown in red is the difference with the normal population distribution of densities. In this case, the abnormality is fixed. There is an additional difference with the usual approach: the defect is not located in pre-set "segments" but is located in the region of the apex, and the size is not determined by the number of segments involved, but by the comparison to total counts and total volume.

are less reducting: the metric is not restricted to the maximum across the segment of the myocardial wall, but all of the myocardial densities can be included (56–59).

5.6. CONCEPTUAL DETOURS

It is important to review the kinetics of ^{201}Tl in the myocardium for historical reasons. We start from the original concept that myocardial perfusion scintigraphy was essentially seen as a method to diagnose or characterize stress ischemia. Basically, one compared the myocardial flow distribution at rest to the distribution during stress (60). Pohost (30, 38) introduced a redistribution image of thallium-201 as a substitute for the resting study. Although he admitted the limitations, of which one was that if not enough thallium was circulating, the redistribution would not occur. Still the redistribution image was quickly (too quickly) accepted as the "real thing" or a strict equivalent of the resting injection.

Redistribution was taken to mean that the deficit in activity, the "defect", actually filled in. Whether it appeared to fill in because the well-perfused regions lost thallium faster, or whether there was a real fill in was not explicitly stated.

Eventually the hypothesis was advanced that the washout (decrease in activity) rate would be higher in well-perfused regions, and less in poorly perfused regions (61–64). Under that hypothesis, the defects do not fill in, the better perfused regions washout faster. Since the image is relative, the filling in is actually a loss of contrast between the well and poorly perfused regions.

In the chapter on compartmental analysis, we consider two compartments connected to the same (third) compartment. If the outflow fractional rate is the same for compartments 1 and 2, and the initial flows remain constant, the concentrations will parallel each other. However, if the initial flow in one of the compartments is elevated and then returns to a basal state, the concentrations will converge. In general, one can state that the higher the original uptake (or initial flow), the faster the "washout". However, in addition, the washout and convergence rates are influenced by plasma concentrations (Figure 5.3).

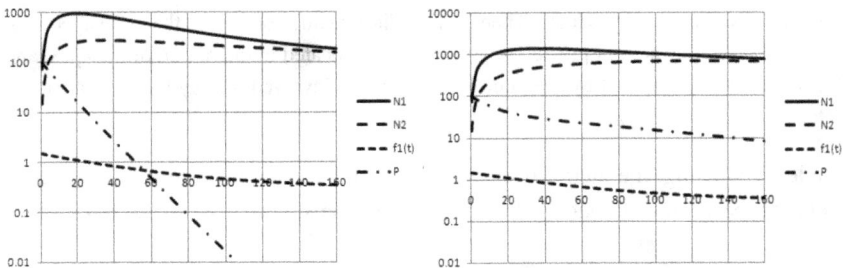

Figure 5.3   The figure illustrates the effect of plasma concentration on two equal volumes of myocardium (in the model of two compartments connected to the same third compartment (plasma). In both cases, the fractional outflow rates are equal (α_{1p} and α_{2p}) and in both cases, the flow (plasma): flow ratio (f_1:f_2) is 1.5:0.3. In both cases, the stress flow returns to normal at the same rate (f_1). But in the case on the left, plasma clearance (p) is swift, while on the right it is slow. The washout from both compartments (N_1 and N_2) is greatly influenced by the plasma clearance in addition to the early concentration. Finally, with higher plasma activity, the concentrations converge faster (see Section 8.5.8).

5.6.1. *The Points to Remember*

- The accumulation of the tracer early is higher in the better perfused studies and remains so for a time, until loss or washout from the tissues become higher than the accumulation.
- The increase in flow due to stress is not maintained for a long time. The model then predicts that eventually, the activities (per gram of tissue) will become equivalent in both the ischemic and normal myocardium.
- The relative washout has been used as an independent sign of ischemia, with the ischemic segments showing slower (relative) washout. The model, however, explains this by the fact that the normal myocardium starts from a higher value. The model is not invalidated by the findings of Nishiyama (62), who studied the effects of coronary flow on thallium uptake and washout. But since he did not separate initial uptake from washout, one cannot conclude that the washout rate is an independent measure of myocardial ischemia.
- Nelson (35) demonstrated that reversibility of defects in delayed ^{201}Tl images is a function of the amount of circulating ^{201}Tl. In his experiment, reversibility rates increased from 15 out of 38 to 27 out of 38 when higher circulating levels were maintained.

5.6.2. *In Addition*

The major papers describing the washout method do not always give separate sensitivity values for stress defects and washout abnormalities (65, 51); but in one paper Garcia (66) does give a hint: Globally speaking the washout was less sensitive than a stress abnormality (75% versus 89%), and equally specific (92%).[m] But the specific gain or loss by the inclusion of washout is not given. Depasquale (67) found that the sensitivity for the identification of LAD, RCA and LCX disease increased from 78% to 81%, 89% to 89% and 65 to 67% respectively by adding washout as an abnormality criterion, but the specificities were equally affected, going from 83% to 74%, 87% to 86% and 95% to 92%. For the identification of LAD, this represents a change in likelihood ratio from 4.6 to 3.1, for RCA from 9.96 to 6.35 and for LCX from 13 to 8.4.[n]

---

[m]Depending on the limits, based on a volunteer normal population.
[n]In Section 7.7 we briefly discussed the irritation habits (1) not to tabulate all the outcome possibilities and (2) to dispense with the need to distinguish between "or" and "and" combinations.

5.6.3. *Eventually People Started to Accept Two Things*

In some cases, redistribution did not result in a normal image. This lack of normalization would be due to the lack of circulating activity; to counteract that, a new injection of the tracer at rest would provide compensation to the deficiency. This second injection at rest was called a re-injection.[o]

Eventually, the realization came that the resting distribution could be abnormal, but that the underperfused myocardium could be viable (see viability). A delayed image after the (re-injection) resting injection could still normalize, and reveal viability (68).[p] The number of papers on the subject trailed on (69), but in the section on viability we will attempt to rationalize to some extent.

5.6.4. *Modified Semiotics*

In a certain way, the semiotics changed dramatically; first because the concept of viability was introduced, and second because the types of information changed according to the procedure. A (partially) arbitrary synopsis is given in Table 5.1.

Table 5.1 Synopsis of the semiotics. The outcome categories are normal, ischemic, infarct and viable. Normal and ischemic are viable by definition. The results of rest injection and "re-injection" are conflated.

Stress	Rest	Redistribution after stress	Redistribution after rest	Category
abnormal	normal			ischemic
abnormal		normal		ischemic
abnormal			normal	ischemic
abnormal		abnormal	abnormal	infarct
abnormal		abnormal		no diagnosis
abnormal		abnormal	normal	viable
abnormal	abnormal	normal		viable
	abnormal		normal	viable
	abnormal		abnormal	infarct

---

[o]I would assume that it was not called a resting injection, because it would indicate that the substitution of the redistribution image for the resting image was a collective mistake.
[p]In Section 5.5, we will interpret "late" redistribution as an expression of cellularity.

5.7. OPERATING CHARACTERISTICS: THE DETECTION OF CORONARY ARTERY DISEASE[q]

5.7.1. *The Arteriogram as the Defining Standard*[r]

For the detection of coronary artery disease, the literature has generally favored the coronary arteriogram as the criterion for the presence of the disease. Even this criterion does vary; some will consider the case positive if there is a 50% stenosis, others if the stenosis is at least 75% of the diameter or area. In general, sensitivity has been found to be > 75% and the specificity > 75%. Sensitivity increases with advanced disease, but is generally supposed to be very sensitive to the adequacy of the intervention (Stress must go to valid end-point: MPHR, ST segment depression, BP drop, arrhythmia) but at least one study challenges that viewpoint (70).

There are a number of problems with the coronary arteriogram as the defining standard. The major one, as we will see (Section 5.7), is that in later times, it was shown that the myocardial perfusion study had prognostic or outcome values independent of the coronary arteriogram. And, indeed, in some circumstances, the myocardial perfusion study was used to define the significance of coronary lesions.

Second, the literature is unclear on the meaning of coronary lesions that do not reach the 50% or 70% threshold. It would not be reasonable, considering the imprecision of the metric, to assume that the limit is binary in those terms. One should expect that if all cases below the 50% threshold are used to define specificity, the specificity would be low if there are a significant number of cases between 30% and 40% (71).

Third, operating characteristics obtained from data in clinical practice are subject to verification bias: Patients with a positive study are more likely to undergo a coronary arteriogram. In the extreme case, if only patients with a positive myocardial perfusion study went on to have a coronary arteriogram, the sensitivity would appear to be 100%, and the specificity 0% (72, 73).[s] To overcome this problem, some authors have favored the use of cohorts of subjects with low probability of CAD to define the specificity (42, 53, 63, 66, 71). To distinguish that approach, they replaced the term specificity with the term "normalcy ratio". And, indeed, in the aggregate for all methods, the normalcy ratio was 0.87 versus 0.74 for the specificity.

---

[q]Operating characteristics have been discussed in Chapter 7.
[r]Often called the "gold standard".
[s]See Section 7.5.

There is a fundamental problem with the normalcy ratio approach: The population is atypical for a population found in a cardiology clinic, or, to put it differently, in the cardiology clinic population, patients do not have either coronary artery disease or nothing. They may have another cardiac condition that may result in an abnormal perfusion study (83–85), including a left bundle branch block (86).

There are methods to overcome verification bias, but they are not usually applied in the myocardial perfusion literature.

5.7.2. *Methodological Problems*

The goal is to define the operating characteristics of myocardial scintigraphy, but this depends on interpretation and (unfortunately) methodology. The methodologies include imaging methods (SPECT versus planar imaging), tracers (see Section 5.2) mainly thallium versus the ^{99m}Tc-labeled tracers sestamibi and tetrofosmin), and the metrics which are based on the methods of quantization (see Section 5.5) and the observed phenomenon (stress/rest, stress redistribution, stress/washout). In Tables 5.2 and 5.3, we show that the results do not fundamentally depend on the methodology,[t] however, the reporting of the results is often flawed in a fundamental way.

In a strange attitude of almost maidenly discretion, most authors do not specify the combination of metrics. In its simplest form, there are a restricted number of metrics and outcomes. The interpretation can be based only on a resting study, which is normal or abnormal. The same is true for a stress study. But if a stress and rest study is performed, the outcome can be normal, a transient abnormality and a fixed abnormality. The number of possible outcomes increases if one also includes washout metrics. Yet, the majority of the authors referenced here do not specify the metric combination.

5.7.3. *Identification of Individual Vessels*

The identification of diseased vessels individually has been tabulated by various authors as a sensitivity for the detection of disease in a vessel. The numbers have to be considered carefully, because they depend on the relative degree of constriction: The stress test is likely to be terminated when ischemia occurs in the domain of the

---

[t] I feel comfortable with the statement, since I introduced some methodologies (Goris, 1976, 1985, 1986, 1987, 1989, 1994, 1999, 2000; Declerck, 1997) that were not shown to change the operating characteristics fundamentally. One is tempted to state that the physiology and physics dominate.

Table 5.2[u] The table illustrates mainly the difference between the normalcy ratio and specificity. The columns "+" and "−" indicate the positive or negative cases. The columns ≤ p yield the probability of having a lower or equal value in a binomial function: For the whole population (all cases and all vessels), the sensitivity was 0.75, and the specificity 0.83 including normalcy ratios. WO is washout, OR is either a transient or fixed defect.

Outcome	Metric	Vessel	+	N	P(S+D+)	p ≤	−	N	P(S−D−)	p ≤
< 1% probability	Stress or WO	Any					50	54	0.926	0.988
< 5%	OR	Any					26	28	0.929	0.963
< 5%	Stress	Any					149	177	0.842	0.692
< 5%	WO only	Any					24	25	0.960	0.991
NCA	OR	Any					169	226	0.748	0.001
NCA	Stress	Any					328	407	0.806	0.111
NCA	Transient	Any					34	44	0.773	0.204
> 50%	Fixed	Any	258	586	0.440	0.000				
> 50%	OR	Any	834	949	0.879	1.000				
> 50%	Stress	Any	274	362	0.757	0.785				
> 50%	Stress or WO	Any	354	458	0.772	0.941				
> 50%	Transient	Any	447	641	0.697	0.009				
> 50%	WO only	Any	36	106	0.338	0.000				
All			**2203**	**3102**	**0.710**		**780**	**961**	**0.812**	

[u]In the tables of this section, the data were culled from Refs. 11, 41, 53, 55, 63, 66, 67, 70, 71, 74–82.

Table 5.3 The tracer and the imaging modality does not seem to influence the outcomes systematically. The metric does: Transient, fixed and resting abnormalities are less sensitive to detect coronary artery disease in general (as opposed to stress ischemia in the absence of myocardial infarction). The columns "+" and "−" indicate the positive or negative cases. The columns ≤ p yield the probability of having a lower or equal value in a binomial function: For the whole population (all cases and all vessels), the sensitivity was 0.75, and the specificity was 0.83.

Tracer	Modality	Metric	Vessel	+	N	P(S+D+)	p ≤	−	N	P(S−D−)	p ≤
MIBI	SPECT	Fixed	Any	252	545	0.462	0.000	5	11	0.455	0.005
MIBI	SPECT	OR	Any	616	695	0.886	1.000	41	55	0.745	0.073
MIBI	SPECT	Stress	Any					30	37	0.811	0.444
MIBI	SPECT	Stress	Any					8	22	0.364	0.000
MIBI	SPECT	Transient	Any	373	545	0.684	0.002	25	33	0.758	0.187
Tetro	SPECT	OR	Any	112	124	0.903	1.000	26	28	0.929	0.963
Thallium	Planar	Fixed	Any	6	41	0.146	0.000				1.000
Thallium	Planar	OR	Any	70	81	0.864	0.998	33	35	0.943	0.988
Thallium	Planar	Rest	Any	31	63	0.492	0.000	20	20	1.000	1.000
Thallium	Planar	Stress	Any	35	63	0.556	0.001	38	40	0.950	0.995
Thallium	Planar	Stress or WO	Any	186	224	0.830	1.000	98	110	0.913	0.972
Thallium	Planar	Transient	Any	76	144	0.528	0.000	9	11	0.818	0.581
Thallium	Planar	WO only	Any	21	80	0.263	0.000				
Thallium	SPECT	Stress	Any	27	29	0.931	0.998	257	294	0.875	0.985
Thallium	SPECT	Stress	Any	18	26	0.705	0.359	151	204	0.740	0.001
Thallium	SPECT	WO only	Any	15	26	0.570	0.052	24	25	0.960	0.991
Tl/Tetro	SPECT	OR	Any	71	89	0.798	0.917	95	136	0.699	0.000
All			**Any**	**1909**	**2775**	**0.68793**		**860**	**1061**	**0.8106**	

Table 5.4 The specificity is low for the LAD and the LCX. The sensitivity is low for the LCX. Generally speaking, the more advance disease (TVD) is detected better than SVD. The finding is paradoxical because the interpretation is based on contrast. NCA: negative coronary arteriogram, LAD: left anterior descending, LCX: left circumflex, RCA: right coronary artery, SVD: single vessle disease, DVD: two vessel disease, TVD: triple vessel disease.

Outcome	Vessel	+	N	P(S+D+)	p ≤	−	N	P(S−D−)	p ≤
< 5%	All					249	284	0.876760563	0.988
NCA	All					326	443	0.735891648	0.000
NCA	LAD					335	427	0.784262295	0.006
NCA	LCX					239	259	0.923243243	1.000
NCA	RCA					279	332	0.841084337	0.714
> 50%	All	1754	2321	0.755708746	0.961				
> 50%	LAD	293	354	0.827683616	1.000				
> 50%	LCX	145	217	0.668202765	0.011				
> 50%	RCA	377	428	0.880841121	1.000				
> 50%	SVD	208	251	0.828685259	1.000				
> 50%	DVD	217	235	0.923404255	1.000				
> 50%	TVD	232	238	0.974789916	1.000				

most affected vessel. The specificity in this context is the ability to state that the vessel is not involved (Table 5.4).

It is important to note that if the lack of specificity is due to the presence of abnormalities unrelated to coronary artery diseases and randomly distributed, then the sensitivity and specificity for vessel detection tend to minimize that effect.

The fact that the sensitivity is higher for triple vessel diseases (TVD) is surprising, because all the methods are essentially based on contrast. In the case of single vessel disease (SVD), one would expect that the vascular domain of the affected vessel be clearly contrasted against the other domains, but in TVD, all domains could be affected.

5.7.4. Type of Stress

No significant differences in sensitivities have been recorded between exercise and pharmacological stress testing (87–90), but in the case of dipyridamole, a higher dose (infused at the same rate for a longer time) increased the number of perfusion defects and transient defects, with an increase in sensitivity from 80% to 87% for 15 patients (91).

One of the reasons for false positive studies is the presence of a left bundle branch block (LBBB). Since the effect of dobutamine is both inotropic and chronotropic, false positive studies are also found in the presence of LBBB (86). The defect was septal and periapical, the technique was planar imaging. It is generally accepted that in the presence of a LBBB, an adenosine or persantine (dipyridamole) challenge is preferable to exercise or dobutamine.

The operating characteristics of the myocardial perfusion studies have to be evaluated in the context of those of the stress ECG. For exercise ECG, Dunn (85) quotes sensitivities ranging from 91% to 53% and specificities ranging from 63% to 93%. In studies in which both myocardial perfusion studies and exercise ECGs are reported, the myocardial perfusion studies have consistently higher sensitivies and specificies. But Dunn does not explicitly address the problem of interdependency in his proposal for a diagnostic pathway. Indeed, in patients with coronary artery disease, 89 out of 104 (85.5%) patients with a positive stress ECG had a transient defect, in comparison with 29 out of 47 (62%) with a negative stress ECG.

5.7.5. *Wall Thickening*

Strangely enough, wall thickening is rarely mentioned in the detection of coronary artery disease in the context of a diagnostic pathway. Theoretically, if a fixed defect is detected, the cause could be an infarct, a hibernating myocardium (see Section 5.10), or an attenuation artifact. In the case of the latter, the function would be maintained. A hibernating or infarcted myocardial segment would (generally[v]) not move normally, but certainly would not demonstrate wall thickening. Using wall motion and wall thickening would therefore increase specificity.

Wall thickening is fundamental. Actively contracting muscles must thicken to shorten. The scintigraphic method tends to lack the spacial resolution to measure the thickness of the myocardial wall precisely. What has been accepted is interesting because the method is based precisely on the lack of resolution of the imaging system (Figure 5.4).

Theoretically, the difficulty resides in the ability to precisely match both flow and kinetic observations to the same segments identified in separate imaging studies. Evaluating both characteristics on the same image is an improvement. And indeed, if at first gating, myocardial perfusion studies were considered a method for improving imaging *per se* (92); planar or SPECT gated perfusion images have been used to evaluate function, either using edge detection (93, 94) or count variation techniques (95, 96), the subject of Figure 5.4.

---

[v]It could be pulled passively by surrounding myocardium.

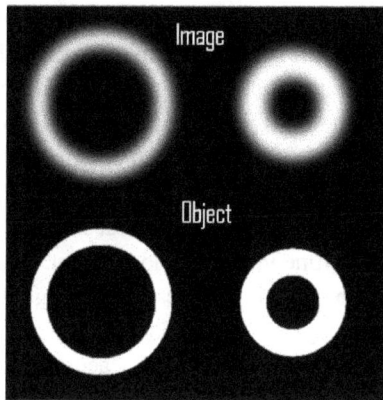

(A)

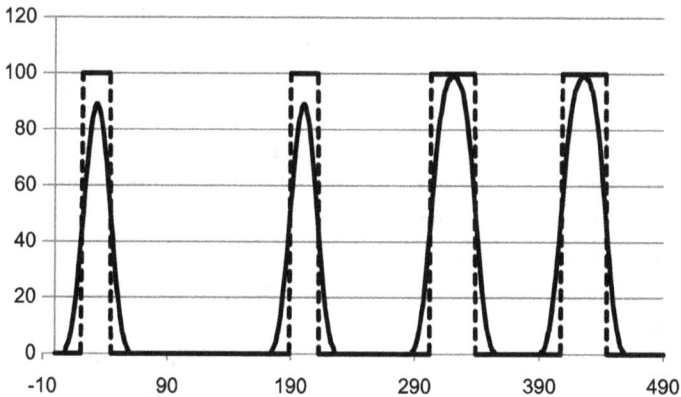

(B)

Figure 5.4 The figure illustrates the estimation of wall thickening based on maximum wall section count increases.[W] In panel A, we see a section of the myocardium in diastole (left) and systole (right) as an image. The image (above) of the object (below) is distorted by the modulation transfer function (MTF). In reality, the wall did thicken but the total wall activity did not change. Panel B shows the count profiles across the wall in the image (full line) and in the object (broken line). The effect of the MTF is that in the thinner wall the maximum counts never reach the actual maximum. They do in the thicker wall. Thickening is transformed to maximum count rate increases (see Section 10.7.5).

[W] It is interesting to note that the best known and most used quantitative techniques (circumferential profiles, bull's eye) are very reductive, because the metric is the maximum value across the myocardial wall. This is also true in the evaluation of wall thickening.

We have proposed (97, 98) a method based on the assumption that in a gated tomographic perfusion image, a segment of the myocardial wall can be characterized by the maximum count rate density in the segment (perfusion), the first moment of the distribution of count rate densities (location), and the second moment of this distribution (thickness). The underlying model assumes that the displacement of the first moment centripetally relative to the center of the left ventricular cavity can be used as a measure of wall motion, and that wall thickening measurements can be based on changes in time in the second moment.

Imaging, following an injection at rest or during maximal stress [7 mCi (0.26 GBq) for the first study, 21 mCi (0.78 GBq) for the second in a one day protocol] is performed as an ECG-gated SPECT acquisition with eight time bins. The acquisition parameters are 30 sec/stop, stop and go, 64 angles over 360 degrees, and a 64 × 64 format.

Tomographic images are reconstructed as 64^3 image volumes (99), normalized for tail drop correction, centered and reoriented. At the end of the reorientation, the ventricle is oriented with the apex downward or pointing south. Non-myocardial structures are masked out, using a truncated ellipsoidal three-dimensional mask. The eight tomographic images are further thresholded to 35% of the maximal myocardial activity in the entire set of eight reconstructed tomographic images.

The masking in combination with thresholding results in eight images in which only myocardial structures have significant non-zero count rate density values. Thresholding, however, is limited so that even underperfused myocardial segments maintain non-zero values.

For each of the time bins, three characteristics of the myocardial wall are mapped in three two-dimensional vectors as follows (97, 99):

The three-dimensional images are sampled along rays or radii, originating in the center of the left ventricular cavity. Each radius is characterized by a longitudinal (a) and latitudinal angle (b). The origin of "b" is the apex, and "b" goes in 32 steps from 0 to 135 degrees, the origin of "a" is the middle of the lateral wall, and "a" varies from 0 to 360 degrees. A value sampled along the radius R(a,b) is stored in the two-dimensional vector (B) at the location (K, L) where K and L are defined as:

$$K = \frac{32b}{135} \cdot \cos{(a)},$$

$$L = \frac{32b}{135} \cdot \sin{(a)}.$$

The vector B is therefore a planar image in which central points represent apical locations and peripheral points represent the basal locations. The anterior wall is mapped on top, the inferior wall at the bottom, the septum in the left-hand side of the image. This vector is exactly comparable to the bull's eye maps described in the literature, except for the fact that the distance from the center represents a latitude "b" in three dimensions, rather than a short axis plane position.

Three values P, D and T are sampled along the radius r(a,b) as follows: If the distribution of count rate densities along R is C(r), the first sampled value is $P = C(r)_{max}$ which is the maximum circumferential count rate density traditionally considered as a measure of regional perfusion.

The second sampled value is the average location of the activity associated with the myocardial wall, along the radius:

$$D = \frac{\int_{r=0}^{r=32} r \cdot C(r) \cdot dr}{\int_{r=0}^{r=32} C(r) \cdot dr}.$$

"D" is the first moment of the count rate distribution along the radius, or the average position of the wall along the radius. The wall's position for each coordinate is therefore defined by the distribution of count rate densities, and not by edge detection.

Finally, the count rate distribution along the radius is further defined by:

$$T = \sqrt{\frac{\int_{r=0}^{r=32} (D - r)^2 \cdot C(r) \cdot dr}{\int_{r=0}^{r=32} C(r) \cdot dr}},$$

where T is the second moment, or the standard deviation of the count distribution around the mean, a measure of wall thickness.

The count rate density distribution describes a unimodal, (more or less) bell-shaped curve. The peak (or maximum of the curve, "P") increases with progressing systole, as does the standard deviation (or the width of the bell), while the whole bell-shaped curve (and hence its average position) moves to the center.

The method presented here is based on the assumption that one can fairly estimate myocardial wall motion as motion directed to the center of the left ventricular cavity. This assumption cannot be completely true, since some torsion of the ventricle is known to occur during contraction. Second, we assume that following the first moment of the count rate density across the myocardial wall is the correct way to estimate wall motion.

Technically, the method is characterized by three factors: First, sampling is radial in space, rather than radial within planes and Cartesian between planes; unless all wall motion is restricted to motion within the planes, comparison of sections at different times of the cardiac cycle becomes uncertain, and more so towards the apex. Second, location and wall thickness are defined by statistical parameters of the count rate distribution, rather than edge detection algorithms.

Third, location and thickness are transformed in densities, located in a vector, not according to the original location, but as a function of sampling angle. This allows one to further analyze the data on the basis of density modulations (e.g. first harmonic analysis (Sections 6.2.3.2 and 10.6) of the density modulation), which cannot be done strictly with the original data, since density modulation assumes that the structures remain mapped in the same pixels. Direct pixel density modulation analysis is probably more appropriate in gated blood pool imaging (100, 101), where the modulation is assumed to be related to volume changes, than in perfusion studies (102), where the density modulations are related to the movement of structures (Sections 6.2.3 and 10.6).

A similar approach was used for wall thickness, but within planes using edge detection (91) or pixel density modulations (92, 93) comparing pixels with their equivalent location on a bull's eye map.

DePuey (103) used the visual interpretation of gated myocardial perfusion images to characterize fixed defects. He found kinetic abnormalities (either wall motion or wall thickening, but otherwise unspecified) in 98 out of 102 fixed defects associated to an infarct. In the case of 78 fixed defects not associated with an infarct, the function was abnormal in 18. The authors assume that those cases represent silent myocardial infarctions, and that the 60 remaining cases are imaging artifacts. It is clear at least that kinetic abnormalities increase the specificity of fixed abnormalities.

5.8. PROGNOSTIC SIGNIFICANCE

One could argue that a sensitivity and specificity of 0.75 and 0.80 respectively is not enough to make a definite diagnosis. Some doubt must remain. However, it is important to remember that the predictive value depends on the prevalence (Table 5.5). Hence the table shows that if the prevalence is 50%, a positive test has a positive predictive value of 79% and a negative predictive value of 76%. If the

Table 5.5

P(D)	P(D−)	P(D+|S+)	P(D−|S−)
0.2	0.8	0.48	0.93
0.3	0.7	0.62	0.88
0.5	0.5	0.79	0.76
0.7	0.3	0.90	0.58
0.8	0.2	0.94	0.44

prevalence is 70%, those values become 90% and 58%. If the prevalence is 0.3, the negative predictive value is 88% (Table 5.5).

However, that is not the whole story. In a review of 3500 cases, Brown (104) found that even in the presence of coronary lesions, the rate of cardiac events in the presence of a normal ^{201}Tl study is less than 1% per year. In a paper published in 1993, Brown (37) found a yearly rate 0.7% of cardiac events in patients with significant coronary lesions, but negative exercise planar 201Tl studies (1 of 75 patients had a non-fatal myocardial infarction). In this cohort of patients, 39 had single, 21 had two and 15 had three vessel diseases. The patients were older, reached a lower heart rate and had more ST segment depressions than the control group of 101 patients without coronary lesions. In addition, he (105) found that the rate of cardiac events correlated with the number of reversible defects, with an incidence of 3%, 0%, 8% and 33% for 1, 2 and more than 3 reversible defects respectively In patients with unstable angina responding to medical treatment and followed for 39 ± 11 months, 26% (6 out of 23) of the patients with transient defect had cardiac events and only 1 out of 29 of those with only fixed defects (106). Finally (107), in another cohort, the number of segment with transient defects was the only significant predictor of future cardiac events.

In a separate study, Hendel (108) found that cardiac events occurred in 30 out of 145 patients with more than one Persantine-induced transient defect, and in 22 out of 329 patients without multiple transient defects.

The prognostic finding is not restricted to myocardial studies with 201Tl. In a cohort of 234 patients, of whom 28 had ST segment depression and 57 had chest pain during stress (exercise or dipyridamole), but who had negative sestamibi SPECT studies, the annualized cardiac event rate was 0.5%/year and two patients underwent coronary revascularization (109).

In patients without a history of previous infarction or CABG, Staniloff (110) found that cardiac death rates or myocardial infarction were best predicted by transient defects (25.4 events/100 patient years), and by profound defects (7.5 events/100 patient years) against a rate of 0.5% when the perfusion study was normal. The length of exercise was a weaker predictor, as was the magnitude of the ST segment depression. However, both variables were strong predictors of interventions (CABG), with a rate of 2.8% for ST depressions lower than 1.0 mm, versus 17.1% with a depression > 2.0 mm. Therapeutic interventions during the observation period obscures the value of the study. If the intervention is taken as a cardiac event, the total number of events increase from 1.28%/100 man years in the case of a normal perfusion study to 58% with reversible defects. For profound defects (fixed or reversible), the total rate becomes 40%.

Assey (111) looked specifically at transient 201Tl defects in patients with and without angina, and found that the prognosis was not better in the absence of anginal pain during stress testing if transient defects are present.

Galvin and Brown (112) were able to demonstrate that the site of an acute myocardial infarction, occurring within 2 years of a myocardial perfusion study, was the site of the transient perfusion defect in 79% of the cases in 14 cases. The final cohort consisted of a mere 34 patients. The global statistics are interesting: there were 1486 consecutive patients with a diagnosis of myocardial infarction. Only 104 of these had a prior myocardial perfusion study. In 30, the infarct site could not be identified, and 8 had undergone interval coronary revascularization. Of the 66 remaining, 24 had a normal myocardial perfusion study, and 8 had fixed defects only. In short, 42 out of 66 infarct had been predicted by a positive myocardial perfusion study. But the interval between the perfusion study and the infarct was 34.3 ± 23.7.

Finally, Dilsizian (113) was able to show that in young patients with a hypertrophic cardiomyopathy, the risk of sudden cardiac arrest or syncope was related to ischemic events, revealed by transient defects in exercise myocardial SPECT.

5.9. PERI-OPERATIVE RISK

In a separate context, the prognostic value of myocardial perfusion studies has been evaluated in the case of patients scheduled for surgery. Leppo (114) looked at 89 consecutive patients scheduled for elective vascular surgery, and studied with dipyridamole ^{201}Tl-myocardial imaging. Taken by themselves, the age, exercise time, peak rate pressure product, percentage maximum predicted heart rate, average number of defects on the scans[x] the frequency of and history of CAD, MI, angina, CHF, or COPD, the frequency of EKG Q waves, the frequency of diabetes, the frequency of ST segment depression or angina during the dipyridamole test, or of ST segment depression or angina during a stress test did not differ significantly in patients who had or did not have a cardiac event[y] after surgery. However, the frequency of abnormal scans (47% versus 93%) and of transient defects (38% versus 93%) was significantly different. Forty-nine patients had an abnormal scan, 28.5% (14 out of 49) had a cardiac event; fifty did not, while 1 out of the 50 (0.5%) did have a cardiac event.

---

[x] Somewhat in contradiction to the number of fixed and transient defects.
[y] MI or death.

Slightly different findings have been reported in a smaller series of 48 patients (115). Cardiac events are death (2), MI (4), angina followed by CABG (2) or stabilization (2), occurring in a total of eight patients. Forty patients did not have a post-operative cardiac event. The age, proportion of males, frequency of chest pain history, previous MI, chest pain or ST depression during dipyridamole injection did not differ between both groups; nor did the number of cases with fixed defects only. But 8 out of 8 had an abnormal scan in the event group versus 20 out of 40 in the non-event group. For a reversible defect, the relative rates are 8 out of 8 and 8 out of 40. Sixteen had dipyridamole-induced transient defects in the myocardial perfusion image, and did not undergo coronary angiography or revascularization but underwent the scheduled surgery. Of those, 50% (8 out of 16) had a post-operative ischemic cardiac event. The frequency was 0 out of 32 in the absence of transient defects. Six patients with transient defects underwent coronary arteriography, and all were positive for severe multivessel disease. Four underwent CABG, later followed by uncomplicated peripheral vascular surgery.

Younis (116) compared the predictive values of dipyridamole thallium myocardial perfusion studies, two-dimensional echocardiography and Goldman classification in the case of non-vascular surgery. Pulmonary edema was included as a "cardiac" event. Pulmonary edema was well predicted by abnormal systolic function detected by echocardiography (1 out of 32 versus 7 out of 21). But myocardial infarction or cardiac death were predicted by transient or fixed perfusion defects only. The Goldman class was not predictive by itself. The combination however is interesting: In the Goldman class I, 0 out of 20 patients with a negative myocardial perfusion study have a cardiac event, 1 out of 4 with a fixed defect, 4 out of 10 with a transient defect. If the Goldman class is ≥ 2, the corresponding values are 3 out of 12, 1 out of 2 and 3 out of 5.

Brown (117) looked at diabetic and non-diabetic uremic patients scheduled for a renal transplant. There were 35 patients who underwent surgery. None had a transient defect in a dipyridamole 201Tl study, 13 had a depressed ejection fraction.

There were no peri-operative cardiac events. Longer follow-ups were available on 65 patients. Three had a transient defect and 3 out of 3 had a cardiac event during follow-up. There were six cardiac events in total with 3 out of 62 patients without a transient defect. There were 23 patients with either a transient defect, or an abnormally low resting ejection fraction. Of the 23, five had a cardiac event. Therefore, 5 out of 6 patients with a cardiac event had either a depressed ejection fraction or a transient defect. In the case of the patients with neither abnormality, the rate of cardiac events was 1 out of 42. The ejection fraction and the perfusion abnormalities are not totally independent findings: in 41 patients with a normal ejection fraction, there was only one with a fixed defect. In 23 patients with a depressed ejection fraction, three had a transient defect and four had a fixed defect.

In general, the number and the degree of abnormality reversibility carries higher risks (118–121).

The data mentioned above can be expressed as the sensitivity, specificity, positive and negative predictive value of the myocardial perfusion study, if the disease is a peri-operative cardiac event. Table 5.6 tabulates the values. In individual reports, except for the paper by Brown, the numbers are small.

Stratifying patients according to their likelihood to benefit from CABG more than from medical treatment is especially important. The CASS study (122) looked at patients with stable angina or without angina following a myocardial infarction, and found no difference between the outcome as a function of the treatment, with all baseline variables equal in both groups, including the ejection fraction (Table 5.6).

5.10. DEFINING VIABILITY

In what follows, we define viable myocardium as myocardium which has either a contractile or perfusion dysfunction that can be shown to be reversed by a vascular restoration.

Viability, therefore, stands in contradistinction to scarring: In the classic paradigm of myocardial perfusion studies, the myocardial scar is underperfused equally at rest and during exercise, and is dysfunctional (akinetic or dyskinetic). Scarred myocardium does not recover function with vascular reconstruction, nor does vascular reconstruction result in higher flow.

It seems obvious that a myocardium with only stress-induced ischemia, but normal resting flow would be viable. This presentation does not, in general, raise the question of viability. The matter is only slightly complicated by the occurrence of stunning: following an ischemic event, the myocardium may remain dysfunctional for some time (123, 124), but recovery is generally spontaneous. In the post-ischemic state when perfusion has returned to the basal state, FDG uptake is enhanced in the ischemic regions only (125) although the FDG uptake has been shown to be suppressed for 30 minutes during the hyperperfusion phase (126).

In short, a stunned myocardium is a myocardium with normal resting flow and contractile dysfunction. The uptake of FDG is increased. The myocardium is also responsive to an inotropic challenge: Kimchi (127) described asynergic segments at

Table 5.6[z]

Reference	Events	Transient #	P(D+|S+) transient	Events	Fixed #	P(D+|S+) fixed	Events	Normal #	P(D+|S+) normal	P(S+|D+) transient	P(S+|D−) transient
114	14	15	0.93	0	5	0.00	1	54	0.02	0.93	0.02
115	8	16	0.50	0	12	0.00	0	20	0.00	1.00	0.20
116	21	27	0.78	8	24	0.33	3	36	0.08	0.66	0.11
117	24	109	0.22	1	33	0.03	3	121	0.02	0.86	0.36
118	9	21	0.43	0	9	0.00	0	30	0.00	1.00	0.24
119	10	71	0.14	1	30	0.03				0.91	0.68
120	8	24	0.33	2	26	0.08				0.80	0.40

[z]Again, most publications gave predictive values, rather than operating characteristics.

rest which became functional during exercise, and were generally free of Q-waves or fixed perfusion abnormalities in thallium imaging. Others utilized post-extra systolic potentiation.

Another state leading to dysfunction is chronic (resting) hypoperfusion. The myocardium apparently goes into a survival mode which is energetically economical, and contraction decreases (hibernation). The modified metabolic state can be shown to be associated with relatively increased sugar utilization, which in turn can be demonstrated by increased or relatively increased FDG uptake.

Hibernating myocardium is, therefore, underperfused and dysfunctional, but has a normal or relatively increased FDG uptake. Takahashi (128), however, found that when the perfusion of the myocardium was less than 45%, there was no increased or relative increase of FDG uptake.

Increased carbohydrate metabolism as indicated by 18-flourodeoxyglucose, is defined by some authors as an absolute increase of FDG uptake, by some as an excess of FDG uptake in comparison to regional blood flow, defined by $^{13}NH_3$ or ^{201}Tl concentration. We have generally accepted that normal FDG concentrations, or relatively increased FDG concentrations, are indicative of the presence of life myocardial tissue (129).

The question of viability would be simple to answer if one could state that scar tissue never contains any myocardial cells, or that hibernating myocardium contains no scar. Put differently, how much myocardium must there be in a myocardial segment for a post-revascularization gain in function to be measurable or significant? The pathophysiological correlate of the meaning of viability is unclear at least in quantitative terms. We will later see that dyskinetic segments which exhibit positive inotropic responses will more likely improve following vascular reconstruction. However, Bodenheimer (130), as an example, found that asynergic myocardial segments which have a positive response to nitroglycerin generally consist of histological normal myocardium, with less than 10% muscle cell loss. A negative response occurs when the loss is larger than 10%, an amount of loss which would not easily be detected by scintigraphic imaging studies of any kind.

In what follows, we will review the data which support the following statements:

1. Normal resting flow predicts viability.

   Normal resting flow is defined as the absence of a perfusion defect following a resting injection of a flow tracer. Normal flow is not defined by redistribution in delayed studies. With normal resting flow, 83% of segments recover following surgery. The contrapositive does not hold: abnormal resting flow does not exclude viability (49% recover).

Table 5.7[aa] In this table, D+ is defined as an improvement in flow or wall motion (any means either one). Redistribution is either after a stress injection or a resting injection. Cellularity is either a positive redistribution or a positive FDG. Transient is either a normal resting flow or a normal redistribution. Under "redistribution after stress", P(S−|D+) indicates that 0.40 of those who will recover have a fixed defect after stress. P(S+|D+) means that 60% of those who recovered after revascularization had redistribution after stress. However, P(S+|D−) indicates that 29% of those who did not recover after intervention did have redistribution. P(D+|D+) indicates that of all the patients with redistribution after stress, 86% recovered after revascularization. Of those who did not have redistribution after stress (P(D−|S−)), 39% had no redistribution. In contrast, if the test was FDG uptake, without FDG uptake 81% did not recover after wall motion. The notation "ANY" means any postoperative improvement (flow or wall motion). PO RWM indicates that the post revascularization test was recovery of resting wall motion.

	Redistribution after stress (ANY)	Redistribution after rest (ANY)	Cellularity stress and FDG (ANY)	Cellularity rest and FDG (ANY)	Rest flow PO RWM	Rest flow PO flow	FDG and PO RWM	Inotropic and PO RWM	Transient PO flow	Transient PO RWM
P(D+)	0.74	0.61	0.69	0.58	0.59	0.70	0.51	0.42	0.75	0.58
P(S−|D+)	0.40	0.28	0.38	0.25	0.61	0.77	0.19	0.15	0.28	0.29
P(S+|D+)	0.60	0.72	0.62	0.75	0.39	0.23	0.81	0.85	0.72	0.71
P(S+|D−)	0.29	0.31	0.31	0.26	0.11	0.03	0.18	0.19	0.32	0.28
P(D+|S+)	0.86	0.78	0.82	0.80	0.83	0.95	0.82	0.76	0.87	0.78
P(D−|S−)	0.39	0.61	0.45	0.68	0.51	0.35	0.81	0.81	0.45	0.65
LR	2.10	2.32	1.99	2.84	3.48	8.32	4.38	4.46	2.24	2.54
N(segments)	1029	556	1441	830	685	484	372	677	685	484

[aa]For Table 5.7, the references are 34, 35, 79, 131–152.

2. The presence of a near normal myocardial mass or normal cellularity predicts viability.

   a. The presence of a near normal myocardial mass can be predicted by re-distribution images following either a stress or resting injection of 201Tl. This prediction however is made more precise in the presence of normal resting wall motion. If there is redistribution after a stress injection, 86% of segments recover flow or normal wall motion. In the case of stress redistribution, the contra-positive does not hold: lack of redistribution does not necessarily exclude viability (61% recover).

   b. The presence of a near normal myocardial mass or cellularity can be predicted by demonstrating glucose metabolism (positive FDG), either at a normal level, increased level, or a level increased compared to the resting flow. A positive FDG study predicts surgical success in 82% of the cases. Absence of FDG activity predicts recovery in only 19% of the cases.

   c. The presence of a near normal myocardial mass can be predicted by demonstrating normal resting wall motion. Success prediction is 85%.

3. The presence of a positive inotropic response is highly predictive of viability for 76% of the cases and the absence of a positive inotropic response failure in 81% of the cases (Table 5.7).

If the criterion for success is a normalization of flow, and the metric is a fixed or transient defect on the stress and redistribution scan, flow improves in 31 of the cases of fixed defects and 85% of the transient defects.

The association between the findings in 201Tl studies with a stress injection and early and late imaging with other findings is variable. Ohtani (144) found that only 17 out of 75 fixed defects in redistribution studies were fixed with a reinjection and that 10 out of 41 partial redistribution were totally reversible with a re-injection. The discrepancy in the case of normal perfusion or transient abnormalities could be explained by stunning (for wall motion), and by the better resolution of PET studies. The study by Naruse (33) is interesting: He compared the ability of different thallium abnormalities to predict viability, or lack of viability. Segments which had a normal stress thallium concentration were almost always viable, but a stress abnormality does not predict lack of viability, nor does a fixed lesion, based on a stress and redistribution study, or a stress and re-injection study. Even fixed abnormalities in a rest and redistribution study are not very predictive of lack of viability in his series. But the severity of the abnormality was more predictive. There were 6 out of 17 (0.35) viable segments with "severe" fixed defects.

It is true that in the dog model with occlusion (followed by a 201Tl injection) and reperfusion (followed by delayed imaging), transient defects are associated with viability and normal (rather than decreased) FDG uptake (153).

Following myocardial infarction and coronary thrombolysis, Franken (154) found that resting wall motion was normal in all 72 cases where resting flow (with MIBI) and fatty acid uptake (BMIPP)[bb] were normal. If the fatty acid uptake was more depressed, 23 out of 29 had abnormal resting wall motion but 15 out of 23 had a positive inotropic response. If both flow and BMIPP uptake were low, 9 out of 9 had resting wall motion abnormalities, and 0 out of 9 had a positive inotropic response. This suggests that a selective depression of BMIPP uptake in the presence of resting dysfunction represents stunned myocardium. In a related paper, a suggestion is made that selective depression of BMIPP is due to delayed recovery (stunning) and that a selective increase in the uptake of the fatty acid is due to the enhanced metabolism induced by passive systolic wall stretch (155).

5.11. INCIDENTAL FINDINGS

Visualization of the right ventricle is not common and has been associated with pulmonary hypertension (156). Cohen (157) studied four groups of patients:

1. eight normals,
2. five patients with angiographically documented coronary artery disease and normal pulmonary artery pressures,
3. ten patients with documented pulmonary hypertension, and
4. eight patients with chronic left ventricular dysfunction and pulmonary hypertension.

The right ventricular free wall was visualized on the thallium-201 myocardial perfusion image in 1 out of 8 normal subjects (group 1) and in only 1 out of 5 patients with coronary artery disease (group 2); the measured wall thickness were 0.5 cm and 0.9 cm respectively. In patients with documented pulmonary hypertension, the right ventricle was visualized on low contrast thallium-201 myocardial perfusion image (18 out of 18). The apparent right ventricular free wall thickness measured from the ungated thallium-201 myocardial perfusion images was 1.7 ± 0.3 cm in group 3 and 1.5 ± 0.2 cm in group 4. Right ventricular hypertrophy was detected by electrocardiography in only 5 of 10 patients in group 3 and only 1 of 8 patients in group 4.

[bb] 123I-beta-methyl-iodophenyl-pentadecanoic acid.

Khaja (158) studied 53 patients. In 33 patients, the right ventricle was visualized clearly (group A). Hemodynamic evidence of right ventricular hypertension with systolic pressure greater than or equal to 30 mmHg was present in 28 out of 33 (85%) of these patients. Other tests were diagnostic for right ventricular enlargement and or pulmonary hypertension as follows: chest X-ray (58%), echocardiogram (36%) and electrocardiogram (15%). In an unselected group of 20 patients (group B) where there was no visualization of the right ventricle, the right ventricular systolic pressure was less than 30 mmHg in all.

Rabinovitch (159) studied patients before and after corrective surgery for cardiac congenital heart defects. A total of 24 patients ranging in age from 7 months to 30 years was studied; 18 were studied before corrective surgery and six after operation. Insignificant right ventricular thallium-201 counts judged as being less than 1% of the injected dose or less than 0.3 of the left ventricular counts were present in six patients all with right ventricular peak systolic pressure less than 30 mmHg. In the remaining 18 patients, there was a good correlation between the right ventricular/left ventricular peak systolic pressure ratio and the right ventricular/left ventricular thallium-201 counts ratio. All patients with right ventricular/left ventricular peak systolic pressure less than 0.5 had right ventricular/left ventricular thallium-201 counts less than 0.4.

REFERENCES

1. Sapirstein LA. Regional blood flow by fractional distribution of indicators. *Am J Physiol* 1958; 193:161–168.
2. Zaret BL, Stenson RW, Martin ND, Strauss HW, Wells HP Jr, McGowan RL, Flamm MD Jr. Potassium 43 myocardial perfusion scanning for the noninvasive evaluation of patients with false positive exercise tests. *Circulation* 1973; 48:1234–1241.
3. Zaret BL, Strauss HW, Martin ND, Wells HP Jr, Flamm MD Jr. Noninvasive myocardial perfusion with radioactive potassium: study of patients at rest, exercise, and during angina pectoris. *N Eng J Med* 1973; 288:809–812.
4. Berman DS, Salel AF, Denardo GL, Mason DT. Noninvasive detection of regional myocardial ischemia using rubidium-81 and the scintillation camera. *Circulation* 1975; 52:619–626.
5. Schelbert HR, Phelps ME, Huang SC, *et al.* N-13 ammonia as an indicator of myocardial blood flow. *Circulation* 1981; 63:1259–1272.
6. Schelbert HR, Phelps ME, Hoffman EJ, *et al.* Regional myocardial perfusion assessed with N-13 labeled ammonia and positron emission computerized axial tomography. *Am J Cardiol* 1979; 43:209–218.
7. Zhao XM, Delbeke D, Sandler MP, Yeoh TK, Votaw JR, Frist WH. Nitrogen-13-ammonia and PET to detect allograft coronary artery disease after heart transplantation: comparison with coronary angiography. *J Nucl Med* 1995; 36:982–987.

8. Okada RD, Glover DK, Nguyen KN, Johnson III G. Technetium-99m Sestamibi kinetics in reperfused canine myocardium. *Eur J Nucl Med* 1995; 22:600–607.

9. Rigo P, Leclerq B, Itti R, Lahiri R, Braat S. Technetium-99m-Tetrofosmin myocardial imaging: a comparison with Thallium-201 and Angiography. *J Nucl Med* 1994; 35:587–593.

10. Tamaki N, Takahashi N, Kawamoto M, Torizuka T, Tadamura E, Yonekura Y, Okuda K, Nohara R, Sasayama S, Konishi J. Myocardial tomography using Technetium-99m-Tetrofosmin to evaluate coronary artery disease. *J Nucl Med* 1994; 35:594–600.

11. Mahmood S, Gunning M, Bomanji JB, Gupta NK, Costa DC, Jarritt PH, Swanton H, Ell PJ. Combined rest thallium-201/stress technetium-99m-tetrofosmin SPECT: feasibility and diagnostic accuracy of a 90-minute protocol. *J Nucl Med* 1995; 36:932–935.

12. Sinusas AJ, Shi Q-X, Saltzberg MT, Vitols P, Jain D, Wackers FJ, Zaret BL. Technetium-99m-Tetrofosmin to assess myocardial blood flow: experimental validation in an intact canine model of ischemia. *J Nucl Med* 1994; 35:664–671.

13. Seldin DW, Johnson LL, Blood DK, Muschel MJ, Smith KF, Wall RM, Cannon PJ. Myocardial perfusion imaging with [99m]technetium-SQ30217: comparison with thallium-201 and coronary anatomy. *J Nucl Med* 1989; 30:312–319.

14. Leppo JA, Meerdink DJ. Comparative myocardial extraction of two technetium-labeled BATO derivatives (SQ30217, SQ32014) and thallium. *J Nucl Med* 1990; 31:67–74.

15. Hendel RC, McSherry B, Karimeddini M, Leppo J. Diagnostic value of a new myocardial perfusion agent, teboroxime (SQ 30, 217), utilizing a rapid planar imaging protocol: preliminary results. *J Am Coll Cardiol* 1990; 16:855–861.

16. Gray WA, Gewitz H. Comparison of ^{99m}Tc-teboroxime with Thallium for myocardial imaging in the presence of a coronary artery stenosis. *Circulation* 1991; 84:1796–1808.

17. Johnson LL. Myocardial perfusion imaging with [99m]Technetium-Teboroxime. *J Nucl Med* 1994; 35:689–692.

18. Nakajima K, Taki J, Bunko H, Matsudaira M. Dynamic acquisition with a three-headed SPECT system: application to [99m]Technetium-SQ30217 myocardial imaging. *J Nucl Med* 1991; 32:1273–1277.

19. Henzlova MJ, Machcac J. Clinical Utility of [99m]Technetium-Teboroxime myocardial washout imaging. *J Nucl Med* 1994; 35:575–579.

20. Blumhardt R, Heyl B, Miller DD, O'Rourke RA. Demonstration of differential poststenotic myocardial [99m]Technetium-teboroxime clearance kinetics after experimental ischemia and hyperemic stress. *J Nucl Med* 1991; 32:2000–2008.

21. Phelps ME, Hoffman EJ, Selin SC, Huang SC, Robinson G, MacDonald N, Schelbert H, Kuhl DE. Investigation of [^{18}F]-2-fluoro 2 deoxyglucose for the measure of myocardial glucose metabolism. *J Nucl Med* 1978; 19:1311–1319.

22. Gropler RJ, Siegel BA, Lee KJ, Moerlein SM, Perry DJ, Bergmann SR, Geltman EM. Nonuniformity in myocardial accumulation of Fluorine-18-fluorodeoxyglucose in normal fasted humans. *J Nucl Med* 1990; 31:1749–1756.

23. Huitink JM, Visser FC, van Lingen A, Groeneveld AB, Bax JJ, van Leeuwen GR, Visser GM, Van Loon MJ, Teule GJ. Visser CA9/2/2010 Feasibility of planar fluorine-18-FDG imaging after recent myocardial infarction to assess myocardial viability. *J Nucl Med* 1995; 36:975–981.

24. Kalff V, Berlangieri SU, Van Every B, Rowe JL, Lambrecht RM, Tochon-Danguy HJ, Egan GF, McKay WJ, Kelly MJ. Is planar thallium-201/fluorine-18 fluorodeoxyglucose imaging a reasonable clinical alternative to positron emission tomographic myocardial viability scanning? *Eur J Nucl Med* 1995; 22:625–632.

25. Martin WH, Delbeke D, Patton JA, Hendrix B, Weinfeld Z, Ohana I, Kessler RM, Sandler MP. FDG-SPECT: correlation with FDG-PET. *J Nucl Med* 1995; 36:988–995.

26. Ebert A, Herzog H, Stoclin GL, Henrich MM, DeGrado TR, Coenen HH, Feinendegen LE. Kinetics of 14(R,S)-Fluorine-18-Fluoro-6- Thia-Heptadecanoic Acid in normal human hearts at rest, during exercise and after Dipyridamole injection. *J Nucl Med* 1994; 35:51–56.

27. Taki J, Nakajima K, Bunko H, Kawasuji M, Tonami N, Hisada K. Twenty-four-hour quantitative Thallium imaging for predicting beneficial revascularization. *Eur J Nucl Med* 1994; 21:1212–1217.

28. Narula J, Khaw BA, Dec GW, Palacios IF, Newell JB, Southern JF, Fallon JT, Strauss HW, Haber E, Yasuda T. Diagnostic accuracy of antimyosin scintigraphy in suspected myocarditis. *J Nucl Cardiol* 1996; 3:371–381.

29. Folke M, Hesse B, Mortensen SA. Pulmonary uptake in Indium-111- antimyosine Fab fragment imaging following human cardiac transplantation. *J Nucl Med* 1994; 35:266–268.

30. Pohost GM, Alpert NM, Ingwall JS, Strauss HW. Thallium redistribution mechanisms and clinical Utility. *Semin Nucl Med* 1980; 10:70–93.

31. Yang LD, Berman DS, Kiat H, Resser KJ, Friedman JD, Rozanski A, Maddahi J. The frequency of late reversibility in SPECT Thallium-201 stress-redistribution studies. *J Am Coll Cardiol* 1990; 15:334–340.

32. Nelson CW, Wilson RA, Angello DA, Palac RT. Effect of thallium-201 blood levels on reversible myocardial defects. *J Nucl Med* 1989; 30:1172–1175.

33. Naruse H, Kondo T, Arii T, Morita M, Ohyanagi M, Iwasaki T, Fukuchi M. Comparative accuracy of various Tl-201 reinjection protocols to detect myocardial viability. *Ann Nucl Med* 1996; 10:119–126.

34. Iskandrian AS, Hakki A, Kane SA, Goel I, Mundth ED, Hakki A-H, Segal BL. Rest and redistribution thallium-201 myocardial scintigraphy to predict improvement in left ventricular function after coronary arterial bypass grafting. *Am J Cardiol* 1993; 51:1312–1316.

35. Bonow RO, Dilsizian V, Cuocolo A, Bacharach SL. Identification of viable myocardium in patients with chronic coronary artery disease and left ventricular dysfunction. Comparison of thallium scintigraphy with reinjection and PET imaging with 18F-fluorodeoxyglucose. *Circulation* 1991; 83:26–37.

36. Gill JB, Ruddy TD, Newell JB, Finkelstein DM, Strauss HW, Boucher CA. Prognostic importance of thallium uptake by the lungs during exercise in coronary artery disease. *N Engl J Med* 1987; 317:1485–1489.

37. Brown KA, Rowen M. Prognostic value of a normal exercise myocardial perfusion imaging study in patients with angiographically significant coronary artery disease. *Am J Cardiol* 1993; 71:865–867.

38. Maddahi J, Berman DS. Reverse redistribution of thallium-201. *J Nucl Med* 1995; 36:1019–1021.

39. Pohost FM, Zir LM, Moore RH, McKusick KA, Guiney TE, Beller GA. Differentiation of transiently ischemic from infarcted myocardium by serial imaging after a single dose of thallium-201. *Circulation* 1977; 55:294–302.
40. Braat SH, Leclercq B, Itti R, Lahiri A, Sridhara B, Rigo P. Myocardial imaging with Technetium-99m-Tetrofosmin: comparison of one-day and two-day protocols. *J Nucl Med* 1994; 35:1581–1585.
41. Van Train KF, Garcia EV, Maddahi J, Areeda J, Cooke CD, Kiat H, Silagan G, Folks R, Friedman J, Matzer L, Germano G, Bateman T, Ziffer J, DePuey EG, Fink-Bennett D, Cloninger K, Berman DS. Multicenter trial validation for qualitative analysis of same-day rest-stress Technetium-99m-Sestamibi myocardial tomograms. *J Nucl Med* 1994; 35:609–618.
42. Heo J, Wolmer I, Kegel J, Iskandrian AS. Sequential dual-isotope SPECT imaging with Thallium-201 and Technetium-99m-Sestamibi. *J Nucl Med* 1994; 35:549–553.
43. Weinmann P, Foult J-M, Le Guludec D, Tamgac F, Rechtman D, Neuman A, Caillat-Vigneron N, Moretti JL. Dual-isotope myocardial imaging: feasibility, advantages and limitations (preliminary report on 231 consecutive patients). *Eur J Nucl Med* 1994; 21:212–215.
44. Berman DS, Kiat H, Van Train K, Friedman JD, Wang FP, Germano G, Berman DS, Kiat H, Van Train K, Friedman JD, Wang FP, Germano G. Dual-isotope myocardial perfusion SPECT with rest thallium-201 and stress Tc-99m sestamibi. *Cardiol Clin* 1994; 12:261–270.
45. Kiat H, Germano G, Friedman J, Van Train K, Silagan G, Wang FP, Maddahi J, Berman D. Comparative feasibility of separate or simultaneous rest Thallium 201 stress Technetium-99m-Sestamibi dual-isotope myocardial perfusion SPECT. *J Nucl Med* 1994; 35:542–548.
46. Segall GM, Davis MJ, Goris ML. Improved specificity of prone versus supine thallium SPECT imaging. *Clin Nucl Med* 1988; 13:915–916.
47. Dakik HA, Vemphaty H, Verani MS. Tolerance, hemodynamic changes, and safety of dobutamine stress perfusion imaging. *J Nucl Cardiol* 1996; 3:410–414.
48. Mertes H, Sawada SG, Ryan T, Segar DS, Kovacs R, Foltz J, Feigenbaum H. Symptoms, adverse effects, and complications associated with dobutamine stress echocardiography. Experience in 1118 patients. *Circulation* 1993; 88:15–19.
49. Goris ML, Daspit SG, McLaughlin P, Kriss JP. Interpolative background subtraction. *J Nucl Med* 1976; 17:744–747.
50. Koster K, Wackers FJ, Mattera JA, Fetterman RC. Quantitative analysis of planar technetium-99m-sestamibi myocardial perfusion images using modified background subtraction. *J Nucl Med* 1990; 31:1400–1408.
51. Burow RD, Pond M, Schafer AW, Becker L. "Circumferential Profiles:" A New Method for Computer Analysis of Thallium-201 Myocardial Perfusion Images. *J Nucl Med* 1979; 20:771–777.
52. Vogel RA, Kirch DL, LeFree MT, Rainwater JO, Jensen DP, Steele PP. Thallium-201 myocardial perfusion scintigraphy: results of standard and multi-pinhole tomographic techniques. *Am J Cardiol* 1979; 43:787–793.
53. Garcia E, Maddahi J, Berman D, Waxman A. Space/Time quantitation of thallium-201 myocardial scintigraphy. *J Nucl Med* 1981; 22:309–317.

54. Goris ML, Boudier S, Briandet PA. Two-dimensional mapping of three dimensional SPECT data: a preliminary step to the quantitation of thallium myocardial perfusion single photon emission tomography. *Am J Physiol Imaging* 1987; 2:176–180.

55. Caldwell JH, Williams DL, Harp GD, Stratton JR, Ritchie JL. Quantitation of size of relative myocardial perfusion defect by single-photon emission computed tomography. *Circulation* 1984; 70:1048–1056.

56. Declerck J, Feldmar J, Goris ML, Betting F. Automatic registration and alignment on a template of cardiac stress and rest SPECT reoriented SPECT images. *IEEE Trans Med Imaging* 1997; 16:727–737.

57. Goris ML, Hotz B, Thirion J-P, Similon P. Factors affecting and computation of myocardial perfusion reference images. *Nucl Med Commun* 1999; 20:627–635.

58. Goris ML, Maladain G, Marque I. Automatic registration of myocardial perfusion studies using a potential based rigid transformation. 2nd International conference of Nuclear Cardiology April 1995, Cannes, France. *J Nucl Cardiol* 1995; 2:S81.

59. Goris ML, Pace WM, Maclean M, Yee A, Kwan A. Three dimensional quantitative analysis of scintigraphic tomographic images after elastic transformation to a template. *Surg Technol Int IX* (2000).

60. Bailey IK, Lawrence SC, Griffith SC, Rouleau J, Strauss HW, Pitt B. Thallium-201 myocardial perfusion imaging at rest and during exercise. Comparative sensitivity to electrocardiography in coronary artery disease. *Circulation* 1977; 55:72–87.

61. Maddahi J, Garcia EV, Berman DS, Waxman A, Swan HJ, Forrester J. Improved noninvasive assessment of coronary artery disease by quantitative analysis of regional stress myocardial distribution and washout of thallium-201. *Circulation* 1981; 65:924–955.

62. Nishiyama H, Adolf RJ, Gabel M, Lukes SJ, Franklin D, Williams CC. Effect of coronary blood flow on thallium-201 uptake and washout. *Circulation* 1982; 65:534–542.

63. Van Train K, Garcia E, Maddahi J, Brown D, Waxman A, Areeda J, Berman D. Improved quantitation of stress/redistribution TL-201 scintigrams and evaluation of normal limits. *IEEE Comput Cardiol* 1982; 311–314.

64. Nieneyer MG, Cramer MJ, van der Wall EE, Verzijlbergen JF, Zwinderman AH, Go LT, Ascoop CAPL, Pauwels EKJ. Value of visual and quantitative analysis of thallium-201 imaging in patients with diagnostic and non-diagnostic exercise electrocardiogram. *Am J Noninvasive Cardiol* 1991; 5:80–87.

65. Van Train KF, Berman DS, Garcia EV, Berger HJ, Sands MJ, Friedman JD, Freeman MR, Pryzlak M, Ashburn WL, Norris SL, Green AM, Maddahi J. Quantitative analysis of stress thallium-201 myocardial scintigrams: a multicenter trial. *J Nucl Med* 1986; 27:17–25.

66. Garcia E, Van Train K, Maddahi J, Prigent F, Friedman J, Areeda J, Waxman A, Berman D. Quantification of rotational thallium-201 myocardial tomography. *J Nucl Med* 1985; 26:17–26.

67. DePasquale EE, Nody AC, DePuey EG, Garcia EV, Pilcher G, Bredlau C, Roubin G, Gober A, Gruentzig A, D'Amato P, Berger HJ. Quantitative rotational thallium-201 tomography for identifying and localizing coronary artery disease. *Circulation* 1988; 77:316–327.

68. Dilsizian V, Freedman SL, Bacharach SL, Perrone-Filardi P, Bonow RO. Regional thallium uptake in irreversible defects. Magnitude of change in thallium activity

after reinjection distinguishes viable from nonviable myocardium. *Circulation* 1992; 85:627–634.

69. Dilsizian V, Perroni-Filardi P, Arrighi JA, Bacharach SL, Quyyumi AA, Freedman NM, Bonow RO. Concordance and discordance between stress-redistribution-reinjection and rest-redistribution thallium imaging for assessing viable myocardium. Comparison with metabolic activity by positron emission tomography. *Circulation* 1993; 88:941–952.

70. Stratman HG, Younis LT, Wittry MD, Amato M, Mark AL, Miller DD. Effects of the stress level achieved during symptom-limited exercise technetium-99m sestamibi tomography on the detection of coronary artery disease. *Clin Cardiol* 1996; 19:787–792.

71. Van Train KF, Maddahi J, Berman DS, Kiat H, Areeda J, Prigent F, Friedman J. Quantitative analysis of tomographic stress thallium-201 myocardial scintigrams: a multicenter trial. *J Nucl Med* 1990; 31:1168–1179.

72. Rozanski A, Diamond GA, Berman D, Forrester JS, Morris D, Swan HJ. The declining specificity of exercise radionuclide ventriculography. *N Engl J Med* 1983; 309:518–522.

73. Diamond GA, Rozanski A, Forrester JS, Morris D, Pollock BH, Staniloff HM, Berman DS, Swan HJ. A model for assessing the sensitivity and specificity of tests subject to selection bias. Application to exercise radionuclide ventriculography for diagnosis of coronary artery disease. *J Chron Dis* 1986; 39:343–355.

74. Levine MG, Ahlberg AW, Mann A, White MP, McGill CC, Mendes de Leon CS, Piriz JM, Waters D, Heller GV. Comparison of exercise, diyridamole, adenosine, and dobutamine stress with the use of TC-99m tetrofosmin tomographic imaging. *J Nucl Med* 1999; 6:389–396.

75. Ahmad M, Dubiel JP, Haibach H. Cold pressor thallium-201 myocardial scintigraphy in the diagnosis of coronary artery disease. *Am J Cardiol* 1982; 50:1253–1257.

76. Botvinick EH, Taradash MR, Shames DM, Parmley WW. Thallium-201 perfusion scintigraphy for the clinical clarification of normal, abnormal and equivocal electrocardiographic stress test. *Am J Cardiol* 1978; 41:43–51.

77. Caldwell JH, Hamilton GW, Sorensen SG, Ritchie JL, Williams DL, Kennedy JW. The detection of coronary artery disease with radionuclide techniques: a comparison of rest-exercise thallium imaging and ejection fraction response. *Circulation* 1980; 61:610–619.

78. Caralis DG, Bailey IB, Kennedy HL, Pitt B. Thallium-201 myocardial imaging in evaluation of asymptomatic individuals with ischemic ST segment depression on exercise electrocardiogram. *Br Heart J* 1972; 42:562–567.

79. Carrel T, Jenni R, Haubolt-Reuter S, von Schulthess, Pasic M, Turina M. Improvement of severely reduced left ventricular function after surgical revascularization in patients with preoperative myocardial infarction. *Eur J Cardiothorac Surg* 1992; 6:479–484.

80. Elhendy A, Sozzi FB, Donburg RT, Bax JJ, Geleijnse ML, Valkema R, Krenning EP, Roeland J. Accuracy of exercise stress technetium 99m sestamibi SPECT imaging in the evaluation of the extent and location of coronary artery disease in patients with an earlier myocardial infarction. *J Nucl Cardiol* 2000; 7:432–438.

81. Liu X-J, Wang X-B, Gao R-L, Lu P, Wang Y-Q. Clinical evaluation of 99mTc-MIBI SPECT in the assessment of coronary artery disease. *Nucl Med Comm* 1992; 13:776–779.

82. Sciammarella MG, Fragasso G, Gerundini P, Maffioli L, Cappelletti A, Margonato A, Savi A, Chierchia S. 99mTc-MIBI single photon emission tomography (SPET) for detecting myocardial ischemia and necrosis in patients with significant coronary artery disease. *Nucl Med Commun* 1992; 13:871–878.

83. McKillop JH, Goris ML. Thallium-201 myocardial imaging in patients with previous cardiac transplantation. *Clin Radiol* 1981; 32:447–449.

84. Folmer SC, Wieling W, Dunning AJ. Myocardial perfusion imaging with thallium-201 to assess left ventricular hypertrophy and regional ischemia in hypertensive patients. *Eur J Clin Invest* 1981; 11:291–297.

85. Dunn RF, Uren RF, Sadick N, Bautovich G, McLaughlin A, Hiroe M, Kelly DT. Comparison of thallium-201 scanning in idiopathic dilated cardiomyopathy and severe coronary artery disease. *Circulation* 1982; 66:804–810.

86. Tighe DA, Hutchinson HG, Park CH, Chung EK, Fishman DL, Raichlen JS. False positive reversible defect during Dobutamine-Thallium imaging in left bundle branch block. *J Nucl Med* 1994; 35:1989–1991.

87. Leppo JA. Dipyridamole-thallium imaging: the lazy man's stress test. *J Nucl Med* 1989; 30:281–287.

88. Gupta N, Esterbrooks DJ, Hilleman DE, Mohiuddin SM. Comparison of adenosine and exercise Thallium-201 single photon emission computed tomography (SPECT) myocardial perfusion imaging. *J Am Coll Cardiol* 1992; 19:248–257.

89. Hays JT, Mahmarian JJ, Cochran AJ, Verani MS. Dobutamine-Thallium-201 tomography for evaluating patients with suspected coronary artery disease unable to undergo exercise or vasodilator pharmacological stress testing. *J Am Coll Cardiol* 1993; 21:1583–1590.

90. Cuocolo A, Soricelli A, Pace L, Nicolai E, Castelli L, Nappi A, Imbriaco M, Morisco C, Ell PJ, Salvatore M. Adenosine Technetium-99m-Methoxy Isobutyl Isonitrile myocardial tomography in patients with coronary artery disease: comparison with exercise. *J Nucl Med* 1994; 35:1110–1115.

91. Lalonde D, Taillefer R, Lambert R, Bisson F, Pietro I, Benjamin C. Thallium-201-Dipyridamole imaging: comparison between a standard dose and a high dose of Dipyridamole in the detection of coronary artery disease. *J Nucl Med* 1994; 35:1245–1253.

92. McKillop JH, Fawcett HD, Baumert JE, McDougall IR, DeBusk RF, Harrison DC, Goris ML. ECG gating of Thallium-201 myocardial images: effect on detection of ischemic heart disease. *J Nucl Med* 1981; 22:219–225.

93. Takeda T, Toyoma H, Ishikawa N, Satoh M, Masuoka T, Ajisaka R, Iida K, Wu J, Sugishita Y, Itai Y. Quantitative phase analysis of myocardial wall thickening by technetium-99m 2-methoxy-isobutyl-isonitrile SPECT. *Ann Nucl Med* 1992; 6:69–78.

94. Mochizuki T, Murase K, Fujirawa Y, Tanada S, Hamamoto K, Tauxe WN. Assessment of systolic thickening with thallium-201 ECG-gated single photon emission computed tomography: a parameter for focal left ventricular function. *J Nucl Med* 1991; 32:1496–1500.

95. Najm YC, Timmis AD, Maisey MN, Ellam SV, Mistry R, Curry PV, Sowton E. The evaluation of ventricular function using gated myocardial imaging with 99mTc sestamibi. *Eur Heart J* 1989; 10:142–148.

96. Marcassa C, Marzullo P, Parodi O, Sambuceti G, L'Abbate A. A new method for noninvasive quantitation of segmental myocardial wall thickening using technetium-99m 2-methoxy-isobutyl-isonitrile scintigraphy — results in normal subjects. *J Nucl Med* 1990; 31:173–177.

97. Goris ML, Thompson CJ, Malone LJ, Franken PR. Modeling the integration of myocardial perfusion and function. *Nucl Med Commun* 1994; 15:9–20.

98. Goris ML, Van Uitert RL. An integral method for the analysis of wall motion in gated myocardial SPECT studies. *Proceedings of the XVIth Conference on Information Processing in Medical Imaging. Lecture Notes in Computer Sciences.* Springer–Verlag 1999; pp. 334–339.

99. Goris ML, Boudier S, Briandet PA. Interrogation and display of single photon emission tomography data as inherently volume data. *Am J Physiol Imaging* 1986; 1:168–180.

100. Graf G, Mester J, Clausen M, Henze E, Bitter F, Heidenreich P, Adam WE. Reconstruction of Fourier coefficients: a fast method to get polar amplitude and phase images of gated SPECT. *J Nucl Med* 1990; 31:1856–1861.

101. Camargo EE, Hironaka FH, Giorgi MC, Soares Junior J, Meneguetti JC, Abe R, Robilotta CC, Munhoz AC, Checchi H, Ramirez JA. Amplitude analysis of stress technetium-99m methoxy isobutylisonitrile images in coronary artery disease. *Eur J Nucl Med* 1992; 19:484–491.

102. Mate E, Mester J, Csernay L, Kuba A, Madani S, Makay A. Three-dimensional presentation of the Fourier amplitude and phase: a fast display method for gated cardiac blood-pool SPECT. *J Nucl Med* 1992; 33:458–462.

103. DePuey EG, Rozanski A. Using gated technetium-99m-seatamibi SPECT to characterize fixed myocardial defects as infarct or artifact. *J Nucl Med* 1995; 36:952–955.

104. Brown KA. Prognostic value of thallium-201 myocardial perfusion imaging. *Circulation* 1991; 83:363–381.

105. Brown KA. The role of stress redistribution thallium-201 myocardial perfusion imaging in evaluating coronary artery disease and perioperative risk. *J Nucl Med* 1994; 35:703–707.

106. Brown KA. Prognostic value of thallium-201 myocardial perfusion imaging in patients with unstable angina who responded to medical treatment. *J Am Coll Cardiol* 1991; 17:1053–1057.

107. Brown KA, Boucher CA, Okada RD, Guiney TE, Newell JB, Strauss HW, Pohost GM. Prognostic value of exercise thallium-201 imaging in patients presenting for evaluation of chest pain. *J Am Coll Cardiol* 1983; 1:994–1001.

108. Hendel RC, Layden JJ, Leppo JA. Prognostic value of dipyridamole-thallium scintigraphy for evaluation of ischemic heart disease. *J Am Coll Cardiol* 1990; 15:109–116.

109. Brown KA, Atland E, Rowen M. Prognostic value of normal technetium-99m-sestamibi cardiac imaging. *J Nucl Med* 1994; 35:554–557.

110. Staniloff HM, Forrester JS, Berman DS, Swan HJC. Prediction of death, myocardial infarction, and worsening chest pain using thallium scintigraphy and exercise electrocardiography. *J Nucl Med* 1986; 27:1842–1848.

111. Assey ME. Prognosis in stable angina pectoris and silent myocardial ischemia. *Am J Cardiol* 1988; 61:19F–21F.

112. Galvin JM, Brown KA. The site of acute myocardial infarction is related to the coronary territory of transient defects on prior myocardial perfusion imaging. *J Nucl Cardiol* 1996; 3:382–388.

113. Dilsizian V, Bonow RO, Epstein SE, Fananapazir L. Myocardial ischemia detected by thallium scintigraphy is frequently related to cardiac arrest and syncope in young patients with hypertrophic cardiomyopathy. *J Am Coll Cardiol* 1993; 22:796–804.

114. Leppo J, Plaja J, Gionet M, Tumolo J, Paraskos JA, Cutler BS. Noninvasive evaluation of cardiac risk before elective vascular surgery. *J Am Coll Cardiol* 1987; 9:269–276.

115. Boucher CA, Brewster DC, Darling RC, Okada RD, Strauss HW, Pohost GM. Determination of cardiac risk by dipyridamole-Thallium Imaging before Peripheral vascular Surgery. *N Engl J Med* 1985; 312:389–394.

116. Younis LT, Byers S, Shaw L, Barth G, Goodgold H, Chaitman BR. Prognostic importance of silent myocardial ischemia detected by intravenous dipyridamole thallium myocardial imagine gin asymptomatic patients with coronary artery disease. *J Am Coll Cardiol* 1989; 14:1635–1641.

117. Brown KA, Rowen M. Extent of jeopardized viable myocardium determined by myocardial perfusion imaging best predicts perioperative cardiac events in patients undergoing non-cardiac surgery. *J Am Coll Cardiol* 1993; 21:325–330.

118. Lette J, Waters, D, Lapoint J, Gagnon A, Picard M, Cerino M, Kerouac M. Usefulness of the severity and extent of reversible perfusion defects during thallium-dipyridamole imaging for cardiac risk assessment before noncardiac surgery. *Am J Cardiol* 1989; 64:276–281.

119. Lane SE, Lewis SM, Pippin JJ, Kosinski EJ, Campbell D, Nesto RW, Hill T. Predictive value of quantitative dipyridamole-thallium scintigraphy in assessing cardiovascular risk after vascular surgery in diabetes mellitus. *Am J Cardiol* 1989; 64:1275–1279.

120. Eagle KA, Singer DE, Brewster DC, Darling RC, Mulley AG, Boucher CA. Dipyridamole-Thallium Scanning in Patients Undergoing Vascular Surgery. *J Am Med Assoc* 1987; 257:2185–2189.

121. Ladenheim ML, Pollock BH, Rozanski A, Berman DS, Staniloff HM, Forrester JS, Diamond GA. Extent and severity of myocardial hypoperfusion a predictors of prognosis in patients with suspected coronary artery disease. *J Am Coll Cardiol* 1986; 7:464–471.

122. CASS Principal Investigators and Associates. Myocardial infarction and mortality in the coronary artery surgery study (CASS) randomized trial. *N Engl J Med* 1984; 310:750–758.

123. Braunwald E, Kloner RA. The stunned myocardium: prolonged postischemic ventricular dysfunction. Late reversibility of tomographic myocardial thallium- 201 defects: an accurate marker of myocardial viability. *J Am Coll Cardiol* 1988; 12:1456–1463.

124. Ellis SG, Henschke CI, Sandor T, Wynne J, Braunwald E, Kloner RA. Time course of functional and biochemical recovery of myocardium salvaged by reperfusion. *J Am Coll Cardiol* 1983; 1:1047–1055.

125. Camici P, Araujo LI, Spinks T, Lammertsma AA, Kaski JC, Shea MJ, Selwyn AP, Jones T, Maseri A. Increased Uptake of 18F-Fluorodeoxyglucose in Postischemic Myocardium of Patients with Exercise-Induced Angina. *Circulation* 1986; 74:81–88.

126. Ratib O, Phelps ME, Huang S-C, Henze E, Selin CE, Schelbert HR. Positron tomography with deoxyglucose for estimating local myocardial glucose metabolism. *J Nucl Med* 1982; 23:577–586.

127. Kimchi A, Rozanski A, Fletcher C, Maddahi J, Swan HJ, Berman DS. Reversal of rest myocardial asynergy during exercise: a radionuclide scintigraphic study. *J Am Coll Cardiol* 1985; 6:1004–1010.

128. Takahashi N, Tamaki N, Kawamoto M, *et al*. Glucose metabolism in relation to perfusion in patients with ischemic heart disease. *Eur J Nucl Med* 1994; 21:292–296.

129. Marshall RC, Tillisch JH, Phelps ME, *et al*. Identification and differentiation of resting myocardial ischemia and infarction in man with positron computer tomography? 180E-labeled fluorodeoxyglucose and N-13-ammonia. *Circulation* 1983; 67:766–778.

130. Bodenheimer MM, Banka VS, Hermann GA, Trout R. Reversible asynergy: histopathologic and electrographic correlations in patients with coronary artery disease. *Circulation* 1976; 53:792–796.

131. Akins CW, Pohost GM, Desanctis R, Block PC. Selection of angina-free patients with severe left ventricular dysfunction for myocardial revascularization. *Am J Cardiol* 1980; 46:695–700.

132. Altehoefer C, vom Dahl J, Biedermann M, Uebis R, Beilin I, Sheehan F, Hanrath P, Buell U. Significance of defect severity in Technetium-99m-MIBI SPECT at rest to assess myocardial viability: comparison with Fluorine-18-FDG. *J Nucl Med* 1994; 35:569–574.

133. Arnese M, Cornel JH, Salustri A, Maat AP, Elhendy A, Reijs AEM, Cate FJT, Keane D, Balk AHMM, Roelandt JRTC, Fioretti PM. Prediction of improvement of regional left ventricular function after surgical revascularization. *Circulation* 1995; 91:2748–2752.

134. Berger CB, Watson DD, Burwell LR, Crosby IK, Wellons HA, Teates CD, Beller GA. Redistribution of thallium at rest in patients with stable and unstable angina and the effect of coronary artery bypass surgery. *Circulation* 1979; 60:1114–1125.

135. Brundage BH, Massie BM. Botvinick Improved regional ventricular function after successful surgical revascularization. *J Am Coll Cardiol* 1984; 3:902–908.

136. Dilsizian V, Rocco TP, Freedman NMT, Leon MB, Bonow RO. Enhanced detection of ischemic but viable myocardium by the reinjection of thallium after stress-redistribution imaging. *N Engl J Med* 1990; 323:141–146.

137. Gibson RS, Watson DD, Taylor GJ, Crosby IK, Taylor GJ, Crosby IK, Wellons HL, Holt ND, Beller GA. Prospective assessment of regional myocardial perfusion before and after coronary revascularization surgery by quantitative thallium-201 scintigraphy. *J Am Coll Cardiol* 1983; 1:804–815.

138. Kiat H, Berman DS, Maddahi J, de Yang L, Van Train K, Rozanski A, Friedman J. Late reversibility of tomographic myocardial thallium-201 defects: an accurate marker of myocardial viability. *J Am Coll Cardiol* 1988; 12:1456–1563.

139. La Canna G, Alfieri O, Giubbini R, Gargano M, Ferrari R, Visioli O. Echocardiography during infusion of dobutamine for identification of reversible dysfunction in patients with chronic coronary artery disease. *J Am Coll Cardiol* 1994; 23:617–626.

140. Liu P, Kiess MC, Okada RD, Block PC, Strauss HW, Pohost GM, Boucher CA. The persistent defect on exercise thallium imaging and its fate after myocardial revascularization: Does it represent scar or ischemia? *Am Heart J* 1985; 110:996–1001.

141. Lucignani G, Paolini G, Landoni C, Zuccari M, Paganelli G, Galli L, Di Credico G, Vanoli G, Rossetti C, Mariani MA, Gilardi MC, Colombo F, Grossi A, Fazio F. Presurgical identification of hibernating myocardium by combined use of Technetium-99m hexokinase 2-methoxyisobutylnitrile single photon emission tomography and Fluorine-18 Fluoro-2-deoxy-d-glucose positron emission tomography in patients with coronary artery disease. *Eur J Nucl Med* 1992; 19:874–881.

142. Marwick T, MacIntyre W, Lafont A, Nemec JJ, Salcedo EE. Metabolic response of hibernating and infarcted myocardium to revascularization: a follow-up study of regional perfusion, function and metabolism. *Circulation* 1992; 85:1347–1353.

143. Mori T, Minamiji K, Kurogane H, Ogawa K, Yoshida Y. Rest-injected thallium-201 imaging for assessing viability of severe asynergic regions. *J Nucl Med* 1991; 32:1718–1724.

144. Ohtani H, Tamaki N, Yonekura Y, Mohiuddin IH, Hirata K, Ban T, Konishi J. Value of thallium-201 reinjection after delayed SPECT imaging for predicting reversible ischemia after coronary artery bypass grafting. *Am J Cardiol* 1990; 66:394–399.

145. Perrone-Filardi P, Pace L, Prastaro M, Piscione F, Betocchi S, Squame F, Vezzuto P, Soricelli A, Indolfi S, Salvatore M. Dobutamine echocardiography predicts improvement of hypoperfused dysfunctional myocardium after revascularization in patients with coronary artery disease. *Circulation* 1995; 91:2556–2565.

146. Popio KA, Gorlin R, Bechtel D, Levine JA. Postextrasystolic potentiation as a predictor of potential myocardial viability: preoperative analyses compared with studies after coronary bypass surgery. *Am J Cardiol* 1977; 39:944–953.

147. Rozanski A, Berman DS, Gray R, Levy R, Raymond M, Maddahi J, Pantaleo N, Waxman AD, Swan HJ, Matloff J. Use of Thallium-201 redistribution scintigraphy in the preoperative differentiation of reversible and nonreversible myocardial asynergy. *Circulation* 1981; 64:936–944.

148. Rozanski A, Berman D, Gray R, Diamond G, Raymond M, Prause J, Maddahi J, Swan HJC, Matloff J. Preoperative prediction of reversible myocardial asynergy by postexercise radionuclide ventriculography. *N Engl J Med* 1982; 307:212–216.

149. Tamaki N, Yonekura Y, Yamashita K, Senda M, Saji H, Konishi Y, Hirata K, Ban T, Konish J. Value of rest-stress myocardial positron tomography using Nitrogen-13 ammonia for the preoperative prediction of reversible asynergy. *J Nucl Med* 1989; 30:1302–1310.

150. Tamaki N, Yonekura Y, Yamashita Y, Saji H, Magati Y, Senda M, Konishi Y, Hirata K, Ban T, Konishi J. Positron emission tomography using fluorine-18 deoxyglucose in evaluation of coronary artery bypass grafting. *Am J Cardiol* 1989; 64:860–865.

151. Tamaki N, Ohtani H, Yamashita K, Magat Y, Yonekura Y, Nohara R, Kambar H, Kawai C, Ban T, Konish J. Metabolic activity in the areas of new fill-in after Thallium-201 reinjection: comparison with positron emission tomography using Fluorine-18-deoxyglucose. *J Nucl Med* 1991; 32:673–678.

152. Tillisch J, Brunken R, Marshall R, Schwaiger, Mandelkern M, Phelps M, Schelbert H. Reversibility of cardiac wall-motion abnormalities predicted by positron tomography. *N Engl J Med* 1986: 314:884–888.

153. Melin JA, Wijns W, Keyeux A, Gume O, Cogneau M, Michel C, Bol A, Robert A, Charlier A, Pouleur H. Assessment of thallium-201 redistribution versus glucose

uptake as predictors of viability after coronary occlusion and reperfusion. *Circulation* 1988; 77:927–934.

154. Franken PR, De Geeter F, Dendale P, Demoor D, Block P, Bossuyt A. Abnormal free fatty acid uptake in subacute myocardial infarction after coronary thrombolysis: correlation with wall motion and inotropic reserve. *J Nucl Med* 1994; 35:1758–1765.

155. De Geeter F, Franken PR, Knapp jr. FF, Bossuyt A. Relationship between blood flow and fatty acid metabolism in subacute myocardial infarction: a study by means of 99mTc-Sestamibi and 123I-P-methyl-iodo-phenylpentadecanoic acid. *Eur J Nucl Med* 1994; 21:283–291.

156. Daspit SG, Stemple DR, Doherty PD, Goris ML. Unusual findings in 201-Thallium myocardial scintigraphy: the "hot heart" sign. *Clin Med* 1977; 2:1–5.

157. Cohen HA, Baird MG, Rouleau JR, Fuhrmann CF, Bailey IK, Summer WR, Strauss HW, Pitt B. Thallium 201 myocardial imaging in patients with pulmonary hypertension. *Circulation* 1976; 54:790–795.

158. Khaja F, Alam M, Goldstein S, Anbe DT, Marks DS. Diagnostic value of visualization of the right ventricle using thallium-201 myocardial imaging. *Circulation* 1979; 59:182–188.

159. Rabinovitch M, Fischer KC, Treves S. Quantitative thallium-201 myocardial imaging in assessing right ventricular pressure in patients with congenital heart defects. *Br Heart J* 1981; 45:198–205.

Chapter **6**

Ventriculography

6.1. INTRODUCTION

Nuclear cardiology emerged in the early seventies with the advent of the mini-computer interfaced to the anger gamma camera. This was a conjunction of two technical advances exploited early and expertly by a small group of investigators and practitioners. First, the anger camera allowed, for the first time, the addition of a dynamic component to scintigraphic images, or conversely the addition of spatial distribution to dynamic studies. Dynamic images had been recorded directly on film or on a video system (1, 2). Those investigators, using relative primitive means, defined two principal aspects of scintigraphic ventriculography: First, counts had to be collected from a region of interest including all of, and restricted to, the left ventricle and that non-cardiac activities within the region of interest (crosstalk) had to be accounted for. Second, recording the digitized data[a] on a computer facil-itated post-processing, and eventual quantification of the data, even though early on analysis was mainly visual (3).

Today, it is difficult to imagine how the time line of applications was com-pressed. The early applications with clinical impact were in the field of shunt (left to right) detection (4–9). The interest in this technique for that application waned rapidly with the introduction of ultrasonography applied to shunting. It did however wax for the detection of coronary artery disease.

The two clinical applications emerging to stay were myocardial perfusion scintigraphy and the evaluation of left ventricular function by either first pass ventriculography (First Pass Nuclear Angiocardiography or FPNA) or ECG-gated

---

[a]It is important to realize that the digitation concerns the x and y coordinates in the camera field of view, and not the scintigraphic events themselves that are digital or discrete to begin with. The representation of the activity in film or rate meter curves corresponds to the transformation of digital to analog data.

scintigraphic ventriculography.[b] One of the principal contributors to the technique must be Steve Bacharach (10, 11).

The first years were mainly spent on validation and on attempts to automate, or at least standardize processing (12–18).

6.2. SCINTIGRAPHIC EVALUATION OF VENTRICULAR FUNCTION

6.2.1. *Physics, Physiopathology and Analysis*

The physics underlying the principle of scintigraphic ventriculography is simple enough. During the ventricular contraction phase, no new blood reaches the ventricle. The concentration of a tracer at the end of diastole stays constant through the end of systole. Since the total amount of tracer in the ventricle is equal to the volume multiplied by the concentration, and since the concentration is constant, ventricular activity is proportional to volume. If the proportionality (k) between count rate and activity remains constant,[c] the end-diastolic count rate (EDCR) is proportional to end-diastolic volume (EDV) and end-systolic count rate (ESCR) is proportional to end-systolic volume (ESV). The ejection fraction (EF) can thus be derived as follows:

$$EF = \frac{EDV - ESV}{EDV} = \frac{kEDV - kESV}{kEDV} = \frac{EDCR - ESCR}{EDCR}.$$

The problem as we shall see lies in the requirement stated in the introduction. The calculation is correct only if all and only the ventricular activity is detected and if tissue crosstalk[d] can be accounted for. In the easiest case, the crosstalk B

---

[b]ECG-gated ventriculography is commonly known as MUGA or multi-gated angiography, an acronym originated as a proprietary acquisition protocol. In this text, we will use the more general term equilibrium-(ECG) gated nuclear angiocardiography or EGNA, to differentiate from first-pass or FPNA. In general, we will use RNV or radionuclide ventriculography.

[c]The assumption has been shown to be incorrect because of the attenuation effect, with significant errors mainly in the case of anterior wall akinesis.

[d]The common nomenclature is background where it should be crosstalk, but the term does not reflect the phenomenon accurately. The term background should be reserved for (white) noise, a signal present anywhere in the image, but not connected to the signal itself. Crosstalk comes in two ways. Channel crosstalk is a signal somehow misdirected, e.g. in a dual isotope study, the signal originating from isotope 1 detected in the channel dedicated to isotope 2 (see Section 10.1.2). Scatter can be considered as channel crosstalk. Scatter appears in a

is constant for systole and diastole. In that case, EDCR = k(EDV + B), ESCR = k(ESV + B). An estimated value for B has to be determined, and any error is reflected in the denominator only:

$$\frac{EDCR - B - (ESCR - B)}{EDCR - B^e} = \frac{k(EDV - ESV)}{kEDV - e},$$

where B^e is the estimated crosstalk and "$e = B - B^e$".

The actual presentation of the problem is different in FPNA from EGNA, as we shall see in Sections 6.2.2 and 6.2.3.

6.2.2. First Pass Nuclear Angiocardiography (FPNA)

In FPNA, a small bolus of solution containing the radiotracer is injected intravenously. The analysis is restricted to the ventricular phase of the bolus. The advantage is that during that time most of the activity is indeed in the left ventricle, and that tissue crosstalk is minimized, because other organs or tissues do not contain much activity. The major advantage is the absence of significant right ventricular activity during the left ventricular phase. This allows for an optimal projection of the left ventricle, without overlap, and in contradistinction to the gated blood pool described below (Section 6.2.3).

The left ventricular activity is captured at a high frequency, such that oscillations in ventricular counts can be measured during the (few) cardiac cycles of the left ventricular phase of the bolus. There are two approaches.

In the first approach, the time activity curve is analyzed directly (19). But this approach would not allow regional analysis. If representative images of the end-diastolic and end-systolic ventricle are wanted, a second approach is used.

Because the count rate is low by necessity,[e] counts obtained from multiple (but generally few) cycles are added up, following synchronization. Originally the synchronization consisted of adding the images corresponding to peaks (for the end-diastolic image) and valleys. Eventually all images of the cardiac cycle, with a temporal resolution of 1/16 of the cardiac cycle were produced, based on

---

location (channel) not dedicated to the origin of the scatter event. Tissue crosstalk arises from overlapping tissues. In planar imaging, tissue crosstalk is ubiquitous, since all organs of interest share a projection plane with overlying and underlying tissues.
[e]There is obviously a limit to the amount of activity that can be injected, hence a relatively low count rate, and the counting time is short, hence relatively low counts. The noise in this context is not white noise or background, but is associated to the signal as Poisson noise.

more sophisticated synchronization schemes[f] or dedicated cameras with a higher sensitivity (20). In this case, the analysis results in a composite cardiac cycle, in which ED and ES images can be analyzed, either on a count-rate basis (see above) or on an area-length basis (21). Analysis on area-length method is close to the contrast method, but suffers from the same model weakness: the left ventricular volume is not well described. Surprisingly, Bodenheimer (21) finds that the correspondence between the first pass EF derived from the count-based method and the area-length method from contrast ventriculography is very good (FPNA EF $= 0.86 \times$ contrast EF $+ 0.09$; r $= 0.81$).

FPNA differs from EGNA on five crucial points:

1. The total acquisition time is short and limited by the first pass of the bolus through the left ventricle.
2. During the recording time, tissue crosstalk is minimal, and anterior or left lateral projections can be obtained with minimal crossover from the right ventricle, atrial and large vessels activity.
3. There is less reliance on perfect synchronization over a large number of cycles. Theoretically, this would allow a more precise measure of the EF at peak exercise.
4. Since the ventricle refills after end-systole, the count rate proportionality with ventricular volume changes according to the variable tracer concentration in the afferent blood; diastolic kinetics cannot be evaluated, but ejection rate can (22).
5. It is difficult to monitor the patient with an EF at each stage of the exercise, and when that is done, one observes that the negative EF changes (a) eventually occur if extreme stress is attained, and (b) that early drops probably indicate more advanced disease (23).

6.2.3. *Equilibrium ECG-Gated Angiocardiography (EGNA)*

6.2.3.1. *Global function*

In EGNA, the tracer is specifically an intravascular tracer, typically labeled autologous red blood cells.[g] The tracer is eventually mixed, and a constant time invariant

---

[f]Synchronization is essential and critical when data from multiple cycles are combined. The effect of poor synchronization is to lower the average end-diastolic counts and increase the end-systolic count rate. Poor synchronization as well as an insufficient temporal resolution results in a lowered ejection fraction.

[g]The tracer is a red blood cell, by definition an intravascular tracer. The label is ^{99m}Tc.

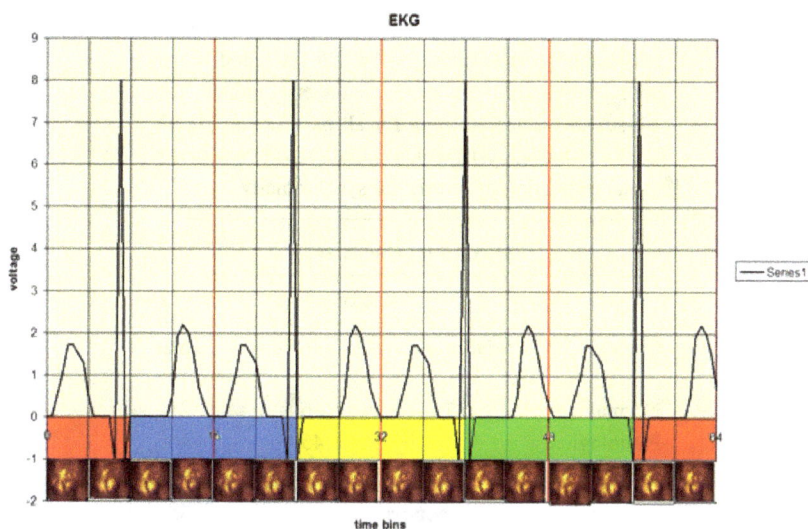

Figure 6.1 Schematic representation of the gated acquisition scheme. In this example, only four time bins are shown. The high peaks represent the QRS complex. The others are the T and P peaks respectively. The QRS triggers the acquisition in four equal time bins in which the data of multiple cycles are summed.

tracer concentration is obtained through the vascular system. This time invariance also applies to the filling phase (unlike in FPNA). This allows the analysis of diastolic dilatation and filling rates (Section 6.2.2).

The acquisition is a cyclic dynamic acquisition, restarted whenever a QRS complex is detected. The data are acquired cumulatively in separate time bins according to a preset division of the RR interval (Figure 6.1). Data acquired in sequential cycles are correspondingly added in the appropriate time bins (24–26).

The ejection fraction (EF) is derived from counts in the left ventricular (LV) region (27).

Adams (25) specifically looked at the concordance with contrast ventriculographic findings, in 2×2 contingency tables. In general, the correspondence with contrast studies is good, except for phase shifts. However, phase shift is analytically not looked at in contrast ventriculography (Section 6.2.3.2 and Table 6.1).[h]

---

[h]This is a good example of the conundrum following from the habit of validating new techniques on the basis of comparisons with old techniques: progress is impossible. The best result is "no worse than".

Table 6.1 The table illustrates the correspondence between the contrast angiography and the gated blood pool studies (25). In 2×2 contingency tables, the chi-square values are high for all parameters, except for the phase analysis, which is more sensitive than the visual inspection of ventricular synchronicity.

Relaxation velocity scan

Contrast	Radionuclide Normal	Pathological	Total
Normal	15	6	21
Pathological	1	45	46
Total	16	51	67
Chi-square			**38**

Phase shift

Contrast	Radionuclide Normal	Phase shift	Total
Normal	35	22	57
Pathological	2	6	8
Total	37	28	65
Chi-square			**3.8**

All parametric

Contrast	Radionuclide Normal	Pathological	Total
Normal	19	2	21
Pathological	4	43	47
Total	23	45	68
Chi-square			**35**

The final image maps a composite cardiac cycle, each frame with a nominal time of RR/n, where n is the division of the RR interval, and an actual acquisition time of $N \times RR/n$, where N is the number of acquired cycles (Figure 6.1). If there is some variation in the RR interval, the last image of the cycle may not have been acquired when the cycle restarts at zero. In that case, the actual acquisition

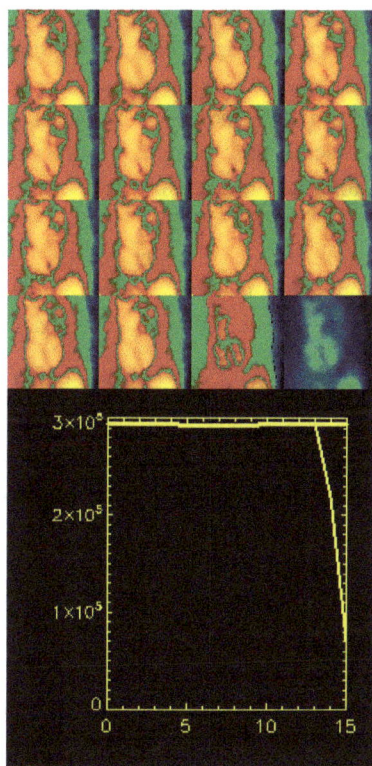

Figure 6.2 The top row shows the uncorrected series of 16 time bins in an EGNA acquisition. The last frame is not visible, because the heart rate was irregular. The total counts in the images illustrate that the acquisition time was shorter at the end of the cycle. The heavy line is after correction for total counts.

time of the last image (or images) of the composite cardiac cycle will be less than $N \times RR/n$. The total counts in those images will be artificially too low. There are different methods to correct for this. The most logical would be to track N for each image, and express everything in count rates rather than total counts.[i] An alternative is to normalize to total counts, as shown in Figure 6.2.

---

[i]Indeed, it is an unfortunate tradition in nuclear medicine to use total counts rather than count rates. The disadvantage is obvious in renography, when multi-phased acquisitions are used (a rapid phase for the arterial phase, a medium phase for accumulation and a slow phase for excretion). Since the display is based on counts rather than count rates, pre-processing is required to display the whole sequence.

The problem of irregular heartbeats is different. In the case of extrasystoles, there are two separate effects: the cycle being acquired when the extra systole occurs is interrupted, and the effect on the data that is discussed in the previous paragraph. However, the next two cardiac cycles can be altered, both in timing and in their mechanic characteristics. Most acquisition software systems have the ability to reject one to two cycles after a shorter than expected RR interval.

In the case of an irregular heartbeat caused by atrial fibrillation, the addition of multiple cycle acquisitions results in a blurring, because the synchronization based on a QRS complex does not guarantee the synchronization of systole for all cycles.

A posteriori resetting the length of the time bins, on the basis of the length of the RR interval is not a solution (28, 29).

In EGNA, the angle of acquisition is chosen to minimize overlap between the ventricles and between the ventricles and the atria. The theoretically optimal acquisition angle is the 45 LAO, slightly modified to have a clear view of the septum, and with a slight caudal tilt to avoid overlap between the left atrium and the left ventricle (Figure 6.3).

The final result of the acquisition is a dynamic image with n frames, count rate densities mapping the activity distribution of the heart, large vessels and surroundings during a composite cardiac cycle. The analysis of this image is both global and regional.

Globally, the ventricles are analyzed by following the total ventricular activity during the cycle. The most straightforward method is to place a region of interest

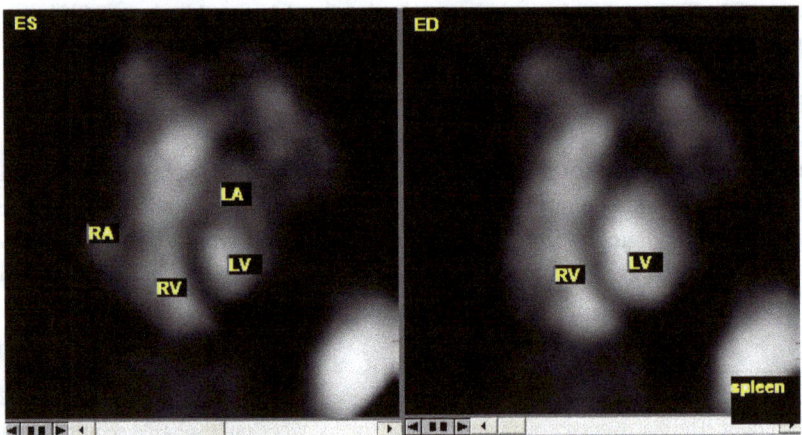

Figure 6.3   The figure illustrates the anatomical structures in end-systole and end-diastole. Note how the atria are more prominent in end-systole.

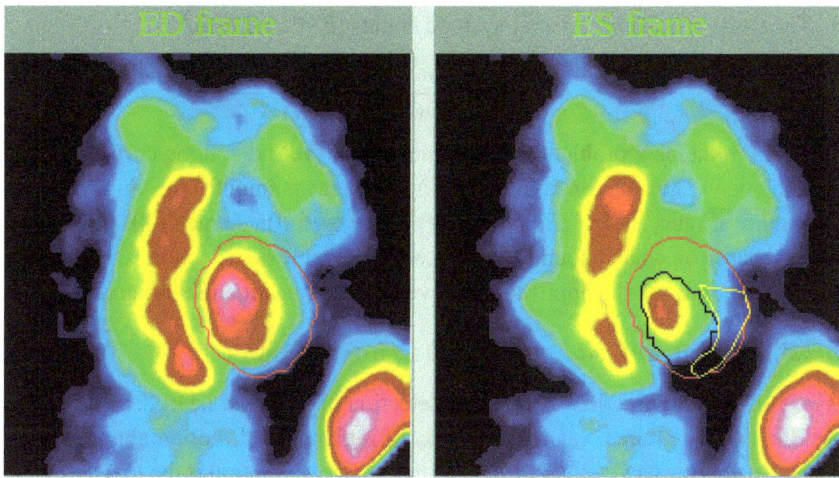

Figure 6.4 Illustration of the regions of interest in ED and ES and a placement of a background region for the correction of the tissue crosstalk.

(ROI) over the left ventricle at end-diastole. Eventually, the consensus was that there is enough movement of the atria within this end-diastolic region to make a separate end-systolic region necessary.[j] For the crosstalk, a separate ROI is placed near the edge of the end-diastolic ROI, from about 3 o'clock to 6 o'clock, or in the same region but between the end-diastolic and end-systolic ROI (Figure 6.4).

The analysis is based on the principle given above; however, the manner in which the crosstalk factor is computed is based on the assumption that there is a constant crosstalk factor in every pixel.

1. First one computes b, the crosstalk factor per pixel by dividing the total counts in the background region B by the number of pixels in the background region nb.
2. Then one subtracts from the end-diastolic counts EDC, b × the number of pixels in the end-diastolic ROI (ned).

---

[j]This approach eventually interferes with the analysis of the curve apart from the determination of the EF. In some cases two curves are produced, one for the determination of the EF, and one for the analysis of the curve. Some have proposed a separate ROI for each frame in the image.

3. The same is done for the end-systolic counts (ESC and nes).[k]

$$EF = \frac{(EDC - b \times ned) - (ESC - b \times nes)}{(EDC - b \times ned)}.$$

There remains a problem if one wants to analyze the volume curve: the data remain noisy. The solution is to find a way to filter (or smooth) the volume curve, even more if rates (filling and emptying) are desired. Bacharach (30) proposed a method based on what amounts to a truncated Fourier series (Section 10.6). In what follows, we will see the application of even more truncation (Section 6.2.3.2).

6.2.3.2. Regional wall motion (phase analysis)

As we shall see in Section 6.2.4.2, the detection of ischemic heart disease, one of the diagnostic features was the detection of regional wall motion abnormalities. The most appropriate method to evaluate regional wall motion is the first harmonic analysis, better known as phase analysis. In short, this analysis yields amplitude and a phase. The amplitude reflects the degree of changes in count rate densities during the cardiac cycle. The phase reflects the timing of the nadir. The analysis is applied to all the pixels in the image (31–34) (Figure 6.5).

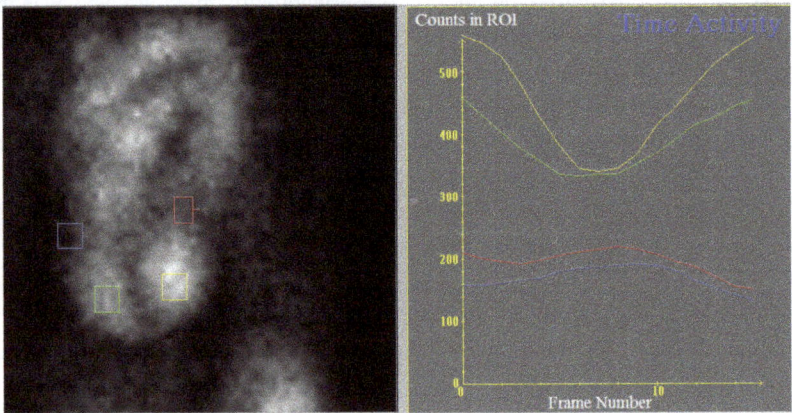

Figure 6.5   The curves were generated from regions of interests over the ventricles. The top (ventricular) and bottom (atrial) ones are out of phase, and this is reflected in the phase image in Figure 6.6. Also, the changes in the ventricular curves are ampler than in the atrial curves, also reflected in the amplitude image in Figure 6.6 (see Section 10.6).

---

[k]The background or crosstalk correction is now applied to the end-diastolic and end-systolic counts separately, because the assumption is that the crosstalk contribution is proportional to the area.

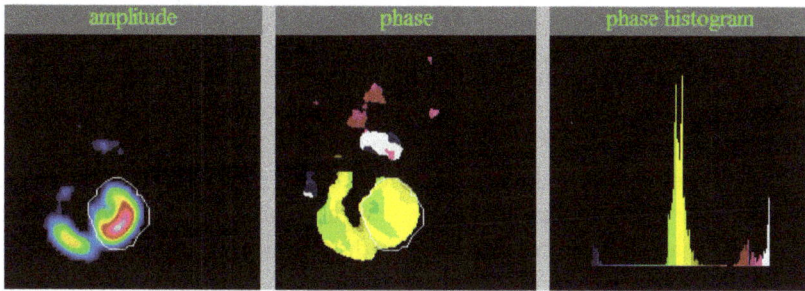

Figure 6.6 The phase histogram shows the number of pixels (in the y-axis) with a particular phase (in the x-axis). The ventricular phase is in the middle (at the time of systole). The atrial and large vessel phases are distributed at both ends of the cycle.

The count rate densities in the right and left ventricular projections show larger amplitudes than those in the atrial and large vessels projection. The nadir occurs just before the mid-cycle. Those in the atrial and large vessels projection have less variation and a maximum around mid-cycle (Figure 6.6).

In the amplitude image, the intensities more or less follow the intensities of the ventricles, with higher densities around the apex and the free wall in the left ventricle. Holman (35) supplemented the amplitude and phase image with the paradox image, which even at the time did not seem to contribute very much to the phase and amplitude images, but which did gain general acceptance, perhaps because it was more direct. The same can be said about the ejection fraction image from Maddox (36, 37).

Both ventricles have the same narrow phase values. The atrial and large vessel regions have low intensities in the amplitude image, and sometimes opposite values. The latter point is better illustrated in the phase histogram.

6.2.4. *Clinical Applications*

6.2.4.1. *Early validations*

One of the problems is that both EGNA and FPNA require a relatively immobile patient at peak exercise, which is near impossible on a treadmill. Foster (38) pointed out that in America at least, functional capacity has been encoded in treadmill exercise terms. However, he finds that the functional capacity computed from a Bruce treadmill protocol and a bicycle protocol are related by Bruce METS = $1.0 \times$ (bike METS) + 1.85.

Originally, the contrast EF was considered the gold standard, and the equivalence tended to be very good, even though the methodology was very different (39, 40).

6.2.4.2. *Detection of coronary artery disease*

Early reported results for the detection of coronary artery disease may have been overoptimistic (39–47) (Table 6.2). There were some reservations. Osbakken (48) improved the results by including the end-systolic volume.

A number of the early validations suffered from the perverse habit of comparing patients with known coronary artery disease with "normal" patients. This approach assumes a binary system (this disease or no disease) not normally encountered in a usual clinical population (see Section 7.6).

A more interesting approach is that of Gibbons (49) who considers the relative contribution of different observations to the diagnosis. To start, working with RH Jones, he does not consider the response of the EF to stress, but the absolute value at peak exercise. Of the radionuclide (FPNA) metrics, the peak exercise EF is the best predictor of chronic coronary artery disease. Following that was the maximum heart rate, and a poorly defined ischemia score. The authors, however,

Table 6.2 Operating characteristics of changes in EF for the detection of CAD.[1] CAD stands for a positive coronary angiogram otherwise not specified. The percentages stand for the degree of stenosis. 3 and LM stand for three vessel disease and the left main. In the aggregate, the sensitivity is 86% and the non-specificity is 31%.

Ref	Year	Patient	Metric	Ischemic	N	P (S+|D+)	Normal	N	P (S+|D−)
39	1979	<50%	EF				0	19	0.00
42	1983	≥ 2 vessel	EF	124	128	0.97			
42	1983	≥ 2 vessel	EF	251	285	0.88			
48	1980	2 vessel	EF	15	20	0.75			
48	1980	3 vessel	EF	29	41	0.71			
42	1983	3 and LM	EF	75	85	0.88			
42	1983	3 and LM	EF	138	150	0.92			
39	1979	≥ 70%	EF	65	73	0.89			
42	1983	CAD	EF	167	208	0.80	49	125	0.39
43	1977	CAD	EF	10	11	0.91			
42	1983	Left Main	EF	11	14	0.79			
42	1983	Left Main	EF	20	24	0.83			
41	1979		EF	44	60	0.73	0	13	0.00
			EF	949	1099	0.86	49	157	0.31

[1]The notations P(X|Y) are explained in Section 7.1.

Table 6.3 Operating characteristic for the detection of CAD. CAD stands for coronary artery disease, RWM for regional wall motion abnormality induced by exercise, SV for single vessel disease. In the aggregate, the sensitivity is 57% and the non-specificity is 0%.

Ref	Year	Patient	Metric	Ischemic	N	P(S+|D+)	Normal	N	P(S+|D−)
48	1980	2 vessel	RWM	7	9	0.78			
48	1980	3 vessel	RWM	11	49	0.22			
43	1977	CAD	RWM	11	11	1.00			
58	1981	CAD	RWM	22	35	0.63			
48	1980	Normal	RWM				0	11	0.00
58	1981	Normal	RWM				0	12	0.00
48	1980	SV	RWM	9	13	0.69			
43	1977	Volunteers	RWM				0	14	0.00
41	1979	CAD	RWM	28	60	0.47	0	13	0.00
39	1979	>70%	RWM	54	73	0.74			
			RWM	142	250	0.57	0	50	0.00

point out that in patients with atypical angina and in women, the specificity decreased. The change in EF was not a significant factor. In fact, Gibbons (49) found that the EF response to exercise was not a reliable finding of coronary artery disease. In this we agreed (15), but we refined the concept by considering the EF change as the fraction of possible change [if the resting EF is $(100 - x)\%$, a decrease is possible only between 0 and $(100 - x)$ and an increase between $(100 - x)$ and 100].

Regional wall motion abnormalities, especially induced by exercise, are more specific than global ejection fraction changes during exercise (Tables 6.2 and 6.3).

6.2.4.3. *Prognostic significance*

Jones (50) described a population treated either medically or surgically (CABG) for coronary artery diseases. In those with abnormal rest and exercise, radionuclide angiography survival was much lower in the medical groups, as was pain relief $(N = 172)$.

Perhaps a more pertinent question at that time; ventriculography and specifically the ejection fraction, was shown to be an important prognostic feature after myocardial infarction, and became crucial in the rehabilitation of myocardial infarction victims.

The resting EF has some predictive value. If the EF is $\leq 30\%$ mortality is 43%, if $\leq 40\%$ it is 14% for more than 12 months follow-up.

DeBusk (51) provided a comprehensive codification, based mainly on the demonstration of residual ischemia. In the end (52), he stratifies patients on the basis of a mortality risk ratio. His conclusions are comparable to those in reports by Hung (53), Gibson (54) and Corbett (55). He tabulates that the risk factors are mainly reversible myocardial perfusion defects, multiple reversible defects, fall in exercise ejection fraction > 5% during submaximal exercise, and failure to increase the exercise EF by at least 5%.

6.2.4.4. *Other applications*

Felipe (56) found diagnostic utility in coronary artery disease, acute myocardial infarction, evaluation of interventional procedure, valvular heart disease, cardiomyopathy, congenital heart disease and evaluation of drug therapy. The multiplicity of applications belies the numbers originally proposed for the specificity of the ejection fraction response.

Valvular disease was evaluated on the basis of equal stroke volumes in R and L ventricles, except in the case of shunting (atrial or pulmonary) or valvular regurgitation. The SV is determined on the basis of net (ED-ES) count differences in LV and RV regions of interest (57). Incidentally, Hecht (58) found that exercise wall motion abnormalities are frequent in patients with valvular disease. Abnormal responses to exercise were also noted in cardiomyopathy (ethanol-induced) and mitral valve prolaps by Lindsay (47).

An interesting application was the definition of the mechanisms of decreased exercise capacity after bed rest (59). The reason is not cardiac, but a preload deficiency. The EF values are actually high.

The positive inotropic response has been discussed in Chapter 5 (60, 61). This response does not indicate coronary artery disease, but does indicate viability (Section 5.10 defining viability).

The detection of doxorubin cardiotoxicity was an interesting application. The first attempt was the serial following of the resting ejection fraction (62). The objection to this approach in children treated for malignancy was the modification of the afterload in young patients with wide variations in general well-being. One way to counteract that effect seemed to be the utilization of exercise testing. Adding the end-exercise ejection fraction increased the sensitivity. A resting EF ≤ 45%, had a sensitivity of 53% and a specificity of 75%. Adding the stress EF increased the sensitivity to 89%, but decreased the specificity to 41% (63). But actually, the maximum stress EF reached had the best correlation with the cumulative dose of doxorubicin (64).

If there was an inherent weakness in the technique, it was the need for an adequate effort. Debusk (65) pointed out the difference between combined static and dynamic, or dynamic effort alone, and found dynamic alone more effective. Brady (66) found a drop in sensitivity from 94% to 62% if the stress was inadequate. On the other hand, the effectiveness of supine and upright bicycle exercise testing does not differ significantly (67). But dynamic effort is not easy to perform with imaging integrated, and that may have been the reason for the replacement of exercise ventriculography by stress (pharmacological) myocardial perfusion. The disadvantage of ventriculography based on myocardial perfusion SPECT is that it cannot be performed during stress, but 3D acquisition eliminates the frustrating problem of tissue crosstalk (68).

6.3. CONCLUSION

Scintigraphic ventriculography is a potentially very powerful tool to study ventricular function in CAD, post-MI patients, pre-CABG patients and patients treated with cardiotoxic drugs. However, the reluctance of practitioners to perform (live) stress testing has degraded the efficacy to a large degree.

REFERENCES

1. Van Dyke D, Anger HO, Sullivan RW, Vetter WR, Yano Y, Parker HG. Cardiac evaluation from radioisotope dynamics. *J Nucl Med* 1972; 13:585–592.
2. Hannan WJ, Hare RJ, Hughes SHC, Scorgie RE, Muir AL. Simplified method of determining left ventricular ejection fraction from a radionuclide bolus. *Eur J Nucl Med* 1977; 2:71–74.
3. Kriss, JP. Cardiovascular: radioisotopic angiocardiography. *Nucl Med Clin Pediatrics* 1975; pp. 69–79.
4. Alazraki NP, Ashburn WL, Hagen A, *et al.* Detection of left-to-right shunts with the scintillation camera pulmonary dilution curve. *J Nucl Med* 1972; 13:142–147.
5. Kriss JP, Enright LP, Hayden WG, *et al.* Radioisotopic angiocardiography: findings in congenital heart disease. *J Nucl Med* 1972; 13:31–40.
6. Jones RH, Sabiston DC, Bates JJ, Anderson PAW, Goodrich JK. Quantitative radionuclide angiocardiography for determination of chamber to chamber transit times. *Am J Cardiol* 1972; 30:855–864.
7. Maltz DL, Treves S. Quantitative radionuclide angiocardiography determination of Qp:Qs in children. *Circulation* 1973; 47:1049–1056.
8. Anderson PAW, Jones RH, Sabiston DC. Quantitation of left-to-right cardiac shunts with radionuclide angiography. *Circulation* 1974; 49:512–516.
9. Alderson PO, Jost RG, Strauss AW, Boonvisut S, Markham J. Radionuclide angiocardiography: improved diagnosis and quantitation of left-to-right shunts using area rations techniques in children. *Circulation* 1974; 51:1136–1143.

10. Bacharach SL, Green MV, Borer JS, Hyde JE, Farkas SP, Johnson GS. Left Ventricular Peak Ejection Rate, Filling Rate, and Ejection Fraction-Frame Rate Requirements at Rest and Exercise: Concise Communication. *J Nucl Med* 1979; 20:189–193.

11. Bacharach SL, Green MV, Borer JS. Instrumentation and data processing in cardiovascular Nuclear Medicine: evaluation of ventricular function. *Sem Nucl Med* 1979; 9:257–273.

12. Goris ML, Wallington J, Baum D, Kriss JP. Nuclear angiocardiography: automated selection of regions of interest for the generation of time-activity curves, and parametric image display and interpretation. *Clin Nucl Med* 1976; 1:99–106.

13. Douglas MA, Green MV, Ostrow HG. Evaluation of automatically generated left ventricular regions of interest in computerized ECG-gated radionuclide angiocardiography. *Comput Cardiol* 1978; 78:201–204.

14. Douglas MA, Green MV. A System for computer Generation of left ventricular masks for use in computerized ECG-gated radionuclide angiocardiography. Nuclear cardiology selected computer aspects. Symposium proceedings Atlanta GA January 22–2. *Soc Nuc Med* 1978; pp. 119–129.

15. Goris ML, Briandet PA, Thomas AJ, McKillop JH, Sneed P, Wiklander DP. A thresholding for radionuclide angiocardiography. *Invest Radiol* 1981; 16:115–119.

16. Goris ML, McKillop JH, Briandet PA. A fully automated determination of the left ventricular region of interest in nuclear angiocardiography. *Cardiovasc Interven Radiol* 1981; 4:117–123.

17. Goris ML, Briandet PA, Huffer E. Automation and operator independent processing of cardiac and pulmonary functions: role, methods and results. *Les Colloques de l'INSERM*: Information processing of medical images. *INSER* 1979; 88:427–445.

18. Hecht HS, Mirell SG, Rolett EL, Blahd WH. Left-ventricular ejection fraction and segmental wall motion by peripheral first-pass radionuclide angiography. *J Nucl Med* 1978; 19:17–23.

19. Schelbert HR, Verba JW, Johnson AD, Brock GW, Alazraki NP, Rose FJ, Ashburn WL. Nontraumatic determination of left ventricular ejection fraction by radionuclide angiocardiography. *Circulation* 1975; 51:902–909.

20. Bates BB, Rerych SK, Jones RH. Exercise techniques for radionuclide angiocardiography. *J Nucl Med Tech* 1978; 6:199–204.

21. Bodenheimer MM, Banka VS, Helfant RH. Nuclear cardiology. I. radionuclide angiographic assessment of left ventricular contraction: uses, limitations and future directions. *Am J Cardiol* 1980; 45:661–673.

22. Marshall RC, Berger HJ, Costin JC, Freedman GS, Wolberg J, Cohen LS, Gottschalk A, Zaret BL. Assessment of cardiac performance with quantitative radionuclide angiocardiography. Sequential left ventricular ejection fraction, left ventricular ejection rate and regional wall motion. *Circulation* 1977; 56:820–829.

23. Goris ML, Hung J, DeBusk RF. Scintigraphic ventriculography and stress testing. *Journal de Biophysique et de Medicine Nucleaire* 1982; 6:227–232.

24. Bacharach SL, Green MV, Borer JS, Douglas MA, Ostrow HG, Johnson GS. A real time system for multi-image gated cardiac studies. *J Nucl Med* 1977; 18:79–84.

25. Adam WE, Tarkowska A, Bitter F, Stauch M, Geffers H. Equilibrium (gated) radionuclide ventriculography. *Cardiovascular Radiology* 1979; 2:161–173.

26. Green MV, Ostrow HG, Douglas MA, Myers RW, Scott RN, Bailey JJ, Johnston GS. High temporal resolution ECG-gated scintigraphic. *J Nucl Med* 1975; 16: 95–98.

27. Green MV, Brody WR, Douglas MA, Borer JS, Ostrow HC, Bacharach SL, Johnston GS. Ejection fraction by count rate from gated images. *J Nucl Med* 1978; 19:880–883.

28. Bacharach SL, Green MV, Borer JS, Ostrow HG, Bonow RO, Farkas SP, Johnston GS. Beat-by-beat validation of ECG gating. *J Nucl Med* 1980; 21:307–313.

29. Goris M. ECG gating does it adequately monitor ventricular contraction (letter to the editor). *J Nucl Med* 1980; 21:1201.

30. Bacharach SL, Green MV, Vitale D, White G, Douglas MA, Bonow Rom Larson SM. Optimum fourier filtering of cardiac data: a minimum-error method: concise communication. *J Nucl Med* 1983; 24:1176–1184.

31. Geffers H, Adam WE, Bitter F, Sigel H, Kampmann H. Data processing and functional imaging in radionuclide ventriculography. In Information processing in medical imaging. Oak Ridge, Biological Computing Technology Information Center, 1977; pp. 322–332.

32. Pavel DG. Detection and quantification of regional wall motion abnormalities using phase analysis of equilibrium gated cardiac studies. *Clin Nucl Med* 1983; 8:315–321.

33. Byrom E, Pavel DG, Swirny S, Myer-Pavel C. Phase images of gated cardiac studies: a standard evaluation procedure. In Esser P (ed): functional mapping of organ systems and other computer topics. *NY Society of Nuclear Medicine* 1981; pp. 129–136.

34. Walton S, Yannikas J, Jarret PH, Brown NJG, Swanton RH, Ell PJ. Phasic abnormalities of LV emptying in coronary artery disease. *Br Heart J* 1981; 46:245–253.

35. Holman BL, Wynne J, Idoine J, Zielonka J, Neil J. The Paradox Image: a noninvasive index of regional left-ventricular dyskinesis. *J Nucl Med* 1979; 20:1237–1242.

36. Maddox DE, Holman BL, Wynne J, Idoine J, Parker JA, Uren R, Neill JM, Cohn PF. Ejection fraction image: a noninvasive index of regional left ventricular wall motion. *Am J Cardiol* 1978; 41:1230–1238.

37. Maddox DE, Wynne J, Uren R, Parker JA, Idoine J, Siegel LC, Neill JN, Cohn PF, Holman BL. regional ejection fraction: a quantitative radionuclide index of regional left ventricular performance. *Circulation* 1979; 59:1001–1009.

38. Foster C, Pollock ML, Rod JL, Dymond DS, Wible G, Schmidt DH. Evaluation of Functional Capacity during Exercise Radionuclide Angiography. *Cardiology* 1983; 70:85–93.

39. Brady TJ, Lo K, Thrall JH, Walton JA, Brymer JF, Pitt B. Exercise radionuclide ejection fraction: correlation with exercise contrast ventriculography. *Radiology* 1979; 132:703–705.

40. Berman DS, Safel AF, DeNardo GL, Bogren HG, Mason DT. Clinical assessment of left ventricular regional contraction patterns and ejection fraction by high resolution gated scintigraphy. *J Nucl Med* 1975; 16:865–874.

41. Berger HJ, Reduto LA, Johnstone DE, Borkowski H, Sands JM, Cohen LS, Langou RA, Gottschalk A, Zaret BL, Pytlick L. Global and regional left ventricular response to bicycle exercise in coronary artery disease. *Am J Med* 1979; 66:13–21.

42. Campos CT, Chu HW, D'Agostino HJ, Jones RH. Comparison of rest and exercise radionuclide angiocardiography and exercise treadmill testing for diagnosis of anatomically extensive coronary artery disease. *Circulation* 1983; 67:1204–1210.

43. Borer JS, Bacharach SL, Green MV, Kent KM, Epstein SE, Johnston GS. Real-time radionuclide cineangiography in the noninvasive of global and regional left ventricular function at rest and during exercise in patients with coronary-artery disease. *N Engl J Med* 1977; 296:839–844.

44. Henning H, Schelbert H, Crawford MH, Karliner JS, Ashburn W, O'Rourke RA. Left ventricular performance assessed by radionuclide angiocardiography and echocardiography in patients with previous myocardial infarction. *Circulation* 1975; 52:1069–1075.

45. Brady,TJ, Thrall JH, Clare JM, Rogers WL, LO K, Pitt B. Exercise radionuclide ventriculography: practical considerations and sensitivity of coronary artery disease detection 1. *Radiology* 1979; 132:697–702.

46. Jones RH, McEwan P, Newman GE, Port S, Rerych SK, Scholz PM, Upton MT, Peter CA, Austin EH, Leong K-H, Gibbons RJ, Cobb FR, Coleman RE, Sabiston DC. Accuracy of diagnosis of coronary artery disease by radionuclide measurement. *Circulation* 1981; 64:586–601.

47. Osbakken MD, Boucher CA, Okada RD, Bingham JB, Strauss HW, Pohost GM. Spectrum of global left ventricular responses to supine exercise: limitation in the use of ejection fraction in identifying patients with coronary artery disease. *Am J Cardiol* 1983; 51: 28–35.

48. Lindsay J Jr, Nolan NG, Goldstein SA, Bacos JM. The usefulness of radionuclide ventriculography for the identification and assessment of patients with coronary artery diseases. *Am Heart Journal* 1980; 99:310–318.

49. Gibbons RJ, Lee KL, Pryor D, Harrel FE, Coleman E, Cobb FR, Rosati RA, Jones RH. The use of radionuclide angiography in the diagnosis of coronary artery disease-a logistic regression analysis. *Circulation* 1983; 68:740–746.

50. Jones RH, Floyd RD, Austin EH, Sabiston DC. The role of radionuclide angiocardiography in the preoperative prediction of pain relief and prolonged survival following coronary artery bypass grafting. *Ann Surg* 1983; 197:743–754.

51. Debusk RF. Position Paper: evaluation of patients after recent acute myocardial infarction. *Ann Intern Med* 1989; 110:485–488.

52. DeBusk RF. Specialized testing after recent acute myocardial Infarction. *Ann Intern Med* 1989; 110:470–481.

53. Hung J, Goris ML, Nash E, Kraemer HC, DeBusk RF. Comparative value of maximal treadmill testing, exercise thallium myocardial perfusion scintigraphy and exercise radionuclide ventriculography for distinguishing high and low risk patients soon after acute myocardial infarction. *Am J Cardiol* 1984; 53:1221–1227.

54. Gibson RS, Watson DD, Craddock GB, Crampton RS, Kaiser DL, Denny MJ, Beller GA. Prediction of cardiac events after uncomplicated myocardial infarction: a prospective study comparing pre-discharge exercise thallium-201 scintigraphy and coronary angiography. *Circulation* 1983; 68:321–336.

55. Corbett JR, Dhemer GJ, Lewis SE, Woodward W, Henderson E, Parkey RW, Blomqvist CG, Willerson JT. The prognostic value of submaximal exercise testing

with radionuclide ventriculography before hospital discharge in patients with recent myocardial infarction. *Circulation* 1981; 64:535–544.

56. Felipe RF, Prpic H, Arndt JW, van der Wall EE, Pauwels EKJ. Role of radionuclide ventriculography in evaluating cardiac function. *Eur J Radiol* 1991; 12:20–29.

57. Handler B, Pavel DG, Pietra R, Swiryn S, Byrom E, Lam W, Rosen KM. Equilibrium radionuclide gated angiography in patients with tricuspid regurgitation. *Am J Cardiol* 1983; 51:305–310.

58. Hecht HS, Hopkins JM. Exercise induced regional wall motion abnormalities on radionuclide angiography. Lack of reliability for detection of coronary artery disease in the presence of valvular heart disease. *Am J Cardiol* 1981; 47:861–865.

59. Hung J, Goldwater D, Convertino VA, McKillop JH, Goris ML, DeBusk RF. Mechanisms for decreased exercise capacity following bed rest in normal middle-aged men. *Am J Cardiol* 1983; 51:344–348.

60. Jansen FH, Van Kroonenburgh MJPG, Van der Wall EE, Valkema R, Zwinderman AH, Blokland JAK, Pauwels EKJ. The diagnostic value of immediate post-exercise left ventricular ejection fraction (LVEF). *Am J Physiol Imaging* 1991; 6:105–109.

61. Horn HR, Teichholz LE, Cohn PF, Herman MV, Gorlin R. Augmentation of left ventricular contraction pattern in coronary artery disease by an inotropic catecholamine. *Circulation* 1974; 44:1063–1067.

62. Alexander J, Dainiak N, Berger HJ, Goldman L, Johnstone D, Duffy T, Schwartz P, Gottschalk A, Zaret B. Serial assessment of doxorubin cardiotoxicity with quantitative radionuclide angiocardiography. *N Engl J Med* 1979; 300:278–283.

63. McKillop JH, Bristow MR, Goris ML, Billingham ME, Bockemuehl K. Sensitivity and specificity of radionuclide ejection fractions in Doxorubicin cardiotoxicity. *Am Heart J* 1983; 106:1048–1056.

64. Pauwels EKJ, Horning SJ, Goris ML. Sequential equilibrium gated radionuclide angiocardiography for the detection of doxorubicin cardiotoxicity. *Radiot Oncol* 1983; 1:83–87.

65. DeBusk RF, Pitts W, Haskell W, Nouston N. Comparison of cardiovascular responses to static-dynamic effort and dynamic effort alone in patients with chronic ischemic heart disease. *Circulation* 1979; 59:977–984.

66. Brady TJ, Thrall JH, Lo K, Pitt B. The importance of adequate exercise in the detection of coronary heart disease by radionuclide ventriculography. *J Nucl Med* 1980; 21:1125–1130.

67. Freeman MR, Berman DS, Staniloff H, Elkayam U, Maddahi J, Swan HJC, Forrester J. Comparison of upright and supine bicycle exercise in the detection and evaluation of extent of coronary artery disease by equilibrium radionuclide ventriculography. *Am Heart J* 1981; 102:182–189.

68. Everaert H, Franken PR, Flamen P, Goris M, Momen A, Bossuyt A. Left ventricular ejection fraction from gated SPECT myocardial perfusion studies: a method based on the radial distribution of count rate density across the myocardial wall. *Eur J Nucl Med* 1996; 12:1628–1633.

Chapter 7

Bayes' Theorem and Related Problems

7.1. BAYES' THEOREM: A TAUTOLOGY

Thomas Bayes (c. 1702–7 April 1761) was a British mathematician and Presbyterian minister, known for having formulated a specific case of the theorem that bears his name: Bayes' theorem, which was published posthumously (1).

Some feel that he became interested in probability while reviewing a work written in 1755 by Thomas Simpson,[a] but others think he learned mathematics and probability while reading a book by de Moivre.[b]

Bayes' theorem is a simple derivation of the tautology I = I (Figure 7.1).

$$I = I,$$

$$\frac{I}{U} = \frac{I}{U},$$

$$\frac{I}{D}\frac{D}{U} = \frac{I}{S}\frac{S}{U}.$$

All we did was divide both sides of the original equation by U, and then for each side dividing and multiplying by the same value, which is the same as multiplying by 1.

---

[a]Thomas Simpson (20 August 1710–14 May 1761) was a British mathematician, inventor and eponym of Simpson's rule to approximate definite integrals. However, this rule was also found 200 years earlier in Johannes Kepler as the so-called Keplersche Fassregel.

[b]Abraham de Moivre, a French mathematician famous for de Moivre's formula that links complex numbers and trigonometry, and for his work on the normal distribution and probability theory.

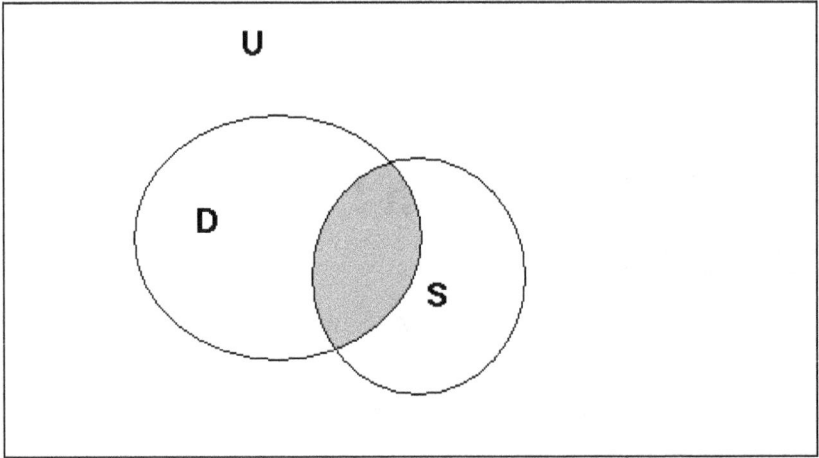

Figure 7.1   The figure represents first, the totality of all possible states (the universum of states), U. Within this universum, there is a population that has a disease (D) and one that has a symptom (S). In gray, there is an intersection of both populations (I) containing the population of those who have both the disease and symptom.

Now consider:

The ratio D:U is the proportion of all people who have the disease; this defines the prevalence of the disease. The usual notation is P(D+), the probability of having the disease. The same holds for S/U = P(S+) the prevalence of the symptom.

I/D is the probability of having the symptom if one belongs to the population that has the disease. It is a conditional probability, symbolically expressed as P(S+ | D+). The same holds for I/S, which is the probability of having the disease if one has the symptom or the conditional probability P(D+ | S+).

Rewriting the last line we have:

$$P(S+\,|\,D+)P(D+) = P(D+\,|\,S+)P(S+).$$

Rearranging, we have:

$$P(D+\,|\,S+) = \frac{P(S+\,|\,D+)P(D+)}{P(S+)}.$$

Now consider the population P(S). It represents the prevalence of the symptom and is composed of those who have the symptoms and the disease, and those who have the symptoms, but not the disease.

$$(S+) = P(S+\,|\,D+)(D+) + P(S+\,|\,D-)(D-),$$

$$\frac{(S+)}{U} = P(S+\,|\,D+)\frac{(D+)}{U} + P(S+\,|\,D-)\frac{(D-)}{U},$$

$$P(S+) = P(S+\,|\,D+)P(D+) + P(S+\,|\,D-)P(D-),$$

$$P(S+) = P(S+\,|\,D+)P(D+) + P(S+\,|\,D-)[1 - P(D+)].$$

The derivation is based on the following definitions:

1. The total amount of those with the symptom and disease is the product of the conditional probability of having the symptom in the presence of disease multiplied by the number of those who have the disease.
2. As shown above, the prevalence of the symptom and of the disease is the number divided by the universum of subjects.
3. The prevalence of those who do not have the disease is (1 – the prevalence of those who have the disease).

The derived and most common formulation of Bayes' Theorem is as follows:

$$P(D+\,|\,S+) = \frac{P(S+\,|\,D+)P(D+)}{P(S+\,|\,D+)P(D+) + P(S+\,|\,D-)[1 - P(D+)]}.$$

Finally, in medicine, the conditional probabilities are named specifically:

1. $P(S+\,|\,D+)$ is the sensitivity.
2. $P(S-\,|\,D-)$ is the specificity.
3. $P(D+\,|\,S+)$ is the positive predictive value (PPV).
4. $P(D-\,|\,S-)$ is the negative predictive value (NPV).
5. $P(S+\,|\,D-)$ is the non-specificity.
6. LR is the likelihood ratio $(LR = P(S+\,|\,D+)/P(S+\,|\,D-))$.

In the formulation of the theorem, it is important to note that the prevalence (on the right) influences the positive predictive value. Only the sensitivity, specificity, and non-specificity are the operating characteristics of a diagnostic test. The predictive values depend on the prevalence. Attention to the Bayes theorem started to be adopted in Nuclear Medicine mainly in the eighties and in Nuclear Cardiology (2–22).

7.2. USING THE LIKELIHOOD RATIO

The usual form of the Bayes theorem has one disadvantage, in that the complete analysis seems to require one to analyze the disease and the absence of disease separately. The likelihood ratio simplifies that problem: It is the ratio of sensitivity over non-specificity or $P(S+\mid D+)/P(S+\mid D-)$.

$$P(D+\mid S+) = \frac{P(S+\mid D+)P(D+)}{P(S+\mid D+)P(D+) + P(S+\mid D-)[1 - P(D+)]},$$

$$P(D+\mid S+) = \frac{\frac{P(S+\mid D+)}{P(S+\mid D-)}P(D+)}{\frac{P(S+\mid D+)}{P(S+\mid D-)}P(D+) + \frac{P(S+\mid D-)}{P(S+\mid D-)}[1 - P(D+)]},$$

$$P(D+\mid S+) = \frac{LR \times P(D+)}{LR \times P(D+) + 1 - P(D+)},$$

$$P(D+\mid S+) = \frac{LR \times P(D+)}{1 + P(D+)(LR - 1)}.$$

Ratios are interesting because they lack symmetry.[c] If the sensitivity is zero, the likelihood ratio is zero. If sensitivity and non-specificity are equal (the test has no diagnostic value), $LR = 1$ if the specificity is a perfect 1, the likelihood ratio is infinite. The three outcomes result to: For $LR = 0$, the positive predictive value is zero (Figure 7.2).

$$P(D+\mid S+) = \frac{0 \times P(D+)}{1 + P(D+)(0 - 1)} = 0.$$

For a non-diagnostic value of $LR = 1$, the positive predictive value is equal to the prevalence (nothing has changed).

$$P(D+\mid S+) = \frac{P(D+)}{1 + P(D+) \times 0} = P(D+).$$

If the specificity is 1, $LR = \infty$, and the positive predictive value is 1:

$$P(D+\mid S+) = \frac{\infty \times P(D+)}{1 + P(D+)(\infty)} = \frac{\infty}{\infty} = 1.$$

7.3. TWO BY TWO CONTINGENCY TABLES

Two by two contingency tables present as follows in Table 7.1.
What it shows is the distribution of a population: those who have or do not have the symptoms, those who have or do not have the disease, and the overlapping classes. In a clinical study, one would classify the patients as having the symptoms, and then see which patients, in either class, have the disease.

There are two questions to resolve: accuracy and verfication bias.

---

[c]The ratio of $2/1 = 2$, the ratio of $1/2 = 0.5$. If a ratio of 1 is the standard, the distance for one ratio is 1, while the other one is 0.5.

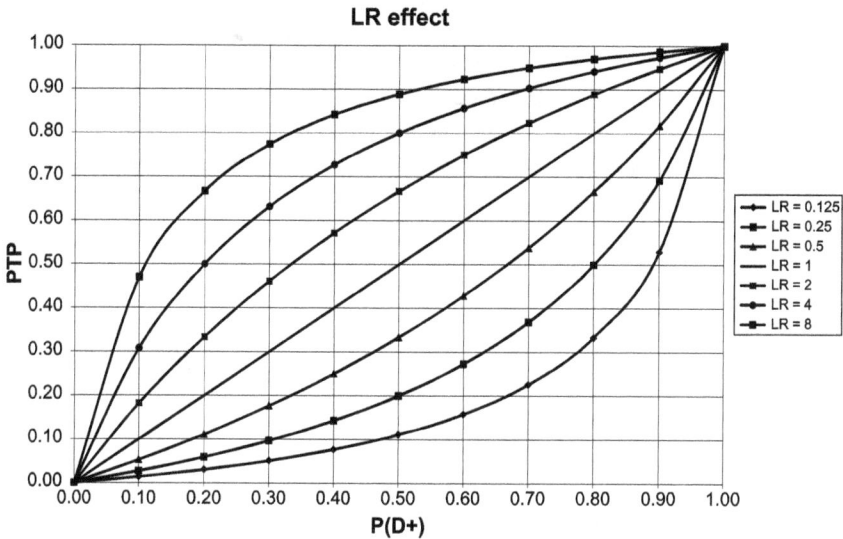

Figure 7.2 The x-axis represents the prevalence or prior probability, while the y-axis represents the positive predictive value. The likelihood ratios are "symmetric" in the sense that 1/2 is made symmetrical to 2/1, and 1/10 to 10/1. The presence of a symptom can make the PPV smaller or larger depending on the LR value.

Table 7.1

	S+	S−	
D+	a	b	a + b
D−	c	d	c + d
	a + c	b + d	a + b + c + d

The total population is N = a + b + c + d.
The prevalence of the disease is (a + b)/N also called prior probability.
The prevalence of the symptom is (a + c)/N.
The positive predictive value (PPV) = a/(a + c).
The negative predictive value (NPV) = d/(b + d).
The sensitivity is a/(a + b).
The specificity is d/(c + d).

7.4. ACCURACY

People have presented the results based on accuracy. In this case, the accuracy would be $(a + d)/N$; it shows the fraction of cases when the classification is correct. The problem with accuracy is that, like the predictive values, it depends on the prevalence. Consider the hypothetical case of a disease with a prevalence of 0.05,[d] and a test that is always negative (worthless) (Table 7.2).

Table 7.2

	S+	S−	Total
D+	0	5	5
D−	0	95	95
Total	0	100	100

The accuracy is $(1 + 94)/100 = 0.95$. This appears good. However,

$P(S+\,|\,D+) = 0.00,$

$P(D+) = 0.05,$

$(1 - P(D+)) = 0.95,$

$P(S+\,|\,D-) = 0.00,$

$P(S+) = 0.00,$

$PPV = $ not defined (0/0).

However, the accuracy is 95% (95/100). Accuracy to characterize a diagnostic test should be avoided (at all cost).[e]

7.5. VERIFICATION BIAS

The proper way to verify the diagnostic value of a test would be to select patients who will have defining tests (e.g. a biopsy), and have them all undergo the test. In general, that is not the case. For myocardial perfusion studies, the usual approach was to test the patient suspected of having coronary artery disease, and then "wait" for the coronary angiogram as a confirmation. What naturally happens is that negative studies tend to be followed less frequently by defining studies, unlike positive

---

[d]For computational reasons it is easier to express all the values as fractions.
[e]It is not avoided nearly enough.

studies. In the extreme, positive studies are verified all the time, whereas negative studies are never. The result is that in contingency tables, specificity tends to decrease, while sensitivity increases (23).

7.5.1. *Eliminating Verification Bias by Applying the Positive and Negative Predictive Values to the Population as a Whole (10, 11, 19)*

Assume a population in which verification is provided more frequently when the symptom is positive. An example would be myocardial perfusion for the diagnosis of coronary artery disease. The defining diagnosis is a coronary angiography.

In the group that had an angiography, the positive predictive value was $P(D+ | S+)$. If the decision to go on to angiography is exclusively based on the positivity of the test (in addition to criteria that apply both to the negatives and positive cases equally) then this value is valid for the population as a whole. The same holds for $P(D+ | S-)$.

However, $P(S+)$ and $P(S-)$ are known for the population as a whole. Hence, an unbiased estimate of $P(S+ | D+)$ can be obtained by substitution.

Note that we could have written Bayes' theorem differently:

$$P(S+ | D+)P(D+) = P(D+ | S+)P(S+),$$

$$P(S+ | D+) = \frac{P(D+ | S+)P(S+)}{P(D+)},$$

$$P(S+ | D+) = \frac{P(D+ | S+) \cdot P(S+)}{P(D+ | S+) \cdot P(S+) + P(D+ | S-) \cdot P(S-)}.$$

Example

In this example, 200 (Table 7.3) patients went on to have a coronary arteriogram.

The relevant numbers extracted from the contingency table are the sensitivity (75%), the non-specificity (13%), the PPV (90%) and the NPV (30%). The total number of patients undergoing a perfusion study was actually 600. In total, there were 200 positive studies and 400 negative ones. Positive studies were oversampled by the defining study (100/200). The negative studies were undersampled (100/200) (Table 7.4).[f]

What we know are the column totals (200, 400 and 600). The fundamental thesis in Diamond's paper (10) is that the PPV and the NPVs do not change. The argument is subtle: The biased selection for arteriography is based exclusively on the positivity.

---

[f]In our example the sampling ratio is 3/1.

Table 7.3

	S+	S−	
D+	90	30	120
D−	10	70	80
	100	100	200

$P(S+ \mid D+) = 0.75$
$P(D+) = 0.60$
$(1 - P(D+)) = 0.40$
$P(S+ \mid D−) = 0.13$
$P(S+) = 0.50$
$P(D+ \mid S+) = 0.90$ (PPV)
$P(D+ \mid S−) = 0.30$
$P(D− \mid S−) = 0.70$ (NPV)

Table 7.4

	S+	S−	
D+	180	120	300
D−	20	280	300
	200	400	600

The analysis of the table yields:
$P(D+ \mid S+) = 0.90$
$P(D+ \mid S−) = 0.30$
$P(D+) = 0.50$
$(1 - P(S+)) = 0.67$
$P(S+) = 0.33$
$P(S+ \mid D+) = 0.60$
$P(S+ \mid D−) = 0.07$

The fact that the patients were referred for the perfusion study makes the population homogeneous in all other aspects.[g]

However (see Table 7.4), if the PVV is the same in the verified and unverified cases, in the second row, the first box value can be computed as 200×0.90 (were 0.90 is the PPV), and in the first row, second box can be computed as 400×0.30).

---

[g]This is very doubtful, since not all positives or negatives are treated equally.

The sensitivity and non-specificity are 0.60 and 0.07 respectively versus the observed values of 0.75 and 0.13.

7.5.2. *Validation of Diagnostic Procedures on Stratified Populations (24)*

In some diseases (e.g. coronary artery disease), the population can be fairly well stratified for risk (e.g. a young female without hypertension or chest pain has a lower probability of having coronary artery disease than an elderly man with hypertension and typical angina). In fact, Diamond *et al.* (4, 8) proposed such a stratification model.

Assume that a population as a whole can be stratified in N groups of progressively increased risks for coronary artery disease. Each group would have its own prevalence $P_i(D+)$. If the diagnostic test is perfect, the prevalence of the symptom $P_i(S+)$ would be equal to $P^i(D+)$.

Again we look for Bayes' theorem:

$$P(S+) = P(S+ \mid D+)P(D+) + P(S+ \mid D-)[1 - P(D+)],$$

$$P(S+) = P(D+)[P(S+ \mid D+) - P(S+ \mid D-)] - P(S+ \mid D-).$$

The rearranged equation in which $P(S+)$ is predicted by $P(D+)$ is actually the equation of a straight line $ax + b$, in which $a = [P(S+ \mid D+) - P(S+ \mid D-)]$ and $b = P(S+ \mid D-)$ and X is the prevalance.

There is an associated observation: b is the non-specificity and corresponds to the intercept. The number of positive tests when the prevalence is actually zero. However, the slope is the sensitivity minus the non-specificity; the prevalence of symptoms does not start at zero. Different possible errors in the derivation of the operating characteristics have been extensively reviewed by Diamond, and are worth studying (10, 11, 13, 19, 20).

7.6. HETEROGENEOUS POPULATIONS

The classical formulation of Bayes' theorem:

$$P(D+ \mid S+) = \frac{P(S+ \mid D+)P(D+)}{P(S+ \mid D+)P(D+) + P(S+ \mid D-)[1 - P(D+)]}.$$

Assume that the population is binary: It is composed of people who do not have the disease (unafflicted) and those who have (afflicted). In actuality, patients in an average clinic are mostly afflicted with something, but not the disease they are concerned about. The unafflicted are not necessarily normal. Typically, in a test that spreads its net a little wide (FDG PET imaging), the aim is to look for malignancy, but FDG uptake is also elevated in infected lymphnodes, pneumonia and other "benign" conditions. If there are $N-1$ benign or not targeted conditions (including totally normal) and 1 targeted condition, the formulation should be rewritten as:

$$P(D_j+\,|\,S+) = \frac{P(S+\,|\,D_j+)P(D_j+)}{\sum_{i=1}^{i=N} P(S+\,|\,D_i+)P(D_i+)}.$$

The denominator would be different for different populations. The primary lesson is that the specificity of FDG PET or FDG PET/CT is independent of the disease targeted, but depends on the population under study.[h]

7.7. MULTIPLE SIGNS AND SYMPTOMS

If the patient undergoes two tests, each of them with known operating characteristics, how should the results be combined?

Let us define $P(A+\,|\,D+)$ and $P(A+\,|\,D-)$, and $P(B+\,|\,D+)$ and $P(B+\,|\,D-)$ as the operating characteristic of test 1 and test 2 respectively. The prevalence is $P(D+)$ to start with. After the first test we have:

$$P(D+\,|\,A+) = (P(A+\,|\,D+)P(D+))/P(A+).$$

After the second test (for which the prior probability is the posterior probability):

$$P(D+\,|\,A+,B+) = \frac{P(B+\,|\,D+)P(D+\,|\,A+)}{P(B+)},$$

$$P(D+\,|\,A+,B+) = \frac{P(B+\,|\,D+)\frac{(P(A+\,|\,D+)P(D+))}{P(A+)}}{P(B+)},$$

$$P(D+\,|\,A+,B+) = \frac{P(B+\,|\,D+)P(A+\,|\,D+)P(D+)}{P(B+)P(A+)}.$$

In general, if we use N tests serially, the expression of Bayes theorem would be:

$$|P(D+\,|\,S_1^N) = \frac{P(D+)\prod_{i=1}^{i=N}(S_i+\,|\,D+)}{\prod_{i=1}^{i=N} p(S_i+)}.$$

---

[h]The literature tends to review FDG PET in the following terms: The sensitivity and specificity of FDG PET in diseases "A". But the specificity is independent of the disease. The title should be: The sensitivity and specificity of FDG PET in a population targeted for disease "A".

One would be tempted to apply Bayes theorem serially, but that would be wrong as the test outcomes may be dependent on each other. Association between symptoms can be detected by chi-square[i] testing. If the association is strong, serial application of Bayes' theorem would be equivalent to applying the results of a single test multiple times and assume that the identical outcomes validate each other.

When reviewing the literature in Chapters 1, 5 and 6, it was noticeable that many authors (and editors for that matter) are uncomfortable with the logical AND and logical OR. In myocardial perfusion, we have stress defect (S) that can be either transient or "fixed", and can be associated with normal or abnormal washout. Normal would be normal for all attributes. There are at least four attributes that can be abnormal. If the criterion is "or", then any abnormality makes the study positive. If the criterion is "and", a particular combination defines the study as positive. But the operating characteristics for all attributes or combination of attributes are different.[j] There are two important factors:

1. If there are two attributes, the combination "and" must have an equal or smaller sensitivity and an equal or higher specificity than the same attributes in an "or" combination.
2. During tabulation of the results (again for two attributes) they should be tabulated as $(-; -), (-; +), (+; -)$ and $(+; +)$, unless there is a need for obfuscation.

7.8. QUANTITATIVE SYMPTOMS AND RECEIVER OPERATING CHARACTERISTICS FUNCTION (ROC FUNCTION)

Not all signs and symptoms are binary. ST segment depressions are expressed (amongst other things) in mm. The metric is the ST segment depression, the value is mm. There could be circumstances where the operating characteristics of a diagnostic test change as the metric value changes. Diamond reviewed such an effect for the electrocardiographic stress test (6, 7). To a test returning a continuous value, one can apply multiple discriminant thresholds and for each define a sensitivity and specificity; the result is a ROC (25–28).

As an example, assume the existence of a test metric, with values ranging from 0 to 10. We could *a priori* call the test positive if the metric value is >1, >2 etc. till >9 since most, not all, normal patients have a value of zero or close to zero.

---

[i]Originally X^2.

[j]Very strangely, in the tabulation of results, the majority of publication reviews are unspecific.

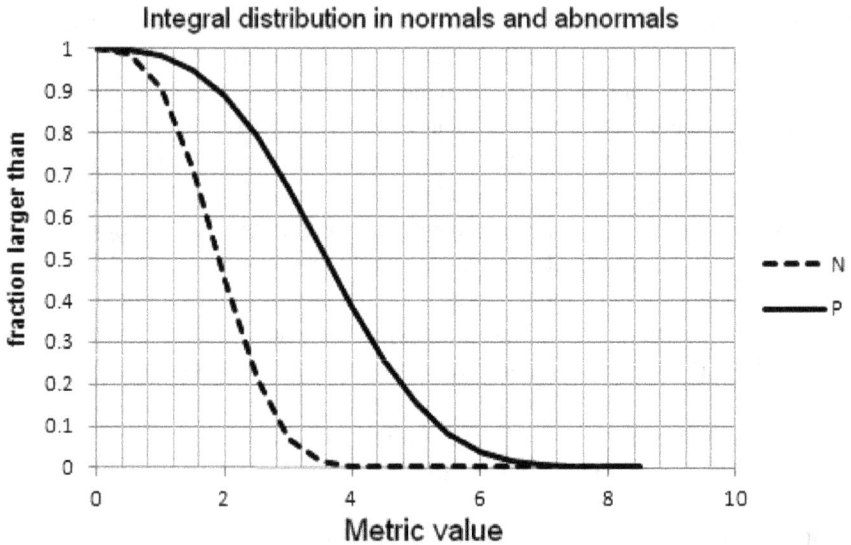

Figure 7.3   The graph represents the percentage of normal or abnormal patients who have a metric value equal or larger than x. In the figure's example, if the metric is 1, only 40% of the unaffected patients have a value larger or equal; however, of the affected patients, 90% would have a value larger or equal.

The underlying basis is as follows: the integral frequency distribution function of the metric value is different for people with and without the disease.

In this particular case, the distribution functions are (Figure 7.3)

$$N = 1.e^{-ax^3},$$

$$P = 1.e^{-bx^3}.$$

Both distribution functions are defined in terms of the metric "x", but the goal is to define P as a function of N. We first redefine x as a function of N : $\ln(N) = -ax^3$. Then, we redefine x as: $x = (\frac{\ln(N)}{-a})^{\frac{1}{3}}$. Finally, we substitute in P : $P = e^{-b(\frac{\ln(N)}{-a})^3}$.

The connection between the "false positive" cases[k] and the "true positive" cases[l] is the metric with values x and the two distribution functions in x.

The test does not necessarily has to have a quantitative metric, but one can be manufactured: The test can be characterized as normal = 0, or abnormal (subjectively) = 1 − 4 (29). Or, if there are many observers reading in a binary mode

---

[k]In the contingency table c/(c + d) or non-specificity (Table 7.1).
[l]In the contingency table a/(a + b) or sensitivity.

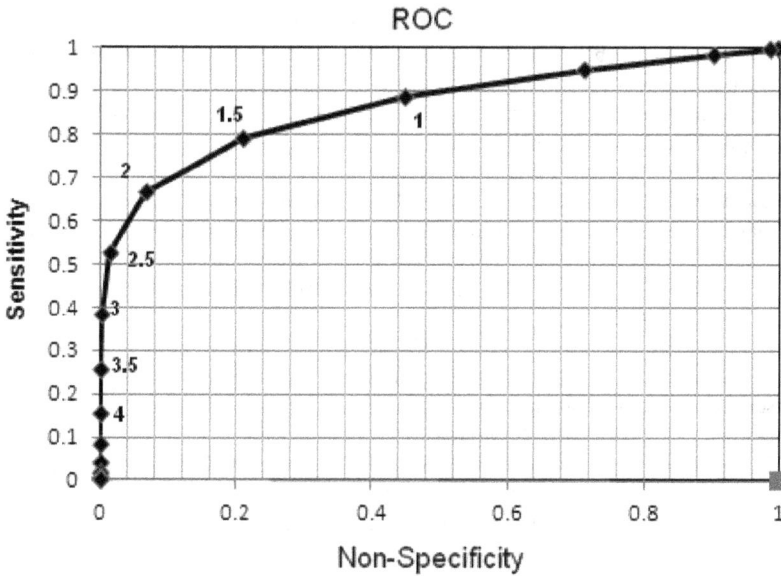

Figure 7.4 ROC function derived from the relationship between the distribution functions of the metric between affected and unaffected subject.

(normal or abnormal) if some are "severe" and others more "tolerant", an ROC function could still be constructed out of each reader sensitivity/specificity pair.

The problem, as we will see, is the interpretation of the function (13, 14), which is sometimes controversial. A "better" test has a larger area under the curve, but subjective interpretations do not generally yield enough data points to define an analytical function, and the area has to be computed graphically (Figure 7.4).

REFERENCES

1. Google.
2. Christopher TD, Konstantinow G, Jones RH. Bayesian analysis of data from radionuclide angiocardiograms for diagnosis of coronary artery disease. *Circulation* 1984; 69:1.
3. Detrano R, Yiannikas J, Salcedo EE, Rincon G, Go RT, Williams G, Leatherman J. Bayesian probability analysis: a prospective demonstration of its clinical utility in diagnosing coronary disease. *Circulation* 1984; 69:3.
4. Diamond GA, Forrester JS. Analysis of probability as an aid in the clinical diagnosis of coronary artery disease. *New Engl J Med* 1979; 300:1350–1358.
5. Diamond GA, Forrester JS, Hirsh M. Application of conditional probability analysis to the clinical diagnosis of coronary artery disease. *J Clin Invest* 1980; 65:1210–1221.

6. Diamond GA, Forrester JS. Improved interpretation of a continuous variable in diagnostic testing: probabilistic analysis of scintigraphic rest and exercise left ventricular ejection fractions for coronary disease detection. *Am Heart J* 1981; 102:189–195.
7. Diamond GA, Hirsch M, Forrester JS, Staniloff HM, Vas R, Halpern SW, Swan HJC. Application of information theory to clinical diagnostic testing: the electrocardiographic stress test. *Circulation* 1981; 63:915–921.
8. Diamond GA, Staniloff HM, Forrester JS, Pollock BH, Swan HJC. Computer assisted diagnosis in the noninvasive evaluation of patients with suspected coronary artery disease. *J Am Coll Cardiol* 1983; 1:444–455.
9. Diamond GA. A clinically relevant classification of chest discomfort. *J Am Coll Cardiol* 1983; 1(2):574–575.
10. Diamond GA, Rozanski A, Forrester JS, Morris D, Pollock BH, Staniloff HM, Berman DS, Swan HJC. A model for assessing the sensitivity and specificity of tests subject to selection bias: application to exercise radionuclide ventriculography for diagnosis of coronary artery disease. *J Chron Dis* 1986; 39:343–355.
11. Diamond GA. Reverend Bayes' silent majority: an alternative factor affecting sensitivity and specificity of exercise electrocardiography. *Am J Cardiol* 1986; 57:1175–1179.
12. Diamond GA, Pollock BH, Work JW. Clinician decisions and computers. *J Am Coll Cardiol* 1987; 9:1385–1396.
13. Diamond GA. ROC Steady: a receiver operating characteristic curve that is invariant relative to selection bias. *Med Decis Making* 1987; 7:238–243.
14. Diamond GA. ROCky III. *Med Decis Making* 1987; 7:247–249.
15. Diamond GA. What is the effect of sampling error on ROC analysis in the face of verification bias? *Med Decis Making* 1987; 7:247–249.
16. Diamond GA. Limited assurances. *Am J Cardiol* 1989; 63:99–100.
17. Diamond GA. How accurate is SPECT thallium scintigraphy? *J Am Coll Cardiol* 1990; 16:1017–1021.
18. Diamond GA. Affirmative actions: can the discriminant accuracy of a test be determined in the face of selection bias? *Med Decis Making* 1991; 11:48–56.
19. Diamond GA. Scotched on the ROCs. *Med Decis Making* 1991; 11:198–200.
20. Diamond GA, Denton TA, Berman DS, Cohen I. Prior restraint: a Bayesian perspective on the optimization of technology utilization for diagnosis of coronary artery disease. *Am J Cardiol* 1995; 76:82–86.
21. Fryback, Dennis G. Bayes' theorem and conditional non independence of data in medical diagnosis. *Comput Biomed Res* 1976; 11:423–434.
22. Fryback, Dennis G. Bayes' theorem and conditional non-independence of data in medical diagnosis. *Comput Biomed Res* 1976; 11:423–434.
23. Rozanski A. The declining specificity of exercise radionuclide. *New Eng J Med* 1983; 309:518–522.
24. Goris ML, Bretille J, Askienazy S, Purcell GP, Savelli V. The validation of diagnostic procedures on stratified populations: application on the quantification of thallium myocardial perfusion scintigraphy. *J Am Physiol Imaging* 1989; 4:11–15.
25. Goodenough DJ, Rossman K, Lusted LB. Radiographic applications of receiver operating characteristics curve. *Radiology* 1975; 110:89–95.
26. Metz CE. Basic principles of ROC analysis. *Semin Nucl Med* 1978; 8:283–298.

27. Metz CE, Goodenough DJ, Rossman K. Evaluation of receiver operating characteristic curve data in terms of information theory with application to radiography. *Radiology* 1973; 109:297–304.

28. Swets JA. ROC analysis applied to the evaluation of medical imaging techniques. *Invest Radiol* 1979; 14:109–121.

29. Hachamovitch R, *et al.* Incremental prognostic value of myocardial perfusion single photon emission computed tomography for the prediction of cardiac death: differential stratification for risk of cardiac death and myocardial infarction. *Circulation* 1979; 97:535–543.

Chapter 8

Compartmental Systems

8.1. TRACER KINETICS AND COMPARTMENTAL SYSTEMS

There are different approaches to the analysis of tracer kinetics (of biological systems). One approach is based on compartmental analysis. The concept of compartment in first order systems is basically that all the elements within a compartment are subjected to the same probability and that this probability is time invariant. The easiest way to understand is to consider a tub filling at one end by a faucet (at constant flow F) and emptying through the drain at the other end (at a constant flow F). It appears obvious that a water molecule just coming out of the faucet is less likely to leave through the drain at that moment than a water molecule that was resident in the tub for a long time; the tub acts as a delay line between faucet and drain.

However, imagine the tub being a whirlpool. The water molecules move so rapidly from one location in the tub to another, such that the new water molecule is just as likely as the veteran water molecule to be near the drain.[a]

If the inflow and outflow are equal (F), a steady state is reached, with a constant total amount of water in the whirlpool (the volume = V); however, not always the same water is in the whirlpool. To distinguish a steady state (in which the volume is constant but the content changes) from a stagnant state (in which the volume also does not change but it is always the same water), one can at a time zero add a very small amount (tracer amount) of an easy-to-measure soluble substance in the whirlpool. What will happen and how to describe it? The whirlpool can be described as a single compartmental system.

In general, compartmental analysis is defined as follows: There are a finite number of spaces (named compartments) in which the substance (tracer) can reside in. Those compartments are connected by the pathways which the tracer can follow

---

[a]This assumes that the outflow rate is relatively low in comparison with the mixing rate.

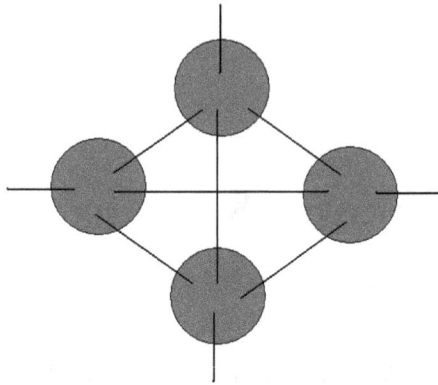

Figure 8.1   Schematic representation of the general (mammillary) compartmental system. Each compartment has connections with all others and to the outside.

to transfer from one compartment to another. Figure 8.1 represents the most general four-compartment system. The two defining characteristics of compartmental systems are:

- The probability that a fraction of the tracer elements goes from compartment i to compartment j per unit of time is time invariant.
- At any given time, the concentration of the tracer within a compartment is spatially constant. Another way to put it is that mixing within a compartment is instantaneous.

The system illustrated in Figure 8.1 is defined by a set of the state equations defining compartment k:

$$\frac{dN_k}{dt} = \sum_{i \neq k} a_{ik}N_i + \sum_{i \neq k} -a_{ki}N_k.$$

- N_k is the number (amount) of tracer elements in compartment k.
- "a_{ki}" is the fraction of the elements in compartment k that transfers to compartment i (it corresponds to a loss). "a_{ki}" is a fractional transfer rate.
- "a_{ik}" is the fraction of the elements in compartment i transferring to compartment k (it corresponds for a gain for compartment k). "a_{ik}" is a fractional rate.
- N_i is the number (amount) of tracer elements in compartment i.
- The rate of change or transfer[b] is $a_{ij}N_j$.

---

[b]As opposed to the fractional rate.

Compartmental systems are prototypes of first order kinetics. In zero order kinetics, the rates are constant. In first order kinetics, the fractional rates are constant but the rates depend on the amount present.

In general, if the biological kinetic system is described by n compartments, the total system will be described by n exponentials, as we will see in Sections 8.4, 8.4.3 and 8.5.4.

We will study the following cases: single compartmental systems and radioactive decay, constant infusion models, catenary systems and two compartmental systems.

8.2. SINGLE COMPARTMENTAL SYSTEMS AND RADIOACTIVE DECAY

8.2.1. *Single Compartment Systems*

Single compartments are defined as follows:

- At time $t = 0$, N_0 molecules of tracer are introduced to the compartment. All the changes of $N(t)$, the total amount still in the system at time t, are due to tracer elements leaving the compartment.
- At all times, the concentration $c(t)$ is constant throughout the compartment and is equal to $N(t)/V$, where V is the volume of the compartment.
- The amount of tracer leaving the system at any time is equal to the flow F multiplied by the concentration $c(t)$.
- The probability that an individual tracer element leaves the compartment is time invariant (regardless of location in the compartment). This probability (λ) has units of time^{-1} and in the example given above, λ is equal to the outflow F divided by the total volume (of water in the whirlpool).
- The actual rate of change is therefore the probability λ multiplying the number of elements present $N(t)$.
- To review:

  a. The rate at which the tracer leaves the system is

  $$\frac{dN}{dt} = -F \cdot c(t),$$

  $$\frac{dN}{dt} = -\frac{F}{V} \cdot V \cdot c(t), \qquad (8.1)$$

  $$\frac{dN}{dt} = -\frac{F}{V} N(t).$$

b. The time invariant probability is the ratio of the time invariant flow over the time invariant volume (in a steady state situation). Hence,

$$\frac{dN}{dt} = -\lambda N. \tag{8.2}$$

Equation 8.2 states that the change in the number of elements per unit of time (dN/dt) is equal to the individual probability λ multiplied by the number of elements present (N). In general, λ is the fractional turnover rate.[c] Equation 8.2 is the state equation and is first order in N. The state equation(s) define(s) the system, together with the initial condition(s). In our example, the initial condition is that before time zero, the compartment does not contain the tracer ($N(t < 0) = 0$), and that after $t = 0$, no more tracer is added.

Rearranging Equation 8.2, we obtain,

$$\frac{dN}{N} = -\lambda \cdot dt. \tag{8.3}$$

To go from the derivative expression to the actual (integral) function, we first integrate both sides,

$$\int_{N(0)}^{N(t)} \frac{dN}{N} = -\lambda \int_{0}^{t} dt. \tag{8.4}$$

The integral over x of dx/x is the natural logarithm of x. The integral over t of dt is t. The integration is from 0 to t. We therefore obtain (Section 10.2),

$$\ln(N)|_{N(0)}^{N(t)} = -\lambda \cdot t|_{0}^{t}. \tag{8.5}$$

When the limits are inserted we obtain;

$$\ln(N(t)) - \ln(N(0)) = -\lambda \cdot t. \tag{8.6}$$

Since the difference between logarithms is equal to the logarithm of the ratio, Equation 8.6 can be rewritten as,

$$\ln\left(\frac{N(t)}{N(0)}\right) = -\lambda \cdot t. \tag{8.7}$$

We now take the exponent of both sides of the equation, keeping in mind that the exponent of the logarithm of x is equal to x. Hence,

$$\frac{N(t)}{N(0)} = e^{-\lambda \cdot t}, \tag{8.8}$$

---

[c]In pulmonary ventilation studies, λ is the fractional ventilation rate $\dot{V}/V$ (Section 2.1.3.1).

which by rearrangement leads to the final equation,

$$N(t) = N_0 \cdot e^{-\lambda \cdot t}. \tag{8.9}$$

Equation 8.9 is the exponential equation which amongst other physical systems describes radioactive decay.

It is unnecessary to follow all the steps that lead from Equation 8.2 to 8.9, but it is important to remember that the state equation is first order[d] in the variable quantity whose kinetics must be defined, and that the result is an exponential function.

If λ is 0.10, it means that during the time interval t and $t + 1$, the amount of tracer will decrease by 10%. The absolute decrease, however, will be larger at earlier times than at later times.

There is one additional characteristic of a single compartmental system, relevant to the concept of effective half-life: If there are many exits from the compartment, the state equation is not affected. One could conceive it as biologically but not mathematically relevant. Consider a tracer that is distributed only in the plasma, is excreted in both kidneys and is accumulated in the liver. If the kinetics are first order, the loss to the left kidney is $f_L F_L c(t)$, on the right $f_R F_R c(t)$ and to the liver $f_H F_H c(t)$. The three organs share the same plasma concentration and $V_p c(t) = N(t)$. F represents plasma flow and f represents extraction efficiency (see Equation 8.1).

$$\frac{dN}{dt} = \frac{f_L F_L}{V_p} N(t) + \frac{f_R F_R}{V_p} N(t) + \frac{f_H F_H}{V_p} N(t),$$

$$\frac{dN}{dt} = \left(\frac{f_L F_L}{V_p} + \frac{f_R F_R}{V_p} + \frac{f_H F_H}{V_p} \right) N(t), \tag{8.10}$$

$$\frac{dN}{dt} = (\lambda_L + \lambda_R + \lambda_H) N(t).$$

The fractional excretion rates are additive.

8.2.2. *Radioactive Decay*

Equation 8.9 is the exponential equation which amongst other physical systems describes radioactive decay. In this form, the equation describes the number of atoms that have not decayed and are present at time t. To express the system in terms of radioactivity rather than number of atoms, we remember that radioactivity is defined as number of disintegrations per unit of time. The number of disintegrations

---

[d]N to the power 1 or N^1.

is equal to the number of atoms disappearing, hence, from Equation 8.9 we define $A(t)$, the radioactivity at time t as $\lambda.N(t)$.

$$\lambda N(t) = \lambda N(0) \cdot e^{-\lambda t},$$

$$A(t) = A(0) \cdot e^{-\lambda \cdot t}.$$

In the case of radioactive decay, the term λ is the decay constant. If the specific activity is the activity per number of atoms, then carrier free radioactive materials with the highest decay constant have the highest specific activity. When specific activity is expressed as mCi/g, the question is more complicated.[e]

8.2.3. Half-Life and Effective Half-Life

It is customary to characterize isotopes not by the decay constant, but by half-life. The period or half-life $T_{1/2}$ is the time needed for the activity to reach half of its original level, and is defined as follows,

$$0.5N(0) = N(0) \cdot e^{-\lambda T_{1/2}},$$

$$\ln(0.5) = -\lambda T_{1/2}.$$

Since the natural logarithm of 0.5 is -0.693,

$$-0.693 = -\lambda T_{1/2},$$

$$T_{1/2} = \frac{0.693}{\lambda}. \tag{8.11}$$

The half-life defined here is the physical half-life. For biological systems, one also defined the biological half-life and the effective half-life. If the kinetics of the substance in a biological system can be described by an exponential function with an exponent b, independent of radioactive decay, the effective kinetics are described by,[f]

$$A(t) = A(0) \cdot e^{-(\lambda+b)t}. \tag{8.12}$$

The effective half-life is derived as follows (the fractional excretion rates or decay constants are additive),

$$T_{effective} = \frac{0.693}{\lambda + b} = \frac{0.693}{\frac{0.693}{T_\lambda} + \frac{0.693}{T_b}} = \frac{1}{\frac{1}{T_\lambda} + \frac{1}{T_b}} = \frac{T_\lambda T_b}{T_\lambda + T_b}. \tag{8.13}$$

---

[e] 1 g of 99m-Tc contains $N_A/99$ atoms, 1 g of 131-I contains $N_A/131$ atoms, where N_A is Avogadro's number.
[f] Because the state equation is $dA/dt = -(\lambda + b)A$. See Equation 8.10.

8.2.4. *Average Life*[g]

The average life or average residency time is generally computed by averaging the exit time Section 10.4.

In this case, $dN/dt = \lambda N$ therefore, the rate (of exit) is:

$$\lambda N e^{-\lambda t}.$$

The average time is:

$$\frac{\lambda N \int_0^\infty t e^{-\lambda t} dt}{\lambda N \int_0^\infty e^{-\lambda t} dt} = \frac{1}{\lambda}. \tag{8.14}$$

The average life is also defined by the area under the curve/initial value:

$$\bar{t} = \frac{A(0) \cdot \int_0^\infty e^{-\lambda \cdot t} \cdot dt}{A(0)} = \frac{1}{\lambda}. \tag{8.15}$$

The relation between half-life and average life is therefore,

$$T_{1/2} = 0.693 \cdot \bar{t}.$$

8.2.5. *Semi-Logarithmic Plots*

To define the decay rate of a pure radioactive isotope, one can count the activity over a number of time intervals, and plot the results $N(t)$. One can also plot the logarithm of $N(t)$ (Section 10.2.1)

$$N(t) = N(0)e^{-\lambda t},$$
$$\ln(N(t)) = \ln(N(0)) - \lambda t. \tag{8.6}$$

This transformation yields the equation of a straight line $y = b + ax$ whose intercept (b) is the logarithm of the initial value, and whose slope (a) is equal to λ. The plot is characterized as a semi-log plot, because the x-axis is linear, and the y-axis is logarithmic.

There is an interesting aspect to the single compartment and plotted in semi-log plot. Consider an intravascular tracer that is cleared from the plasma by the liver, spleen and bone marrow (which would be the case for a colloidal substance, e.g. ^{99m}Tc-sulfur colloid).

The kinetics would be well described by a single exponential, with λ the fractional uptake in liver, spleen and bone marrow. If the plasma is sampled at

---

[g]The average life is used in dosimetry as the residency time or $\mu CiHr/\mu Ci$ (Section 4.2.1) and in non-compartmental models as transit time (Section 9.1.1).

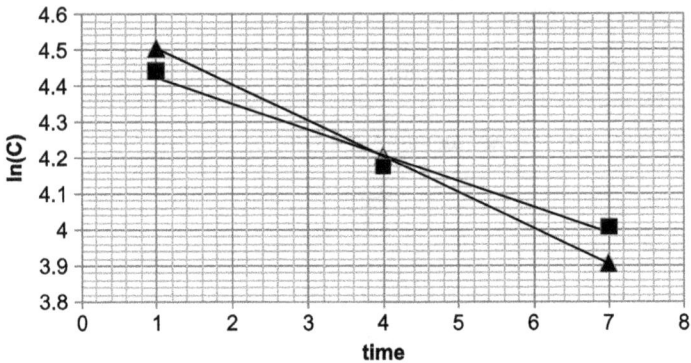

Figure 8.2   The figure shows a semi-log plot of three concentrations. The triangles are a noiseless exponential. The squares are the same values plus noise. For the noiseless data, the logarithmic intercept value is 4.6, the linear value is 100 (I), the fractional clearance rate (λ) is 0.1. If the injected amount was 10 000 (D), the volume would be 100 (V), and the flow (F) would be 10. The corresponding values for the noisy data are respectively 4.49, 89.8 (I), 0.07 (λ), 111.3 (V) and the flow $F = 8.07$. Since the flow is λV, and the noise decreased λ, but increased V, in a single exponential fits the error is somewhat mitigated. This characteristic is exploited in the determination of the glomerular filtration by using only the slow component of the concentration curve (Section 1.7).

three time points, one could obtain three concentration values (C_1, C_2, C_3). If the concentrations are transformed to their logarithm, they would be aligned in a straight line. The exponent of the value of that line at time zero, C_0 (the intercept), would correspond to the injected amount D divided by the plasma volume V. Hence, $V = D/C_0$. The plasma flow to the liver, spleen and marrow would be λV (Figure 8.2).

The analysis of a single compartmental system does not seem to be very relevant except in the description of radioactive decay and by derivation, the definition of half-life, average life (which will be used in internal dosimetry) and effective half-life. However, this simple derivation was used in early analysis of liver blood flow with radio-tracers and the kinetics of sodium as related to renal function (1, 2). In addition, it served us to become familiar with the formality of exponential functions, and will in a few of the following cases, be the basis to jump to more complex systems (see also Section 1.7.2 and Figure 1.12).

8.2.6. *A Simple Application: Liver Blood Flow*

Dobson *et al.* (1, 2) were interested in arterial liver blood flow. From experiments in mice, they noticed that the reticuloendothelial cells lining the sinusoidals in the liver capture 100% of all the colloid passing through the hepatic vessels. Since the collodial substance does not leave the plasma and is not excreted by the kidneys, they considered that the clearance from plasma was only to the liver with minor contributions from clearance to the spleen and bone marrow. Indeed, when they plotted the concentration of the colloid in the plasma, they found the data to be well fitted by a single exponential: $C_t = C_0 e^{-at}$. If the plasma volume is V (ml), and the flow to the liver, spleen and bone marrow is F (ml/min), the fractional clearance from the plasma has to be $a = F/V (ml^{-1})$. If the plasma volume V (ml) is known, the flow to the liver (spleen and bone marrow) is equal to aV (ml/min) (Figure 8.2).

8.3. CONSTANT INFUSION MODEL

A particular case of a tracer kinetic model is the single compartment constant infusion model. The model is relevant in the discussion of glomerular filtration (Section 1.7.1) and lung ventilation imaging (Section 2.1.3).

The tracer is infused into the compartment at a constant rate k(g/min). The volume or size of the compartment is V(ml). The total amount of tracer in the compartment at time $t = A(t)$. The exit from the compartment is first order: the outflow from the compartment is F. The amount of A leaving the compartment is $Fc(t) = F\frac{A}{V} = \frac{F}{V}A$, or the flow to volume ratio multiplying the concentration. If $F/V = a$, the state equation is (Figure 8.3)

$$\frac{dA}{dt} = k - aA. \tag{8.16}$$

The unit for aA is g/(min). For convenience, we assume the initial condition to be $A_{(0)} = 0$.

The derivation of the integral function A(t) is straightforward,

$$\frac{dA}{dt}e^{+at} + ae^{+at}A = ke^{+at}. \tag{8.17}$$

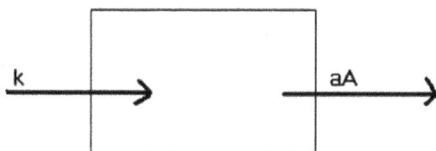

Figure 8.3 The tracer is introduced at a constant rate (g/min or mCi/min) but leaves the compartment at a rate proportional to the amount present in the compartment aA. The value a is the time invariant fractional rate.

At this time, one observes that the argument on the left is a partial derivative, or the derivative of a product (Section 10.3). The integration of both sides yields

$$Ae^{at}|_0^t = \frac{k}{a}e^{at}|_0^t,$$

$$A_{(t)}e^{at} - A_{(0)}e^0 = \frac{k}{a}\left(e^{at} - e^0\right),^{\text{h}}$$

$$A_{(t)}e^{at} = \frac{k}{a}\left(e^{at} - 1\right).$$

Finally,

$$A(t) = \frac{k}{a}(1 - e^{-at}). \tag{8.18}$$

The function A approaches a constant or equilibrium value, when $dA/dt = 0$,[i] supposedly at $t = \infty$ (Figure 8.4).

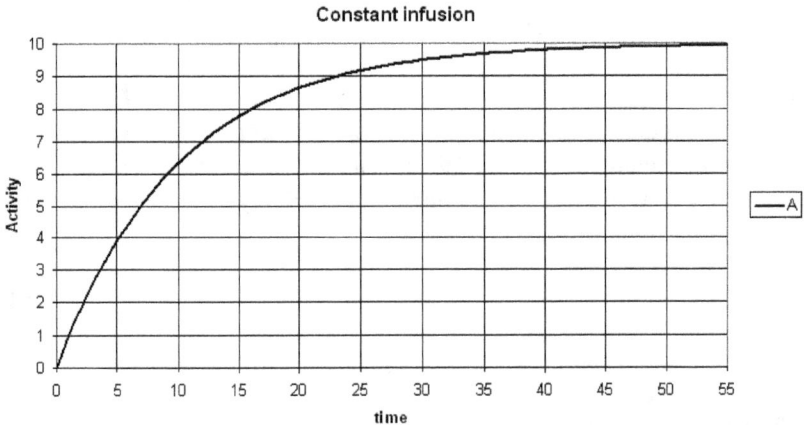

Constant infusion

Figure 8.4 Equation 8.18 has value 0 at time 0, because $e^0 = 1$, and the term $(1 - e^{-at})$ becomes $(1 - 1)$. At $t = \infty$, $e^{-\infty} = 0$, and $A(\infty) = k/a$. The figure shows the evolution of A in time for $k = 1$ and $a = 0.1$.

If $dA/dt = 0$, then $0 = k - aA(\infty)$ and therefore, $k = aA(\infty)$.

$$k = aVc(\infty),$$

$$\frac{k}{c(\infty)} = aV,$$

---

[h]The initial conditions state that $A_{(0)} = 0$ and we know that $e^0 = 1$.
[i]By definition, if there is zero change, equilibrium is reached.

$$\frac{k}{c(\infty)} = \frac{F}{V}V,$$

$$\frac{k}{c(\infty)} = F. \tag{8.19}$$

The constant k is the infusion rate and therefore would have units g/min or milli-Curie/min. The equilibrium concentration would be g/ml or mCi/ml and the flow F should be ml/min.

Indeed,

$$k\left(\frac{g}{min}\right) \times \frac{1}{c(\infty)} \left(\frac{1}{g/ml}\right) = F\left(\frac{ml}{min}\right).^{j}$$

When we discuss glomerular filtration, we will find that the continuous infusion method necessarily results in a GFR expressed in ml/min which is not a favorable unit, because it begs a correction for the subject size (Section 1.7.1).

8.4. CATENARY SYSTEMS

Catenary systems are first order systems in which the connection is from compartment "I" to compartment "$i + 1$" unidirectionally. There are three principles to remember.

- The output function is a function of the input function convoluted by the transit function (Section 10.7.3)
- If only for that reason, the output function has an apparent rate that cannot be faster than the rate of the input function.
- If the transit function has no mixing, the system acts as a delay line, and the output function is the input function.

In cathenary systems, multiple systems are connected but in a unidimensional manner. The tracer leaving compartment i enters compartment $i + 1$, and there is no return from $i + 1$ to i (Figure 8.5).

For each compartment, the state equation is as follows:

$$\frac{dN_i}{dt} = -a_{i,i+1} \cdot N_i + a_{i-1,i} \cdot N_{i-1}.$$

We will explicitly solve a two-compartmental catenary system, with an initial condition of $N_{1(0)} = D$ (for total dose) and $N_{2(0)} = 0$.

---

[j]It is useful after long and complex derivations to check the "dimensions" or "units" of the results.

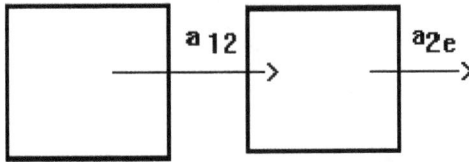

Figure 8.5   Catenary systems: Two compartmental example.

There are two state equations:

$$\frac{dN_1}{dt} = -a_{12} \cdot N_1,$$

$$\frac{dN_2}{dt} = +a_{12} \cdot N_1 - a_{2e} \cdot N_2.$$

The first compartment has a state equation of a single compartment system. Therefore,

$$N_1(t) = N_1(0)e^{-a_{12}t}. \tag{8.12}$$

In the state equation for compartment 2, the integral solution for compartment 1 is substituted:

$$\frac{dN_2}{dt} = +a_{12} \cdot N_1(0) \cdot e^{-a_{12} \cdot t} - a_{2e} \cdot N_2. \tag{8.20}$$

By rearranging Equation 8.20,

$$\frac{dN_2}{dt} + a_{2e} \cdot N_2 = +a_{12} \cdot N_1(0) \cdot e^{-a_{12} \cdot t}.$$

Again, we multiply both sides by an exponential with a_{2e},[k]

$$\frac{dN_2}{dt} \cdot e^{+a_{2e} \cdot t} + a_{2e} \cdot e^{+a_{2e} \cdot t} \cdot N_2 = +a_{12} \cdot N_1(0) \cdot e^{(a_{2e}-a_{12}) \cdot t}.$$

By integrating both sides, and remembering that $N_2(0) = 0$ we obtain,

$$N_2(t) \cdot e^{+a_{2e} \cdot t} = a_{12}N_1(0) \int_0^t e^{(a_{2e}-a_{12}) \cdot t} \cdot dt,$$

---

[k]See partial derivatives in Section 10.3.

$$N_2(t) \cdot e^{+a_{2e} \cdot t} = \frac{a_{12}}{(a_{2e} - a_{12})} N_1(0) \cdot \left[e^{(a_{2e} - a_{12}) \cdot t} - 1. \right],$$

$$N_2(t) = \frac{a_{12}}{(a_{2e} - a_{12})} N_1(0) \cdot \left[e^{-a_{12} \cdot t} - e^{-a_{2e} \cdot t} \right]. \tag{8.21}$$

The result for N_2 is a sum of two exponentials, multiplied by $N_1(0)$, or the injected dose D, and a ratio of the fractional turnover rates. In this formalism, we assumed that $a_{2e} > a_{12}$, the ratio of fractional turnover rates is positive and, except at t = 0, when both exponential terms are equal to 1, the exponent in a_{2e} is always smaller than the one in a_{12}. Hence, $N_2(t)$ is zero or positive.

If $a_{2e} < a_{12}$, the ratio of the fractional turnover rates becomes negative, and it is customary to rewrite the equation by reversing the exponential terms and the terms in the denominator of the coefficient ratio:

$$N_2(t) = \frac{\alpha_{12}}{(\alpha_{12} - \alpha_{2e})} N_1(0)(e^{-\alpha_{2e} t} - e^{-\alpha_{12} t}). \tag{8.22}$$

The ratio and the sum of exponentials in both cases remain positive. Not only that, but in the long run, when t becomes large, the function is always dominated by the slowest component. The general rule is that the apparent kinetics in systems in series are dominated by the kinetics of the slowest component. A consequence exists in the interpretation of renograms with excretable tracers. An immediate application is the Bateman equation (Section 8.4.1).

8.4.1. *Generators and the Bateman Equation*

In the case of generators or parent—daughter relationships, we consider activities rather than number of elements. The basic relationship is $A = \lambda N$. Set λ_1 is the decay constant of the generator or mother isotope, and λ_2 is the decay constant of the daughter. If $\lambda_1 < \lambda_2$, the equation is written as,[1]

$$A_2(t) = \frac{\lambda_2 \cdot A_1(0)}{(\lambda_2 - \lambda_1)} \cdot \left[e^{-\lambda_1 \cdot t} - e^{-\lambda_2 \cdot t} \right]. \tag{8.23}$$

At t = 0, or immediately after the generator has been eluted, the sum of the two exponentials become $(1 - 1)$. The initial value of the daughter isotope is zero. If the difference between λ_1 and λ_2 is significant, there will be a time when $e^{-\lambda t}$ becomes much smaller than the first term in λ_1. Therefore, as time proceeds the

---

[1]The more general solution (also known as the "Bateman Equation") does not assume that $A_2(0) = 0$. In that case, a term is added of the form $A_2(0) \cdot e^{-\lambda_2 t}$.

equation becomes

$$A_2(t) = \frac{\lambda_2 \cdot A_1(0)}{(\lambda_2 - \lambda_1)} \cdot e^{-\lambda_1 \cdot t}.$$

The equation is then a mono-exponential function with a fractional rate corresponding to that of the slow component, in this case the mother isotope or the generator.

The order of the coefficients is important: If the order is $(\lambda_2 - \lambda_1)$, the order is $(e^{-\lambda_1 t} - e^{-\lambda_2 t})$, but if $\lambda_1 > \lambda_2$ the order is $e^{-\lambda_2 t} - e^{-\lambda_1 t}$ and as time progresses the mono-exponential has the rate of the daughter isotope.

Three terms have been defined: secular equilibrium, transient equilibrium and no equilibrium.

The secular equilibrium occurs when $\lambda_2 \gg \lambda_1$ (the daughter isotope has a significantly shorter half-life that the mother one) in such a way that in relation to t, $\lambda_1 \approx 0$. Bateman's Equation reduces to

$$A_2(t) = A_1(0) \cdot \left[1 - e^{-\lambda_2 t}\right].$$

As time progresses, the activity of the daughter becomes equal to that of the parent at time $t = \infty$.

Transient equilibrium occurs if the half-life of the daughter is shorter than that of the parent isotope $(\lambda_2 > \lambda_1)$, which in turn, however, is not near zero. There are three consequences:

- The ratio of decay constants multiplying the initial parent activity is larger than 1. There will eventually be more daughter than parent.

$$\frac{\lambda_2}{(\lambda_2 - \lambda_1)} > 1.$$

- When the time "t" becomes appreciable, the daughter's activity decreases with the decay rate of the parent. This happens because the second term in Bateman's equation becomes zero or near zero:

$$A_2(t) = \frac{\lambda_2 \cdot A_1(0)}{(\lambda_2 - \lambda_1)} \cdot [e^{-\lambda_1 \cdot t} - 0].$$

- Equilibrium is reached for an instant when there is exactly as much daughter as parent.

No equilibrium occurs when $\lambda_1 > \lambda_2$. After a time, there is only daughter left, decaying at its own rate

$$A_2(t) = \frac{\lambda_2 \cdot A_1(0)}{(\lambda_1 - \lambda_2)} \cdot [e^{-\lambda_2 t} - 0].$$

We have not discussed the case were $\lambda_1 = \lambda_2$, but this will be elaborated in the next section.

For two compartments in series, we have demonstrated that the slow component ends up dominating the kinetics of the second component. The well-known application in nuclear medicine is the Bateman equation describing generators. The issue will be visited again in the discussion of the renogram, where a slow "excretion" phase could be due, not to obstruction, but counterintuitively, to low global renal function and the resulting slow plasma clearance (Figure 8.6).

8.4.2. *Multiple Compartments with Identical Fractional Transfer Rates*

There is a special case in which multiple compartments in series have identical fractional transfer rates (in this case "a").

We first look at compartment 2. The derivation is the same as the one we used before, except that $a_{12} = a_{22e}$.

$$\frac{dN_2}{dt} = +a_{12} \cdot N_1(0) \cdot e^{-a_{12} \cdot t} - a_{2e} \cdot N_2, \qquad (8.24)$$

is reduced to

$$\frac{dN_2}{dt} + aN_2 = aN_{1(0)}e^{-at}.$$

When both sides are multiplied by e^{+at}, this becomes

$$\frac{dN_2}{dt}e^{at} + aN_2e^{at} = aN_{1(0)}e^{(a-a)t} = aN_{1(0)}.$$

On the right side, the exponent term is reduced to 1. However, the integral introduces a term in "t". The integration on both sides yields

$$N_2e^{at} = aN_{1(0)} \int_0^t dt,$$

$$N_{2(t)} = atN_{1(0)}e^{-at}. \qquad (8.25)$$

For compartment 3, we start with a^2: $\frac{dN_3}{dt} = a^2tN_{1(0)}e^{-at} - aN_3$ and eventually we have:

$$N_{3(t)} = \frac{a^2t^2}{2}N_{1(0)}e^{-at}.$$

It is easy to show that in the end:

$$N_1(t) = \frac{\alpha^{n-1}t^{n-1}}{(n-1)!}Qe^{-\alpha t}, \qquad (8.26)$$

where Q is the injected dose and therefore $= N_1(0)$, and $(n-1)!$ is a factorial. If $n = 5$, the factorial is $(1 \times 2 \times 3 \times 4 \times 5)$.[m]

---

[m]$0! = 1$.

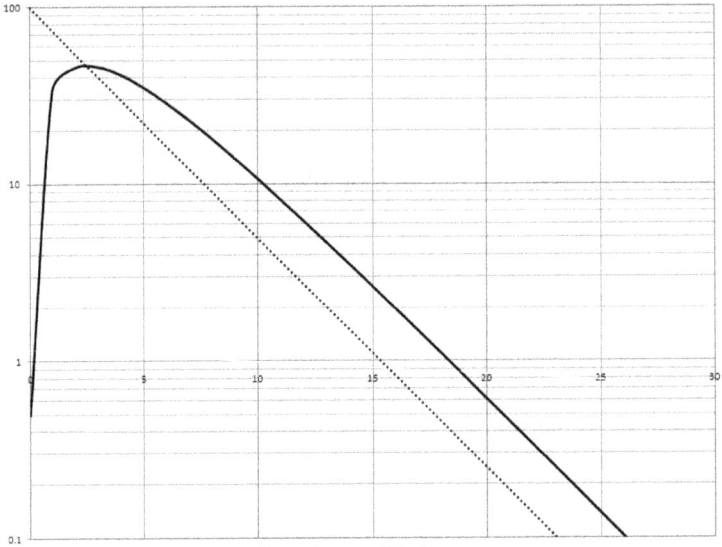

Transient equilibrium:

$$A_2(t) = \frac{\lambda_2 \cdot A_1(0)}{(\lambda_2 - \lambda_1)} \cdot \left[e^{-\lambda_1 \cdot t} - 0 \right]$$

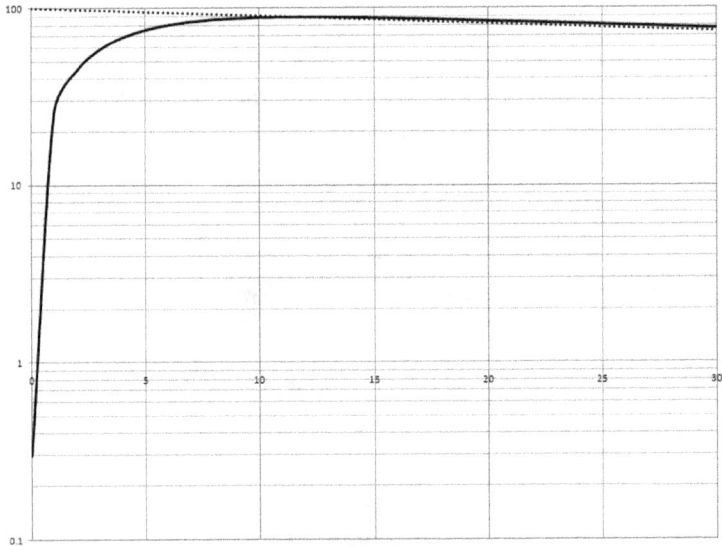

Secular equilibrium:

$$A_2(t) = A_1(0) \cdot \left[1 - e^{-\lambda_2 t} \right]$$

Figure 8.6   The figure illustrates the three cases discussed above.

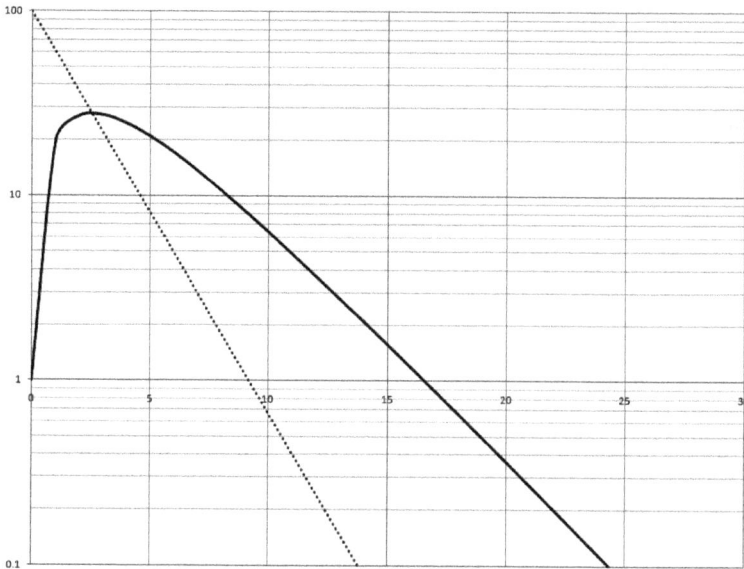

No equilibrium:

$$A_2(t) = \frac{\lambda_2 \cdot A_1(0)}{(\lambda_1 - \lambda_2)} \cdot \left[e^{-\lambda_2 t} - 0 \right]$$

Figure 8.6 (*Continued*)

The fina formulation is actually that of a gamma function (Section 10.2.2). The name, gamma function, comes from the integral

$$\int_0^\infty x^{n-1} e^{-x} dx = \Gamma(n),$$

or

$$\int_0^\infty z^n x^{n-1} e^{-zx} dx = \Gamma(n),$$

where $\Gamma(1) = 1$ and $\Gamma(n = 1) = n\Gamma(n)$ if $n > 0$ or n! if n is an integer (see Section 10.2.2 and Figure 8.7).

The function describes what would happen to a bolus in an arterial system, in which fl w and diameter remain constant, but there is a fi ed difference in velocity between the center and the periphery.

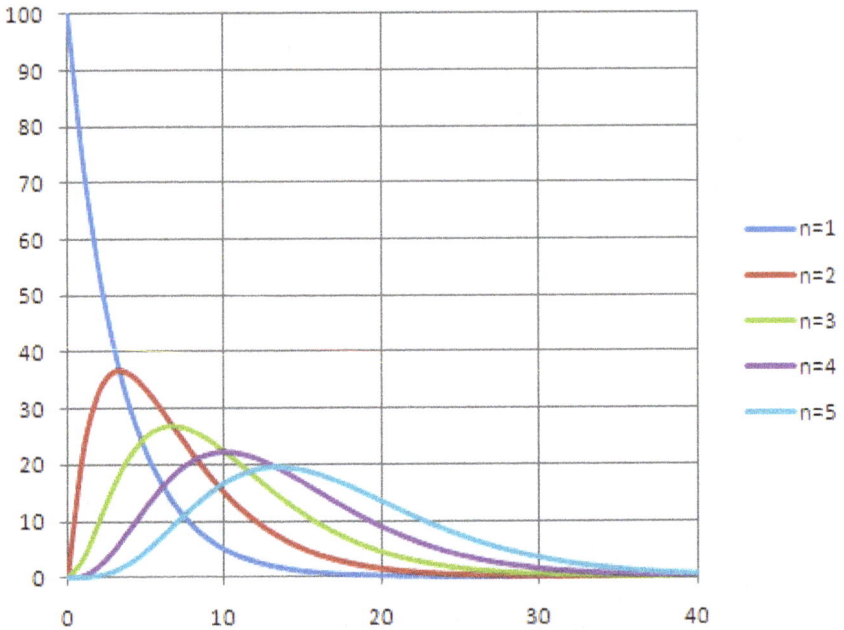

Figure 8.7 The figur shows the kinetics of fi e systems in series with the same fractional transfer rates. As the activity progresses, the "bolus" becomes flatte and wider. The system has interesting features. First, according to the definitio of compartments, at $t = 0 + dt$, there already is activity in the nth compartment. There is no delay in compartments. However, if delay is introduced, the result is similar to lagged normal density curves proposed by Bassingthwaighte (3, 4) as a model of arterial dilution.

8.5. TWO-COMPARTMENTAL SYSTEMS

8.5.1. *The System*

- Like all compartmental systems, the transit from one system to the other is define by a time invariant probability, e.g. the transfer from compartment 1 (e.g. plasma) to compartment 2 (e.g. extracellular fluid except plasma) is the fractional transfer rate multiplied by the amount present in compartment 1.
- The fact that there is a compartment 3 is not contradictory. The model is based on the assumption that tracer entering 3 does not return to 1. In a model describing the kinetics of a renal tracer, compartment 3 would be both kidneys.
- The concentration at any time is constant throughout the compartments.

- The generalized model would also include a transfer from N2 to N3, but in the case of renal tracers as in most cases, there is no irreversible uptake in N3, except from the plasma.
- Again, the system is characterized by the initial conditions and by a set of differential equations describing changes (the state equations).
- The first equation expresses that changes in the quantity of tracer in compartment 1 (N_1) are due to losses to compartments 3 and 2, and gains from the tracer returning from compartment 2. The coefficients a_{ij} are constant (time invariant) and are the fraction of N_i (the content in compartment i) that is transferred to compartment j.

$$\frac{dN_1}{dt} = -(\alpha_{13} + \alpha_{12}) + \alpha_{21}N_2. \tag{8.27}$$

- The second equation expresses that changes in the quantity of tracers in compartment 2 (N_2) are due to losses from compartment 2 to compartment 1 and gains from transfer from compartment 1 to compartment 2.

$$\frac{dN_2}{dt} = \alpha_{12}N_1 - \alpha_{21}N_2. \tag{8.28}$$

- The coefficients a_{ij} are the fractional transfer rates from i to j. Because the system is in a steady state, the flow F_{12} from 1 to 2 should be equal to the flow from 2 to 1. If the concentration in compartment 1 at time t is $C_{1(t)}$, the transfer rate is $FC_{1(t)}$. But $C_{1(t)} = N_{1(t)}/V_1$, where V_1 is the volume of compartment 1. It is clear that $FC_{1(t)} = F_{12}N_{1(t)}/V_1$ and that $\alpha_{12} = F_{12}/V_1$. Therefore if $F_{12} = F_{21}$, the ratio of the fractional transfer rates are the inverse of the ratio of the volumes:

$$\frac{\alpha_{12}}{\alpha_{21}} = \frac{V_2}{V_1}.$$

- The initial conditions result from a single introduction of a dose D of the tracer in compartment 1 at t = 0.

$$N_1(0) = D,$$

$$N_2(0) = 0,$$

$$N_3(0) = 0.$$

8.5.2. *Integral Solution*

We are looking for the integral solution of the two differential equations. The integral solution will provide a set of functions describing the evolution of N_1 and N_2, as a function of time $N_1(t)$ and $N_2(t)$. We start with Equations 8.27 and 8.28.

The first step is to eliminate the mixture of integrals (N_i) and derivatives dN_i/dt. We will do this through a Laplace transform, represented here by "Λ" (Section 10.7.1.).

$$\Lambda\left[\tfrac{dN_1}{dt}\right] = -(\alpha_{13} + \alpha_{12})\Lambda_{(N_1)} + \alpha_{21}\Lambda_{(N_2)},$$

$$\Lambda\left[\tfrac{dN_2}{dt}\right] = \alpha_{12}\Lambda_{(N_1)} - \alpha_{21}\Lambda_{(N_2)}. \tag{8.29}$$

Remembering the Laplace transform of a first derivative (Section 10.7.1),

$$s\Lambda_{[N_1]} - N_1(0) = -(\alpha_{12} + \alpha_{13})\Lambda_{[N_1]} + \alpha_{21}\Lambda_{[N_2]},$$

$$s\Lambda_{[N_2]} - N_2(0) = \alpha_{12}\Lambda_{[N_1]} - \alpha_{21}\Lambda_{[N_2]}. \tag{8.30}$$

After rearranging, we have either the integral (Ni) at time zero without coefficients or the Laplacian of N_1 with coefficients.

$$(s + \alpha_{12} + \alpha_{13})\Lambda_{[N_1]} - \alpha_{21}\Lambda_{[N_2]} = N_1(0),$$

$$-\alpha_{12}\Lambda_{[N_1]} + (s + \alpha_{21})\Lambda_{[N_2]} = N_2(0). \tag{8.31}$$

The result is a set of two linear equations with two unknowns ($\Lambda_{[N1]}$ and $\Lambda_{[N2]}$). N_1 at $t = 0$ is D (the injected amount) and $N_2 = 0$.

The set of equations is shown in matrix algebra format (Section 10.1.1.).

$$\begin{bmatrix} (s + \alpha_{12} + \alpha_{13}) & -\alpha_{21} \\ -\alpha_{12} & s + \alpha_{21} \end{bmatrix} \bullet \begin{bmatrix} \Lambda_{[N_1]} \\ \Lambda_{[N_2]} \end{bmatrix} = \begin{bmatrix} D \\ 0 \end{bmatrix}. \tag{8.32}$$

The solution for $\Lambda_{[N1]}$ is a determinant ratio which, when rearranged, shows "s" with power 0, 1 and 2.

$$\Lambda_{N_1} = \frac{\begin{vmatrix} D & -\alpha_{21} \\ 0 & s + \alpha_{21} \end{vmatrix}}{\begin{vmatrix} s + \alpha_{12} + \alpha_{13} & -\alpha_{21} \\ -\alpha_{12} & s + \alpha_{21} \end{vmatrix}},$$

$$\Lambda_{[N_1]} = \frac{(s + \alpha_{21})D}{(s + \alpha_{12} + \alpha_{13})(s + \alpha_{21}) - \alpha_{12}\alpha_{21}}, \tag{8.33}$$

$$\Lambda_{[N_1]} = \frac{D(s + \alpha_{21})}{s^2 + (\alpha_{12} + \alpha_{13} + \alpha_{21})s + \alpha_{13}\alpha_{21}}.$$

To progress, we make an abrupt transition here. We know that the Laplace transform of a single exponential is a simple ratio.

$$\Lambda_{[Ne^{-\lambda t}]} = \frac{N}{s + \lambda}.$$

Consider a sum of two exponentials,

$$Ae^{-at} + Be^{-bt}. \tag{8.34}$$

The Laplacian of the sum is equal to the sum of the laplacians

$$\Lambda_{[Ae^{-at}+Be^{-bt}]} = \frac{A}{s + a} + \frac{B}{s + b},$$

$$\Lambda_{[Ae^{-at}+Be^{-bt}]} = \frac{A(s + b) + B(s + a)}{s^2 + (a + b)s + ab}, \tag{8.35}$$

$$\Lambda_{[Ae^{-at}+Be^{-bt}]} = \frac{(A + B)s + (Ab + Ba)}{s^2 + (a + b)s + ab}.$$

Rearranging Equation 8.35, it is easy to derive the values of a_{ij} in terms of α and β by the comparison of the coefficients with equal order of s.

$$\frac{(A + B)s + (Ab + Ba)}{s^2 + (a + b)s + ab} \quad \text{compared to} \quad \frac{Ds + \alpha_{21}D}{s^2 + (\alpha_{12} + \alpha_{13} + \alpha_{21})s + \alpha_{13}\alpha_{21}}.$$

This provides a set of equivalences:

$$(A + B) \cdot s = D \cdot s,$$
$$(Ab + Ba) = \alpha_{21}D,$$
$$(a + b)s = (\alpha_{12} + \alpha_{13} + \alpha_{21}) \cdot s, \tag{8.36a}$$
$$ab = \alpha_{13}\alpha_{21}.$$

The goal (in general) is to define the coefficients $\alpha_{12}, \alpha_{21}, \alpha_{13}$, the fractional transfer rates.

$$D = (A + B),$$
$$\alpha_{21} = \frac{Ab + Ba}{(A + B)},$$
$$\alpha_{13} = \frac{ab}{a_{21}} = \frac{ab(A + B)}{Ab + Ba}, \tag{8.36b}$$
$$\alpha_{12} = a + b - \alpha_{13} - \alpha_{21}.[n]$$

---

[n]The Equations 10.36a and 10.36b are in fact the same set of equivalences.

In most situations, but not all, "a_{13}" is the physiological parameter to define. In the case of a renal tracer, a_{13} would be the fractional renal uptake from the plasma.

8.5.3. Observed Values

In most cases, the easiest compartment to sample is the plasma, but the whole plasma activity cannot be observed uniquely (all of it and only it). The exponentials $Ae^{-at} + Be^{-bt}$ have to be derived from the concentration of the tracer in plasma samples. The metric is concentration and what is observed therefore is D/V_1 and N_1/V_1 and consequently, $A/V_1 = C_A$ and $B/V_1 = C_B$. The observed integral function is $C_Ae^{-at} + C_Be^{-bt}$.

However, the derivation of a_{13} is not affected, as shown here

$$\alpha_{13} = \frac{ab \cdot (A + B)}{(Ab + Ba)} = \frac{ab\frac{(A+B)}{V_1}}{\frac{(Ab+Ba)}{V_1}} = \frac{ab(C_A + C_B)}{(C_Ab + C_Ba)}. \tag{8.37}$$

8.5.4. Effect on the Exponentials

In the previous section, we used the coefficients of the observed exponential functions to derive the parameters of the biological system, mainly α_{13}. There is some benefits to look at the problem in the opposite direction. It has been stated and many people accept that in the sum of two exponentials, the fast component reflects the physiological factor of interest (renal function, bone uptake), and the slow one reflects mixing between the two compartments. In fact, both component reflect all physiological parameters ($\alpha_{12}\alpha_{21}\alpha_{13}$).

Consider the equivalences from the previous section:

First, $ab = \alpha_{13}\alpha_{21}$ which defines b in terms of a.

$$b = \frac{\alpha_{13}\alpha_{21}}{a}.$$

Second,

$$a + b = (\alpha_{12} + \alpha_{13} + \alpha_{21}).$$

And with substitution,

$$a + \frac{\alpha_{13}\alpha_{21}}{a} - (\alpha_{12} + \alpha_{13} + \alpha_{21}) = 0.$$

This reduces to a quadratic equation

$$a^2 - (\alpha_{12} + \alpha_{13} + \alpha_{21})a + \alpha_{13}\alpha_{21} = 0.$$

The solution of a quadratic equation $ax^2 + bx + c$ is given by: $x = \frac{-b \mp \sqrt{b^2 - 4ac}}{2a}$. In our case, this means that:

$$a = \frac{(\alpha_{12} + \alpha_{13} + \alpha_{21}) + \sqrt{(\alpha_{12} + \alpha_{13} + \alpha_{21})^2 - 4\alpha_{13}\alpha_{21}}}{2} \qquad (8.38a)$$

$$b = \frac{(\alpha_{12} + \alpha_{13} + \alpha_{21}) - \sqrt{(\alpha_{12} + \alpha_{13} + \alpha_{21})^2 - 4\alpha_{13}\alpha_{21}}}{2} \qquad (8.38b)$$

In addition $Ab + Ba = \alpha_{21}D$, and hence

$$Ab + (D - A)a = \alpha_{21}D$$

$$A(b - a) = (\alpha_{21} - a)D$$

$$A = \frac{(\alpha_{21} - a)}{(b - a)}D \qquad (8.39a)$$

$$B = D - A = D - \frac{(\alpha_{21} - a)}{(b - a)}D = \frac{D(b - a) - D(\alpha_{21} - a)}{b - a} = \frac{(b - \alpha_{21})}{b - a}D$$

$$(8.39b)$$

Going back to Equation 8.34, $Ae^{-at} + Be^{-bt}$ and the derivations to 8.38 and 8.40a and 8.38b, we conclude that all physiological parameters influence all coefficients and exponents of the observed sum of exponential functions. In short,

$$Ae^{-at} + Be^{-bt} = D\left[\frac{(\alpha_{21} - a)}{(b - a)}e^{at} + \frac{(b - \alpha_{21})}{(b - a)}e^{bt}\right].^{\circ} \qquad (8.40)$$

Later we will see an application in which the effective renal plasma flow is derived from a single blood sample and the plasma volume. On the face of it, this is unlikely. However, assuming that α_{12} and α_{21} remain constant, what is the effect of the changes in α_{13} (Figure 8.8 and Table 8.1)?

8.5.5. *Another View: Looking at Compartment 2*

The first compartment is solved by using the matrix solution for two equations with two unknowns by way of the determinant ratio (see Equation 8.29):

The result was an equivalence between the coefficients of a sum of two exponentials and the parameters of the physiological system, namely the injected dose and the fractional transfer rates.

$^{\circ}$For clarity, we use the coefficients a and b rather than their long expression in the fractional transfer rates α_{ij}.

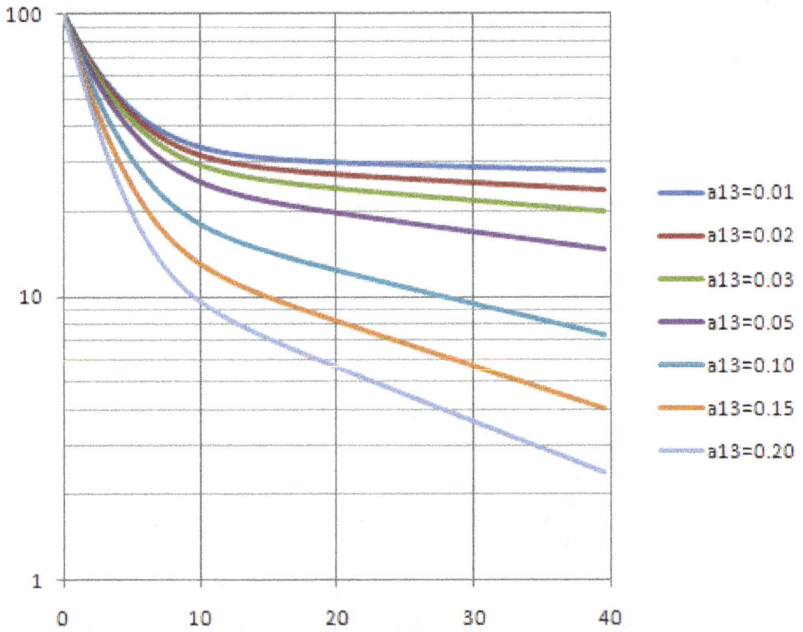

Figure 8.8 Plots of the two exponentials for seven values of the fractional transfer rate α_{13}. The scale is semi-logarithmic. See single sample technique in Section 1.6.

Table 8.1 The table illustrates the changes in the observed values (two-exponentials) when the fractional transfer rates α_{12} and α_{21} remain constant, but α_{13} increases. Note that all four parameters (A, B, a and b) change. The more relevant observation is the value of $N_1(30)$, which is related to a_{13} by the equation $\ln(N_1(30)) = 3.4 + 11\alpha_{13}$.

$\alpha 13$	N1(30)	A	B	a	b
0.01	28.87	68.12	31.88	0.31	0.00
0.02	25.09	73.43	26.57	0.34	0.01
0.03	21.89	78.87	21.13	0.37	0.03
0.05	16.86	69.53	30.47	0.31	0.01
0.10	9.33	70.88	29.12	0.32	0.01
0.15	5.59	83.11	16.89	0.41	0.04
0.20	3.58	86.38	13.62	0.46	0.04

The solution for compartment 2 also comes from the matrix solution (see Section 10.1.1).

$$\Lambda_{N_2} = \frac{\begin{vmatrix} (s+\alpha_{12}+\alpha_{13}) & D \\ -\alpha_{12} & 0 \end{vmatrix}}{\begin{vmatrix} s+\alpha_{12}+\alpha_{13} & -\alpha_{21} \\ -\alpha_{12} & s+\alpha_{21} \end{vmatrix}}.$$

Assuming that the solution again is of the type $Ae^{-at} + Be^{-bt}$, we have the equivalence now between $\dfrac{(A+B)s+(Ab+Ba)}{s^2+(a+b)s+ab}$ and $\dfrac{\alpha_{12}D}{s^2+(\alpha_{12}+\alpha_{13}+\alpha_{21})s+\alpha_{13}\alpha_{21}}$.

With the consequence that

$$A+B=0,$$

$$Ab+Ba=\alpha_{12}D,$$

$$a+b=(\alpha_{12}+\alpha_{13}+\alpha_{21}),$$

$$ab=\alpha_{13}\alpha_{21},$$

$$A=-B,$$

$$A(b-a)=\alpha_{12}D,$$

$$A=\frac{\alpha_{12}D}{(b-a)},$$

$$B=\frac{\alpha_{12}D}{(a-b)}.$$

What both compartments have in common are the definitions of the exponent in terms of the fractional transfer rates,

$$b=\frac{\alpha_{13}\alpha_{12}}{a},$$

$$a+\frac{\alpha_{13}\alpha_{12}}{a}=(\alpha_{12}+\alpha_{13}+\alpha_{21}),$$

$$a^2-(\alpha_{12}+\alpha_{13}+\alpha_{21})a+\alpha_{13}\alpha_{12}=0,$$

$$a=\frac{(\alpha_{12}+\alpha_{13}+\alpha_{21})+\sqrt{(\alpha_{12}+\alpha_{13}+\alpha_{21})^2-4\alpha_{13}\alpha_{21}}}{2}, \qquad \text{[see 8.38a]}$$

$$b=(\alpha_{12}+\alpha_{13}+\alpha_{21})-a,$$

$$b=\frac{(\alpha_{12}+\alpha_{13}+\alpha_{21})-\sqrt{(\alpha_{12}+\alpha_{13}+\alpha_{21})^2-4\alpha_{13}\alpha_{21}}}{2}. \qquad \text{[see 8.38a]}$$

The solution for compartment 1 was given by

$$N_1(t)=\frac{D}{b-a}[(\alpha_{21}-a)e^{-at}+(b-\alpha_{21})e^{-bt}]. \qquad (8.41)$$

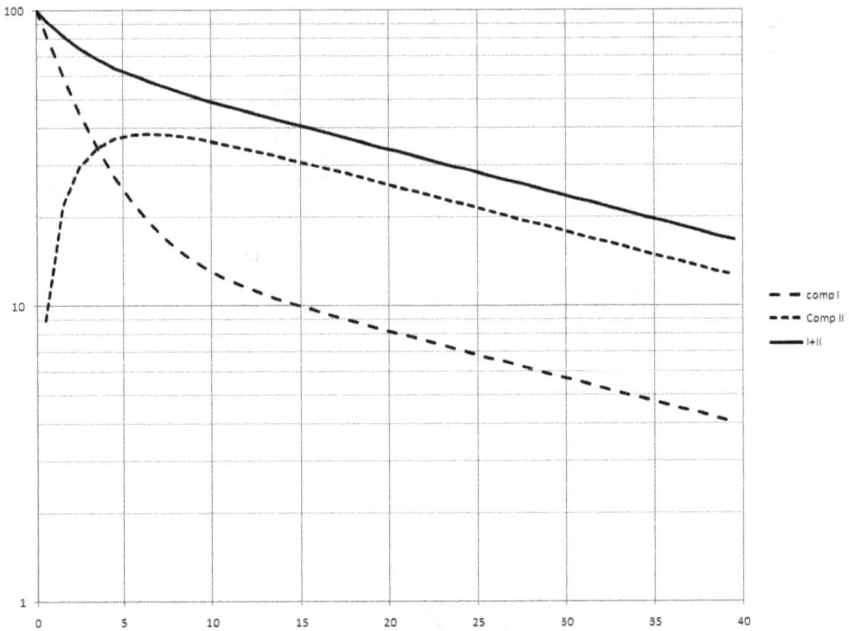

Figure 8.9   The functions $N_1(t)$ and $N_2(t)$ and $N_1(t)+N_2(t)$ are plotted, on a semi-log plot. The physiological parameters in this case are $\alpha_{12} = 0.2$, $\alpha_{21} = 0.1$, $\alpha_{13} = 0.15$. $D = 100$. The slopes a and b are common to N_1 and N_2 and are 0.41 and 0.036 respectively. For N_1, A = 83.1 and B = 16.9. For N_2, A = $-$B = $-$52.98. When the fast component (a = 0.41) is exhausted, the slopes become parallel on the semi-logarithmic scale. An observer measuring both compartments simultaneously would not observe a single exponential until that happens (see MIRD).

For compartment 2 the solution is (Figure 8.9)

$$N_2(t) = \frac{\alpha_{12}D}{(b-a)}(e^{-at} - e^{-bt}). \tag{8.42}$$

All the coefficients and exponents are common to both departments. The sum of the activities in both compartments $N_1(t) + N_2(t)$ is given by

$$\frac{D}{(b-a)}(ae^{-at} + be^{-bt}).$$

We could have approached it differently, using the partial derivative method. The state equation for compartment 2 is:

$$\frac{dN_2}{dt} = -\alpha_{21}N_2 + \alpha_{12}N_1,$$

$$\frac{dN_2}{dt}e^{+\alpha_{21}t} + \alpha_{21}e^{+\alpha_{21}t}N_2 = \alpha_{12}e^{\alpha_{21}t}N_1,$$

$$N_2(t)e^{+\alpha_{21}t} = \alpha_{12}\frac{D}{b-a}\left[(\alpha_{21}-a)\int_0^t e^{(\alpha_{21}-a)t} - (\alpha_{21}-b)\int_0^t e^{(\alpha_{21}-bt)}\right],$$

$$N_2(t)e^{+\alpha_{21}t} = \alpha_{12}\frac{D}{b-a}\left[\frac{(\alpha_{21}-a)}{(\alpha_{21}-a)}(e^{(\alpha_{21}-a)t}-1) - \frac{(\alpha_{21}-b)}{(\alpha_{21}-b)}(e^{\alpha_{21}-bt}-1)\right],$$

$$N_2(t) = \alpha_{12}\frac{D}{b-a}[(e^{-at}-e^{-\alpha_{21}t}) - (e^{-bt}-e^{-\alpha_{21}t})],$$

$$N_2(t) = \alpha_{12}\frac{D}{b-a}(e^{-at}-e^{-bt}).^{\text{p}}$$

It is worth noting that the exponents of the exponentials are the same for both compartments. There is no additional fractional transfer rate to provide an additional exponent.

8.5.6. When α_{13} is Equal to Zero

There is a special case when $a_{13}=0$. Physically, the kinetics are restricted to mixing between two compartments. In that case, the Laplacian derived from the state equations would have yielded:

$$\Lambda_{[N_1]} = \frac{D(s+\alpha_{21})}{s^2+(\alpha_{12}+\alpha_{21})s},$$

to be compared to

$$\frac{(A+B)s+(Ab+Ba)}{s^2+(a+b)s+ab},$$

derived from the two exponentials:

$$Ae^{-at}+Be^{-bt}.$$

The equivalences are best started by considering that ab in the denominator is equal to zero. Also

$$A+B = D,$$

$$\alpha_{21}D = Ab+Ba,$$

$$\alpha_{12}+\alpha_{21} = a+b,$$

$$ab = 0.^{\text{q}}$$

---

[p]Because $\alpha_{13}\alpha_{12}=0$.
[q]Because $\alpha_{13}\alpha_{21}=0$.

If $b = 0$,[r] this reduces to $a_{21}D = Ba$, $\alpha_{12} + \alpha_{21} = a$ and $A = D - B$. From there we have, $\frac{a_{21}}{a_{12}+a_{21}}D = B$. The fractional transfer rates are actually F/V, and the actual flows have to be equal in both directions ($F_{12} = F_{21}$). It is easy to derive that

$$A = \frac{V_2}{V_1 + V_2}D,$$

$$B = \frac{V_1}{V_1 + V_2}D.$$

Hence,

$$N_{1(t)} = \frac{D}{(V_1 + V_2)}(V_2 e^{-(a_{12}+a_{21})t} + V_1).$$

Compartment 2 contains everything that is left from compartment 1,

$$N_{2(t)} = D - \frac{D}{(V_1 + V_2)}(V_2 e^{-(a_{12}+a_{21})t} + V_1).$$

If we look at $N_{1(t)}$ at $t = 0$, the exponent part is equal to 1, and the part between brackets is $V_2 + V_1$. Therefore at $t = 0$, the activity in compartment 1 is the initial dose. At $t = \infty$ (therefore at equilibrium), the exponential part is equal to zero and the activity in 1 is given by

$$N_{1(\infty)} = \frac{DV_1}{(V_1 + V_2)}.$$

The concentration must be the same in both compartments, and is defined by $D/(V_1 + V_2)$. $N_{1(\infty)} = C_1 V_1$.

In the same way, at $t = 0$, the activity in compartment 2 is zero:

$$N_{2(t)} = D - \frac{D}{(V_1 + V_2)}(V_2 + V_1).$$

But at $t = \infty$, the activity is $N_{2(t)} = D - \frac{DV_1}{(V_1+V_2)}$ or $\frac{D(V_1+V_2)-DV_1}{V_1+V_2} = \frac{DV_2}{V_1+V_2}$.

Again, the final amount in compartment 2 is the common concentration multiplied by the volume of compartment 2.

If $\alpha_{13} = 0$, the case is finally reduced to a dilution case.

8.5.7. A Special Case: Two Compartments Connected to Common Compartment with no Return

The case relates to DMSA in renal evaluations, to the first part of the renogram and to an extent (Sections 1.2.2 and 5.2.1), to the early part myocardial perfusion with thallium or for all parts with non-redistributing cardiac flow tracers.

---

[r]It could be a that is equal to zero, but it has to be either a or b, and in the end it does not matter which.

Consider two set of tissues (e.g. two kidneys). Both accumulates the tracer from the plasma with different extraction efficiencies. For the right kidney, the blood flow expressed as a fraction of the total cardiac output would be F_R, and the reciprocal on the left F_L. The same applies to the extraction efficiencies f_R and f_L. Since there is no return to the plasma compartment, if the tracer remains in the plasma, the state equation for the plasma is

$$\frac{dA}{dt} = -(F_R f_R + F_L f_L)A,$$

and the solution is

$$A(t) = A_0 e^{-(F_R f_R + F_L F_L)}.$$

To simplify, we set $(F_R f_R + F_L f_L) = \lambda$.

The uptake in the right kidney is the fraction of the cardiac output going to the right kidney multiplied by the extraction efficiency: $\frac{dR}{dt} = F_R f_R A(t)$ and for the left $\frac{dL}{dt} = F_L f_L A(t)$. The difference between the two are the coefficient Ff, but the function $A(t)$ is identical for both kidneys, and both renal curves have an

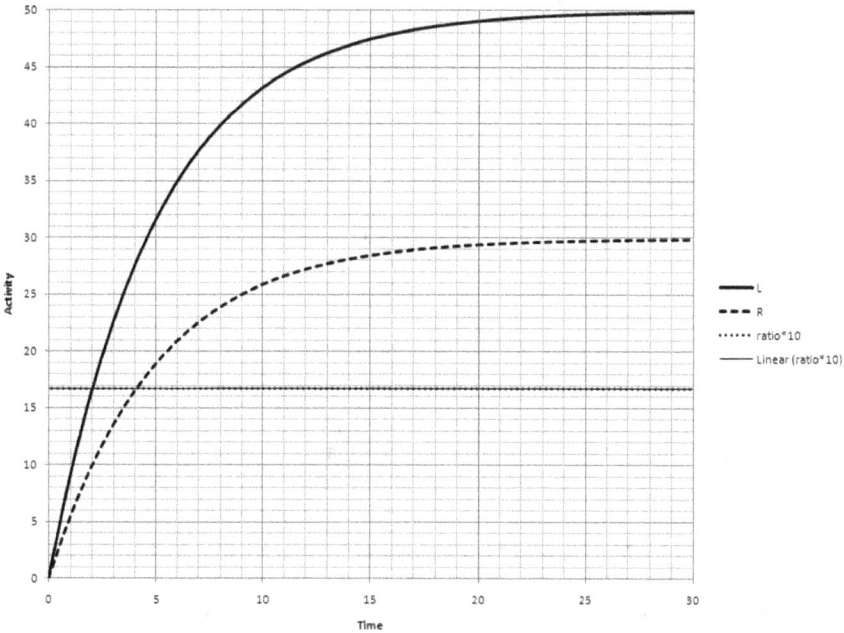

Figure 8.10 The graph represents the activity and the ratio between the activities if the Ff ratio is 16.7. The ratio between the activities remains 16.7 at all times. The uptake curve reflects the reciprocal of the plasma activity curve.

identical functional form (see Figure 8.10)

$$R = Ff\frac{A_0}{\lambda}(1 - e^{-\lambda t}).$$

8.5.8. *A Special Case: Two Compartments Connected to Common Compartment with Return*

In this section, we consider two compartments exchanging tracers with a common compartment. The common compartment may be in contact with multiple other compartments, but we will discuss an example where the common compartment's kinetics is well described by a sum of two exponentials. The common compartment would be the plasma. In this case, we express the kinetics in plasma concentrations.

$$c_{p(t)} = Ae^{-at} + Be^{-bt}.$$

The two other compartments are perfused with a flow F1 and F2, and extract from the plasma a fraction (a) proportional to the concentration. The fractional uptake rate is respectively $f_1 = aF1$ and $f_2 = aF2$. (The assumption is that the tracer is very diffusible and the diffusion in the tissues happens almost instantaneously (Figure 8.11).) The return rates are α_{1p} and α_{2p}. The state equation for

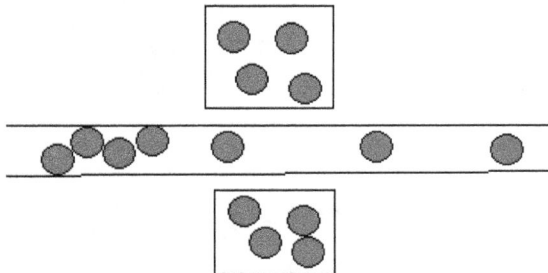

Figure 8.11   Illustration of a flow tracer diffusing rapidly (at first pass) from the vascular system, but remaining (lost) in the extravascular (or intracellular) spaces.

Figure 8.12   In this example (left panel) A = 50, a = 0.1, B = 50, b = 0.02, $f_1 = 0.5$, $f_2 = 0.25$ and $\alpha_{1p} = \alpha_{2p} = 0.01$. The flow remains constant. The functions $N_{1(t)}$ and $N_{2(t)}$ remain parallel at all times. If the flow is not constant, but slowly decreases to return to resting flow, inspection reveals (right panel) that at early times, the flow to the tissues dominates the distribution to the tissues, but at later times a component comes in that reflects redistribution,[s] without an effect of flow. The concept is important in myocardial perfusion studies with thallium-201.

---

[s]And also washout, but this will be revisited in Section 5.6.

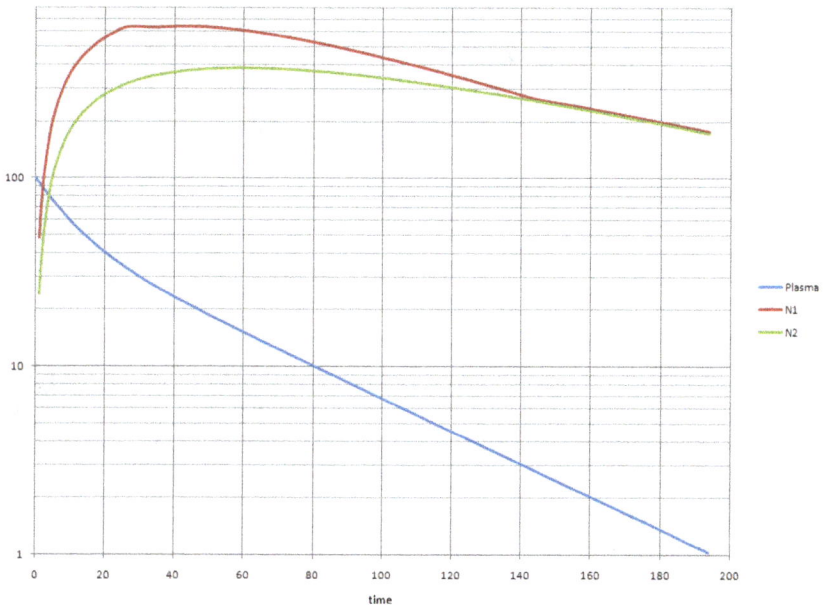

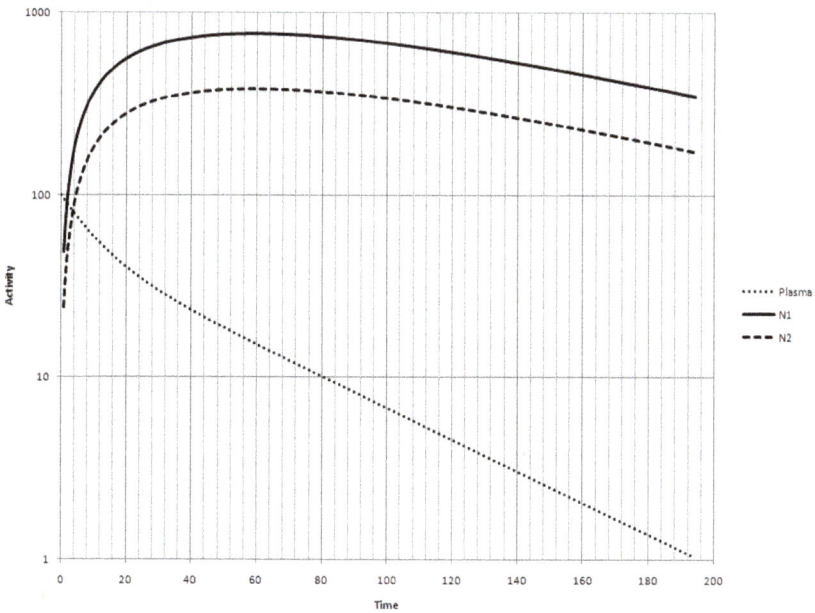

Figure 8.12 (*Continued*)

compartment 1 is

$$\frac{dN_1}{dt} = f_1 c_{p(t)} - \alpha_{1p} N_1.$$

The derivation is simple enough (see above and partial derivatives in Section 10.3).

$$\frac{dN_1}{dt} e^{\alpha_{1p}t} + \alpha_{1p} N_1 e^{\alpha_{1p}t} = f_1 c_{(t)} e^{\alpha_{1p}t},$$

$$N_{1(t)} e^{\alpha_{1P}t} = f_1 \left[\frac{A}{(\alpha_{1P} - a)} (e^{(\alpha_{1P} - a)t} - 1) + \frac{B}{(\alpha_{1P} - b)} (e^{(\alpha_{1P} - b)t} - 1) \right],$$

$$N_{1(t)} = f_1 \left[\frac{A}{(\alpha_{1P} - a)} (e^{-at} - e^{-\alpha_{1P}t}) + \frac{B}{(\alpha_{1P} - b)} (e^{-bt} - e^{\alpha_{1P}t}) \right],$$

For $N_{2(t)}$, the equation is identical but for the substitution of α_{2p} for α_{1p} and f_2 for f_1. If $\alpha_{1p} = \alpha_{2p}$, then the two curves parallel each other and are relatively scaled by f_1/f_2.

In some circumstances, the flow is not constant. The typical example would be after the injection of a cardiac tracer (e.g. thallium) during stress. Consider two myocardial regions: one is able to accommodate increased blood flow, the other not (see Section 5.6). The increased in (stress) flow is only temporary, and (quickly) returns to the resting rate. Formally for $N_{1(t)}$, the expression is $N_{1(t)} = f_{1(t)} \left[\frac{A}{(\alpha_{1P} - a)} (e^{-at} - e^{-\alpha_{1P}t}) + \frac{B}{(\alpha_{1P} - b)} (e^{-bt} - e^{\alpha_{1P}t}) \right]$ because f_1 varies over time (Figure 8.12).

REFERENCES

1. Dobson EL, Warner GF, Finney CR, Johnston ME. The measurement of liver circulation by means of the colloid disappearance rate: I. Liver blood flow in normal young men. *Circulation* 1954; 7:690–695.
2. Dobson EL, Warner GF. Measurement of regional sodium turnover rates and their application to the estimation of regional blood flow. *Am J Physiol* 1957; 189:269–276.
3. Bassingthwaighte JB, Ackerman FH, Wood EH. Applications of the lagged normal density curve as a model for arterial dilution curves. *Circulation Res* 1966; 18:398–418.
4. Bassingthwaighte JB, Wang CY, Chan IS. Blood-tissue exchange via transport and transformation by capillary endothelial cells. *Circulation Res* 1989; 65:997–1020.

Chapter 9

Non-Compartmental Models

9.1. DENSITY DISTRIBUTION OF TRANSIT TIMES

9.1.1. *Sampling the Output Function*

The model for this approach is a system defined by flow and volume, i.e. a vascular network. There are no mixing assumptions, but the existing assumptions are stringent (1, 2):

1. Stationarity of flow and volume during the time of the experiment.
2. The flow of tracer is representative of the flow of fluid.
3. There are no stagnant pools (nothing is captured in the system[a]).
4. There is no recirculation.

If an amount "Q" of tracer is injected at time $t = 0$, all of Q has to leave the system between time $t = 0$ and $t = \infty$, since there are no stagnant pools. The (stationary) flow F at the exit carries the tracer exiting the system. The amount of tracer leaving the system at time t is given by: $F.c(t)$, where $c(t)$ is the (average) concentration of the tracer in the outflow tract's volume.

The prototype of the non-compartmental system is the vascular network: The system consists of a single input, connected to a single output, and connected by vascular pathways of different lengths (Figure 9.1).

If each vascular connection has a flow "f_i", the total flow "F" at the input "F_{in}" and at the output "F_{out}" is the sum of the flows f_i:

$$F_{in} = \sum_i f_i = F_{out}.$$

---

[a]In contradistinction with the pool considered for the Patlak plot method.

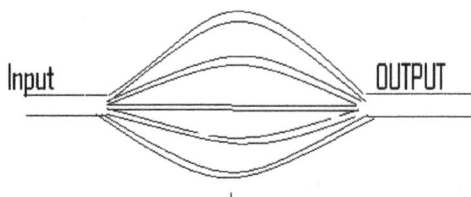

Figure 9.1   The figure is a schematic representation of a vascular "unit" with one input artery connected through a network of vessels to a single (venous) output. An anatomical model is the kidney, with a single renal artery and a single renal vein. Sampling both for a renal tracer allows the definition of an extraction efficiency. The difference with the kidney is that there should be no trapping or exit from the basic system (Sections 1.1.1 and 1.2.2).

Each vascular pathway has a volume V_i. The total volume of the system is the sum of the component volumes:

$$V = \sum_i V_i.$$

The analysis of such a system is based on the simple proposition that if an elementary volume element "dv_i" enters pathway "i" at time t_{in}, this volume element will reach the end of the pathway, at a time t_{out}, such that $t_{out} - t_{in} = t_i$. The definition of t_i in terms of flow and volumes[b] is $t_i = \frac{v_i}{f_i}$ where v_i and f_i are the volume of and the flow through the pathway "i" respectively (Section 1.5.1).

An observer, sampling at the output, would see a certain amount of tracer leave between $t = 0$ and $t = \infty$. Per unit of time, the amount of tracer leaving is equal to the flow F multiplied by the concentration $c(t)$. If all of the tracer is introduced at time $t = 0$, the distribution of exit times as a function of time is the distribution of the transit times of the tracer, and reflects the distribution of the transit times of the elementary volumes (see Section 10.7.3). The distribution of transit times divided by the total Q (i.e. normalized), is the density distribution of transit times.

Looking back at the model's assumptions:

1. Between time zero and time $= \infty$, all of the tracer must eventually leave the system (there are no stagnant pools).
2. The flow is constant.
3. The tracer enters and leaves the system only once (there is no recirculation).

---

[b]We have used this definition in the discussion of diuresis renography: The relation $t = V/F$ is equivalent to $t = d/v$, where d is the distance and v is the velocity.

The three conditions together define the identity $F \int_0^\infty c(t)dt = Q$ and a density distribution of transit times $h(t) = [Fc(t)]/Q$. The density distribution of transit times is a normalized frequency distribution.

By definition, $h(t)$ has two characteristics:

1. $\int_0^\infty h(t) \cdot dt = 1$.
2. If $H(t) = \int_0^t h(t)dt$, $H(\infty) = 1$.
3. Finally, referring to the definition of averages (Section 10.4):

$$\int_0^\infty t \cdot h(t) \cdot dt = \bar{t}, \tag{9.1}$$

where $\bar{t}$ is the average or mean transit time. Going back to the observed values, we note the equivalences:

$$\int_0^\infty h(t) \cdot dt = \int_0^\infty \frac{F \cdot c(t)}{Q} \cdot dt = \frac{\int_0^\infty F \cdot c(t) \cdot dt}{Q} = \frac{Q}{Q} = 1. \tag{9.2}$$

Therefore,

$$\bar{t} = \frac{\int_0^\infty tFc(t)dt}{\int_0^\infty Fc(t)dt} = \frac{\int_0^\infty tc(t)dt}{\int_0^\infty c(t)dt}. \tag{9.3}$$

Averages are of dubious significance, but in this analysis, the average time physically represents the proportion between volume and flow (see note above). There is, however, a question on how the average works in the case of the vascular network. Each pathway has its own transit time, defined as $t_i = v_i/v_i$.

A priori the ratio V/F is not the sum of the ratios defined by individual pathways (Section 10.5):

$$\frac{V}{F} = \frac{\sum v_i}{\sum f_i} \neq \sum \frac{v_i}{f_i}.$$

However, if we look at the distribution of transit times, the situation is as follows: The tracer distributes between the pathways, in proportion to the flow in those pathways. The fraction of tracer in pathway "i" is the flow in pathway divided by the sum of all the flows. The time t_i is "seen" with a frequency defined by the amount of tracer going through pathway "i". The solution is therefore based on the fact that $f_i / \sum f_i$ is actually a density distribution of the transit times. Thus,

$$\bar{t} = \sum t_i \left(\frac{f_i}{\sum f_j} \right).$$

By substitution, we can derive the following:

$$\bar{t} = \sum_i \left(\frac{v_i}{f_i} \frac{f_i}{\sum f_j} \right) = \sum_i \frac{v_i}{\sum f_j} = \sum_i \frac{v_i}{F} = \frac{1}{F} \sum_i v_i = \frac{V}{F}. \qquad (9.4)$$

Therefore, the relation between the average transit time and the ratio of volume over flow remains (see also Section 10.4 on averages).

9.1.2. Compartmental Analog

Single compartmental systems or catenary compartmental systems are a subset of non-compartmental models since there is an assumption of stationarity of flow and volume during the time of the experiment, the flow of tracer is representative of the flow of fluid, there are no stagnant pools and there is no recirculation (unlike in mamillary systems).

The kinetics of a single compartmental system are described by the exponential function $N_1(t) = N_{10}e^{-\lambda t}$ with the initial condition that at time zero, the total amount in the compartment is N_{10} and the state equation $dN_1/dt = -\lambda N_1$.

An observer looking at the output from the compartment would observe an output described by $\lambda N_0 e^{-\lambda t}$. The exponent λ is the volume divided by the flow, the amount in the compartment is the concentration c_1 multiplied by the volume V_1, hence the intermediate steps are

$$\lambda = \frac{F}{V_1},$$

$$N_1(t) = c_1(t)V_1(t).$$

The final step is the expression of the output function in terms of the (constant) flow and the variable concentration.

$$\lambda N_{10}e^{-\lambda t} = \frac{F}{V_1}(V_1 c_{10})e^{-\lambda t} = Fc_{10}e^{-\lambda t} = Fc_1(t).$$

In this case, $h(t) = \frac{N_0 e^{-\lambda t}}{N_0}$ and the mean transit time is therefore

$$\bar{t} = \frac{\int_0^\infty te^{-e\lambda t}dt}{\int_0^\infty e^{-\lambda t}} = \frac{\Gamma(2)/\lambda^2}{1/\lambda} = \frac{1}{\lambda}^c,$$

---

[c] One needs to know that $\int_0^\infty te^{-\lambda t}dt = \frac{\Gamma(2)}{\lambda^2}$ and that $\Gamma(n+1) = n\Gamma(n)$, if $n > 0$, and $\Gamma(n) = n!$ if n is a positive integer. Hence $\Gamma(2) = \Gamma(1+1) = 1\Gamma(1) = n! = 1$ (Section 10.2.2).

which was the definition of the mean or average time and

$$\bar{t} = \frac{1}{\lambda} = \frac{V}{F}. \tag{9.5}$$

9.1.3. *Residency Times: Sampling the Compartment*

It is important to remember that $h(t)$ is observed at the exit or outflow of the system. If, on the other hand, one observes the system itself, one observes the activity $q(t)$ remaining in the system.

Assuming that the total amount of tracer Q was introduced at time $t = 0$, at any time t, the amount remaining in the system is the total amount Q minus the total which has left up to that time.

$$q(t) = Q - F \cdot \int_0^t c(t) \cdot dt.$$

Expressing it in terms of the density distribution of transit times[d] yields:

$$q(t) = Q - Q \frac{\int_0^t Fc(t)dt}{Q},$$

$$q(t) = Q \left[1. - \int_0^t h(t) \cdot dt \right].$$

Substituting the integral form $H(t) = \int_0^t h(t)dt$, we rewrite $q(t) = Q[1. - H(t)]$. Then we integrate the compartment's time-activity function (also referred to as area under the curve: $\int_0^\infty q(t)dt = Q \int_0^\infty [1 - H(t)]dt$. The next step is obtained using the partial derivative (see Section 10.3):

If we take the derivative of $t[1. - H(t)]$, we obtain:

$$\frac{d}{dt}[t \cdot (1. - H(t))] = (1. - H(t)) - t \cdot \frac{d}{dt}H(t).$$

The solution contains a derivative of the integral $H(t)$ which is $h(t)$

$$\frac{d}{dt}[t \cdot (1. - H(t))] = (1. - H(t)) - t \cdot h(t).$$

Rearranging the terms, we have:

$$(1. - H(t)) = \frac{d}{dt}[t \cdot (1. - H(t))] + t \cdot h(t).$$

Integrating yields:

$$\int_0^\infty [1. - H(t)]dt = t[1. - H(t)] + \int_0^\infty th(t)dt.$$

---

[d] $h(t) = \frac{F \cdot c(t)}{Q}$.

Since at t = 0, the first term is $0 \times (1 - H(t)) = 0$, and at $t = \infty$, $H(\infty) = 1$ and $(1 - H(t)) = 0$, the result is

$$\int_0^\infty q(t)dt = Q \int_0^\infty th(t)dt \quad \text{or} \quad \frac{\int_0^\infty q(t)dt}{Q} = \bar{t}. \tag{9.6}$$

In this model, the average transit time is in fact the average residency time. The vulgar expression is the normalized area under the curve or the area under the curve divided by the activity at time t = 0.

9.1.4. Compartmental Analog

9.1.4.1. Single compartment

The analogy is trivial. Going back to the notation we have used before, we have $q(t) = N(t) = N(0) \cdot e^{-\lambda \cdot t}$ and $Q = N(0)$. The integral now becomes:

$$\bar{t} = \frac{N(0) \int_0^\infty e^{-\lambda \cdot t} dt}{N(0)} = \int_0^\infty e^{-\lambda \cdot t} \cdot dt = \frac{1}{\lambda},$$

which was the definition of the mean transit time[e] given in the prior section.

9.1.4.2. For the two-compartment system

In this case, the situation is complicated by the fact that it has been suggested that one can apply the integral method to the first compartment. But that approach would violate the non-recirculation clause, since the tracer leaves compartment 1 to enter compartment 2 and eventually reappear in compartment 1.

We will first derive the exact solution, and then show that the integral method applied on compartment 1 is actually an application of the analysis of the output function.

The physical assumption is that one observes the total amount of tracer in both compartments, that is $N1(t) + N2(t)$. In the case of a renal tracer, this would be the whole body activity with the exception of the renal, collecting system and bladder activity.

We have seen in Section 8.5.5 that the solutions for compartments 1 and 2 are given by the following equations.

---

[e]Actually the mean residency time.

The solution for compartment 1 was given by

$$N_1(t) = \frac{D}{b-a}[(\alpha_{21} - a)e^{-at} + (b - \alpha_{21})e^{-bt}]. \tag{8.40}$$

For compartment 2, the solution is:

$$N_2(t) = \frac{\alpha_{12} D}{(b-a)}(e^{-at} - e^{-bt}). \tag{8.41}$$

By adding the coefficients with equal exponents, we obtain

$$N_1(t) + N_2(t) = D\left[\frac{-a + \alpha_{12} + \alpha_{21}}{b - a}e^{-at} + \frac{b - \alpha_{12} - \alpha_{21}}{b - a}e^{-bt}\right].$$

The integral becomes

$$\int_0^\infty [N_1(t) + N_2(t)]dt$$

$$= D\left[\frac{-a + \alpha_{12} + \alpha_{21}}{(b - a)a} + \frac{b - \alpha_{12} - \alpha_{21}}{(b - a)b}\right] \tag{9.7}$$

And the term in parenthesis can be reduced to

$$D \cdot \frac{V_2 + V_1}{\alpha_{13} \cdot V_1}. \tag{9.8}$$

If we go back to the initial definition of the mean transit time we obtain

$$\bar{t} = \frac{\int_0^\infty (N_1(t) + N_2(t))dt}{D} = \frac{1}{\alpha_{13}} \cdot \frac{V_1 + V_2}{V_1}. \tag{9.9}$$

For memory, we note that a_{1e} was defined as F/V_1. Therefore, we have

$$\bar{t} = \frac{V_1}{F_{13}} \times \frac{V_1 + V_2}{V_1} = \frac{V_1 + V_2}{F_{13}}.$$

The mean transit time for the system as a whole is therefore the reciprocal of the flow from compartment 1 to the outside, divided by the total volume of both compartments.

9.2. GASTRIC EMPTYING

The major problem with the density distribution of transit times is the limitation of the reasonable observation time. To overcome this problem, one needs a model. Gastric emptying studies are typical, because it is difficult to attach a single model to it.

Observation confirms that the system is not first order (single exponential emptying), nor in fact zero order (linear kinetics). There definitely appears that there is a lag time, or an initial slow component.

The first question is to answer in the absence of a model, if there is a single parameter, or small and manageable number of parameters that adequately describe the gastric emptying function. In general, there has been a focus on the half-emptying time.

Physiologically one could imagine a first order system only if there was a reason for the stomach to release a set fraction of its contents per unit of time. In that case, the function would be a single exponential, totally described by either the fractional rate λ, the half-life $T_{1/2}$ or the average residency time $\bar{t}$ (see Sections 8.2.1–8.2.3).

$$g(t) = A^{-\lambda t}, \tag{8.9}$$

$$T_{1/2} = \frac{0.693}{\lambda} = 1.44\,\bar{t}. \tag{8.11}$$

It is however difficult to imagine, except for liquid meals perhaps, considering that the contents have to mixed and influenced (macerated) by the gastric juices. One function described by a single parameter, but with an explicit lag-time is the power exponential function:

$$g(t) = Ae^{-\lambda t^2},$$

$$\frac{1}{2}A = Ae^{-\lambda (T_{1/2})^2},$$

$$\ln(0.5) = -\lambda (T_{1/2})^2,$$

$$T_{1/2} = \sqrt{\frac{0.693}{\lambda}}.$$

The power-exponential curve has the advantage that it is described by a single parameter λ, from which the half-life and residency time can be derived, but the lag-time, if physiologically important, cannot be independent from λ. If the lag time is defined as the time it takes for the function to drop to 90% of the time 0 value,[f] then the lag time is defined by (Figure 9.2)

$$T_{0.9} = \sqrt{\frac{0.105}{\lambda}}.$$

---

[f]Elastoff (1982) rightly points out that it is difficult to even define t = 0.

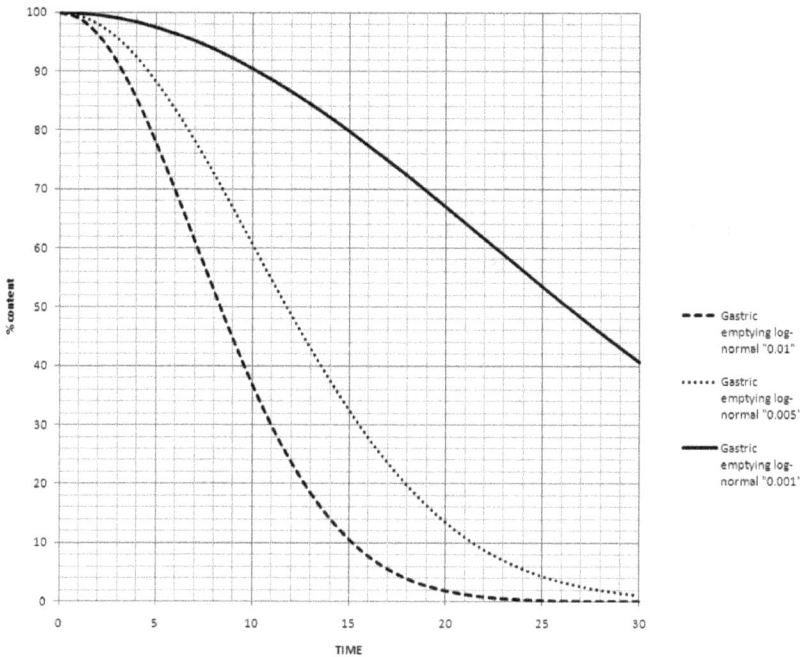

Figure 9.2 Three examples of the log normal gastric emptying curves with the values of $\lambda \, \text{min}^{-1}$ as indicated. The corresponding lag times are 3, 4 and 10 minutes.

Elashoff (3) repeats the requirements for the model or functional form:

1. minimize the number of parameters,
2. the parameters should be clearly related to the shape of the curve,
3. the function should be adapted to many types of patients and emptying patterns, and finally
4. the curve should extrapolate beyond the observation time. A final requirement harks back to the definition of $t = 0$.

His formal proposal is to fit the data to a function:

$$f = 2^{-\left(\frac{t}{T_{1/2}}\right)^{\beta}}.$$ (9.10)

Generalizing would yield:

$$G(t) = Ae^{-(\alpha t)^{\beta}},$$ (9.11)

a function with two parameters and that can be linearized.[g]

---

[g]Fitting after linearization has some disadvantages as pointed out by the authors.

Siegel (4) proposes a functional form that formalizes the lag phase more precisely. He posits that the functional form is

$$G(t) = (1 - (1 - e^{-\alpha t}))^{\beta}. \qquad (9.12)$$

The main point of his presentation is that β is the intercept of the function $A(t) = Ae^{-\alpha t}$ which is defined by fitting the tail end of the total curve. The lag time is then defined as the time when the functions $Ae^{-\alpha t}$ and $G(t) = (1 - (1 - e^{-\alpha t}))^{\beta}$ actually merge. The problem is that this point in time is not easy to define (Figures 9.3 and 9.4).

The requirements set by Elashoff and a push for standardization eventually led to a consensus between nuclear medicine and gastroenterology (5). First, a standard meal was defined, which is not new,[h] but somewhat awkward. Second,

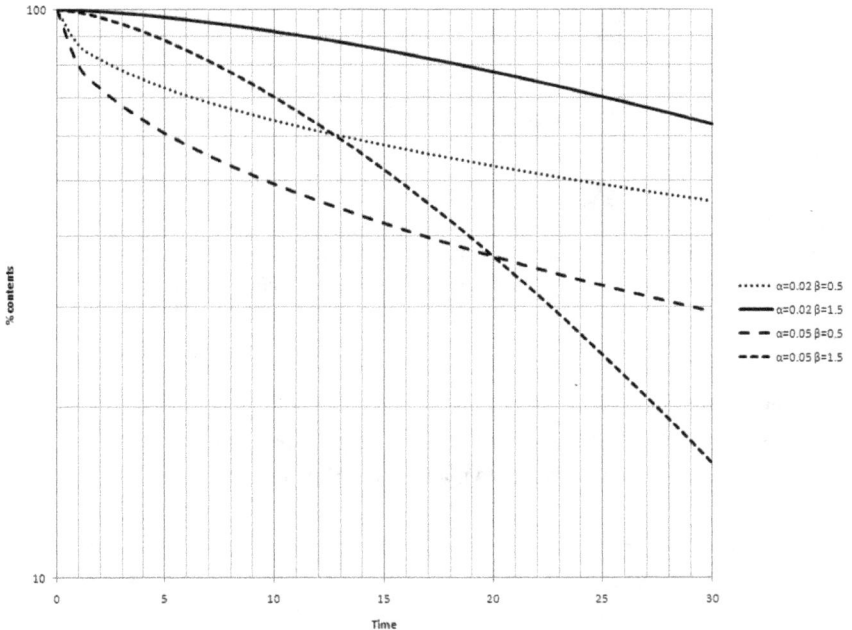

Figure 9.3 Elastoff function, with the parameters as indicated. The half emptying values are 23, >30, 9, 15 and the lag times <1, 11, <1, 4. The parameters are relatively independent of each other.

---

[h]Most of my patients referred for gastric emptying studies were infants, and, if they had been able to take a standard meal, they would not have been referred for a gastric emptying study. Most adults (not all) are able to take it.

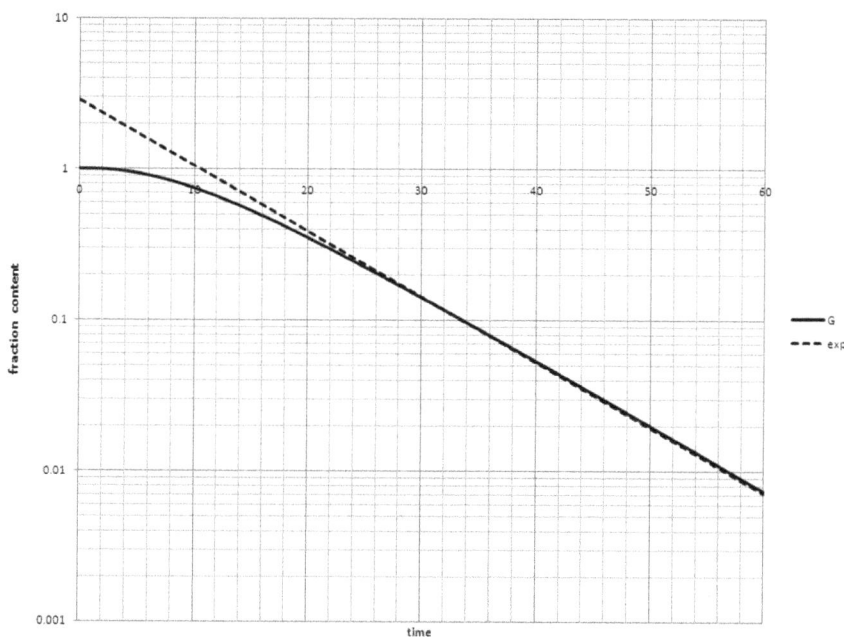

Figure 9.4   The functions A(t) and G(t) appear to merge in a satisfactory manner at t = 20. However, while $\beta = 3$, the intercept A(0) is 2.88. And in fact, closer inspection shows that even at 60 minutes the two functions are not superimposed.

the observation time is extended to 4 hours. Finally there is no model, but normal limits for the five (0–4) hourly observations individually. This defeats the effort of having a few parameters defining the whole study. The consensus paper does not define how one would deal with a mixture of normal data points and abnormal data points. One would not even know if and how the results at different time points correlate.

9.3. RED BLOOD CELLS SURVIVAL TIMES

In the normal case, the survival time of red blood cells is 120 days. The circulating red cells are cohorts of different ages (in days). The kinetics are zero order. If at time t = 0 we re-inject red blood cells (RBC) taken from the patient and labeled together, we would have, in the re-injected RBCs, 120 cohorts aged 1–120. The state equation is

$$\frac{dN}{dt} = -\frac{N_0}{120}.$$

To generalize, set the survival time = T, then

$$\frac{dN}{dt} = -\frac{N_0}{T}. \tag{9.13}$$

or if we set k = 1/T, then

$$\frac{dN}{dt} = -kN_0,$$

$$dN = -kdt, \tag{9.14}$$

$$N(t) = N_0 - N_0 kt,$$

$$N(t) = N_0(1 - kt).$$

If the derivation of Equation 9.14 is exact, the time to reach 50% of the original values is given by

$$0.5 = 1 - \left(\frac{1}{120}\right)T_{1/2},$$

$$T_{1/2} = 0.5 \times 120 = 60 \text{ days}.$$

The original work had been done by Winchell (6), Shapiro (7) and Landaw (8), who had injected heme labeled with ^{14}C (carbon-14), and recuperated carbon monoxide (^{14}CO). At 120 days, the expiratory gases of the subject contained a spike of ^{14}CO.

In the clinic the method was hard and was replaced by ^{51}Cr (chromium) labeling. The problem was that the label tended to elute (9), and a measure of ^{51}Cr activity is actually defined by a more complex state equation. The elution rate is estimated at 0.012 day^{-1}.

The usual method is to assume that the two losses of the label can be combined to a single loss rate (1/120 + 0.012 = 0.0203) and applied to a first order system; in which case the normal value would be a half-life of 34 days. However that assumes the state equation to be first order, which it is not. If we keep k as 1/(life span) and λ as the fractional dilution rate, then the state equation is as follows:

$$\frac{dN}{dt} = N_0 - kN_0 - \lambda N_t. \tag{9.15}$$

Note that k is applied to the initial value (N_0) and λ to the present value (N).

In the end, the liberty taken by most practitioners, by assuming that k and λ are additive and can be used as in a first order system, does not change the results very much. The normal value with the usual (incorrect) method is 34 days. However the "normal" value in infants is shorter (20 days) (10) and that should be taken into account in compatibility studies (11) (Figure 9.5).

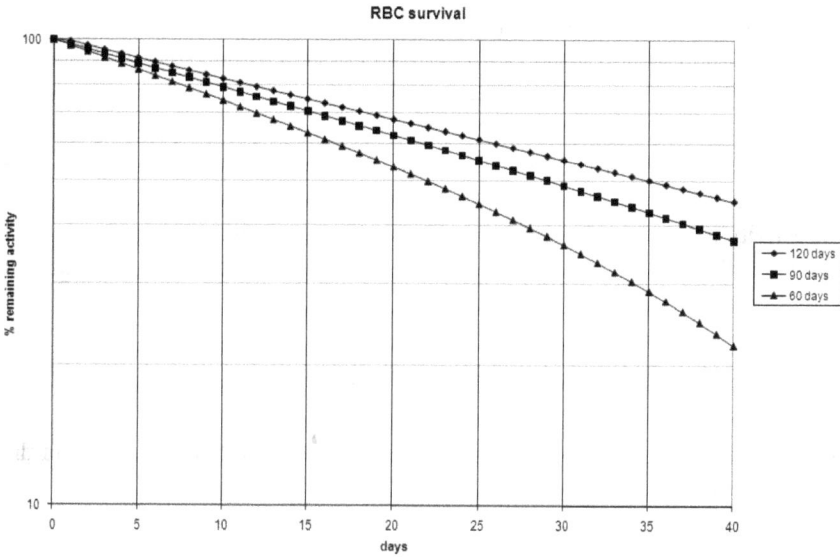

RBC survival

Figure 9.5 The functional shape of the retention curve is shown for k = 1/120, 1/90 and 1/60 and for $\lambda = 0.012$ as shown in Equation 9.15. If those curves are analyzed (as is the custom) by fitting an exponential, the resulting life time would have been 34, 28 and 19 respectively. The correct values would have been 35, 28 and 22.

9.4. THE PATLAK METHOD APPLIED TO KIDNEYS

This section properly belongs to compartmental models, except for the fact that the solution is not exactly analytical and the observational conditions are particular. The assumptions are (12, 13):

a. The whole organ or compartment of interest can be observed and the whole content can be measured.

b. The transfer from plasma to the compartment is irreversible.

If the fractional transfer rate is represented by the lumpen constant K, the transfer rate is given by:

$$\frac{dA}{dt} = KC_p(t). \tag{9.16}$$

In this case, K is essentially the plasma flow to the compartment multiplied by the plasma concentration $C_p(t)$ at time t. If the activity remains in the organ (if there is no negative term to the state equation), then

$$A(t) = K \int_0^t C_p(t)dt.^i \qquad (9.17)$$

Observationally, one would easily "see" all of the compartment, but not only the compartment. In superposition, one would also see part of the plasma volume and the activity it contains $(A_p(t) = V_p \times C_p(t))^j$ and part of the extravascular volume and the activity it contains $(A_e(t) = V_e \times C_e(t)).^k$ The result is that the observed activity curve is now

$$A(t) = K \int_0^t C_p(t)dt + V_e C_e(t) + V_p C_p(t). \qquad (9.18)$$

At this point a stringent condition is introduced: IFF^l the transfer rate from the plasma to extravascular is very rapid, then $C_e(t) = C_p(t)$. Therefore,

$$A(t) = K \int_0^t C_p(t)dt + (V_e + V_p)C_p(t).$$

We assume that $C_p(t)$ is known, and divide both sides of the equation by $C_p(t)$:

$$\frac{A(t)}{C_p(t)} = K \frac{\int_0^t C_p(t)dt}{C_p(t)} + (V_e + V_p). \qquad (9.19)$$

However, in general $C_p(t)$ is not known, or if known, is not measured with the identical efficiency of the measurement of $A(t).^m$ To overcome the problem, we make all observations from the same probe or device.

A region of interest is placed outside of the object of interest (e.g. kidney) but on a plasma-rich region. The volume in that region is $(V_e^b + V_p^b)$ but the activity is $A_b = (V_e^b + V_p^b)C_p(t)$ where A_b represents the activity in this outside region, observed with the same efficiency as A, the renal region. Equation 9.19 can be

---

^{i}If the plasma concentration function $C_p(t)$ is known, then K can be derived by $K = \frac{A(\infty)}{\int_0^\infty C_p(t)dt}$.

^{j}The volume V_p is not the plasma volume, but the part of the plasma volume observed within the field of view.

^{k}Note that the volumes remain constant, but the concentrations vary with time.

^{l}IFF is a notation signifying "if and only if".

^{m}The plasma would be sampled and the sample counted in a well counter, the kidney is monitored with an external probe or imaging device.

rewritten as:

$$\frac{A(t)}{(V_e^b + V_p^b)C_p(t)} = K \frac{\int_0^t C_p(t)dt}{(V_e^b + V_p^b)C_p(t)} + \frac{(V_e + V_p)}{(V_e^b + V_p^b)},$$

$$\frac{A(t)}{A_b(t)} = K \frac{\int_0^t C_p(t)dt}{A_b(t)} + \frac{(V_e + V_p)}{(V_e^b + V_p^b)}. \qquad (9.20)$$

Equation 9.20 is in fact the equation of a straight line $y = ax + b$, where

$$y = \frac{A(t)}{A_b(t)},$$

$$a = K,$$

$$b = \frac{(V_e + V_p)}{(V_e^b + V_p^b)},$$

$$x = \frac{\int_0^t C_p(t)dt}{A_b(t)}.$$

However, Equation 9.20 still contains two types of observations (blood sampling and external counting), but can be modified by multiplying the term representing "x" by the volume of the non-target region:

$$\frac{A(t)}{A_b(t)} = K \frac{(V_e^b + V_p^b)\int_0^t C_p(t)dt}{(V_e^b + V_p^b)A_b(t)} + \frac{(V_e + V_p)}{(V_e^b + V_p^b)},$$

and finally,

$$\frac{A(t)}{A_b(t)} = \frac{K}{(V_e^b + V_p^b)} \frac{\int_0^t A_b(t)dt}{A_b(t)} + \frac{(V_e + V_p)}{(V_e^b + V_p^b)}. \qquad (9.21)$$

With exclusive external counting, the solution is not in terms of K, but the ratio of K over the non-target volume. It should be noted that the term representing "b" in the linear equation (the intercept) is not the background.

The main point of Equation 9.21 is that the ratio of the target activity over the non-target activity plotted against (normalized) time, eventually is a straight line whose slope is a function of the flow (and uptake efficiency). The normalized time is the ratio of the integral of the non-target activity over the non-target activity.

9.5. STEWART HAMILTON AND THE CARDIAC OUTPUT

The system is the heart (LV) during a first pass of a bolus injection of activity Q. The assumption is that there is a phase (the LV phase of the first pass), when the activity A(t) is passing through the LV (of volume V) and can be observed whole and by itself. In that case, the "area under the curve does apply to the LV activity (see Section 8.2.4).

$$\bar{t} = \frac{V}{F} = \frac{\int_0^\infty A(t)dt}{Q}. \tag{8.15}$$

Rearranging the terms we have:

$$F = \frac{QV}{\int_0^\infty A(t)dt},$$

and finally

$$F = \frac{Q}{\int_0^\infty C_r(t)dt} \tag{9.22}$$

where $C_r(t)$ is the "real" average concentration in the left ventricle (14, 15).

The observables are a count rate $c_o(t)$ related to the concentration by a constant k. When the activity has equilibrated in the plasma, the constant k is still valid. The constant is the ratio of the count rate at equilibrium over the real concentration at equilibrium.

By dilution principle, the plasma volume is the total dose divided by the equilibrium concentration (if the tracer is a plasma tracer[n])

$$C_o(t) = kC_r(t).$$

$$k = \frac{C_o(\infty)}{C_r(\infty)}.$$

$$V_p = \frac{Q}{C_r(\infty)}.$$

If there was a plasma sample at equilibrium, the cardiac output is given by:

$$F = \frac{Q}{k \int_0^\infty C_o(t)dt}. \tag{9.23}$$

If there is not, the cardiac output is expressed in fractions of the plasma volume (14, 15):

$$F = \frac{V_p C_o(\infty)}{\int_0^\infty C_o(t)dt},$$

$$\frac{F}{V_p} = \frac{C_o(\infty)}{\int_0^\infty C_o(t)dt}. \tag{9.24}$$

The important factor of the last two examples is that one has to deal with the observed rather than the theoretical variables and that there is no analytical solution needed for the analysis. Nothing is said about $C_o(t)$, except for one thing: The function is extrapolated so that recirculation would not be included in the integral.

---

[n]Or intravascular volume, i.e. if labeled red blood cells are used.

9.6. COMPETITIVE SYSTEMS

In Section 5.2.1, perfusion tracers are discussed. The general equation is as follows.

$$A_i(t) = \frac{F_i}{CO} \int_0^t c(t)dt, \tag{9.25}$$

where A_i is the activity in organ i, CO is the cardiac output and $c(t)$ is the plasma concentration of the tracer. It should be noted that the value of t is problematic: The equation is valid only if at time t no tracer has left the organ yet. But the main point is that all systems (early on) drink from the same well (16–18).

The same is true for competitive systems. A typical competitive system is found in ^{18}F-fluorodeoxyglucose PET. In that case,

$$A_i(t) = K \int_0^t c(t)dt, \tag{9.26}$$

where K is a combination of flow and avidity for glucose. The important factor is the integral over the plasma concentration. As an illustration, in the absence of renal function, $c(t)$ would be slower to decrease than if renal function was hyper normal.[o] In the same sense, if a particular lesion in a first study has $SUV = n$ but in the presence of a large amount of glucose avid tissue (a large tumor mass), and if in the second study that mass has disappeared, then the SUV would be higher than n if the biological activity of the lesion has not changed (K remains constant, but $c(t)$ is now slower to decrease).

REFERENCES

1. Meier P, Zierler KL. On the theory of the indicator-dilution method for measurement of blood flow and volume. *J Appl Physiol* 1954; 6:731–744.
2. Zierler KL. Equations for measuring blood flow by external monitoring of radioisotopes. *Circulation* 1965; 16:309–321.
3. Elashoff JD, Reedy TJ, Meyer JH. Analysis of gastric emptying data. *Gastroenterology* 1982; 83:1306–1312.
4. Siegel JA, Urbain JL, Adler LP, Charkes ND, Maurer AH, Krevsky B, Knight LC, Fisher RS, Malmud LS. Biphasic nature of gastric emptying. *Gut* 1988; 29:85–89.
5. Abell TL, Camilleri M, Donohoe K, Hasler WL, Lin HC, Maurer AH, McCallum RW, Nowak T, Nusynowitz ML, Parkman HP, Shreve P, Szarka LA, Snape WJ Jr, Ziessman HA. Consensus recommendations for gastric emptying scintigraphy: a joint report of

---

[o]The Standard Uptake Value or SUV computes the organ activity as a fraction of the decay corrected injected dose and the weight or body surface area of the patient. If there is no renal function, the average SUV should be equal to 1.

the American neurogastroenterology and motility society and the society of nuclear medicine. *Am J Gastroenterol* 2007; 102:1–11.

6. Winchell HS. Quantitation of red cell and heme production and destruction using radioisotope kinetics. *Prog Med* 1968; 2:85–112.

7. Shapiro SI, Landaw SA, Winchell HS, Williams MC. Independence of mechanical fragility and red blood cell age in the rat. *Proc Soc Exp Biol Med* 1969; 131: 1206–1209.

8. Landaw SA. Endogenous production of carbon monoxide: the human body as a cause of air pollution. *Ann Intern Med* 1969; 70:1275–1276.

9. Pearson HA, Spencer RP. Hematological Studies in Pediatrics, in James, Wagner, Cooke (eds.) *Pediatric Nuclear Medicine* (1974) W.B.Saunders Co, Philadelphia, London, Toronto.

10. Pearson HA. Life span of the fetal red blood cell. *J Pediatr* 1967; 70:166–171.

11. Silvergleid AJ, Wells RF, Hafleigh EB, Korn G, Kellner JJ, Grumet FC. Compatibility test using 51-chromium-labeled red. *Transfusion* 1978; 18:8–14.

12. Patlak CS, Blasberg RG. Graphical evaluation of blood-to-brain transfer constants from multiple-time uptake data. Generalizations. *J Cereb Blood Flow Metab* 1985; 5: 584–590.

13. Schmidt KC, Turkheimer FE. Kinetic modeling in positron emission tomography. *Q J Nucl Med* 2002; 46(1):70–85.

14. Profant M, Vyska K, Eckhardt U. The Stewart-Hamilton equations for the indicator dilution method. *Siam J Appl Math* 1978; 34:666–675.

15. Valentinuzzi ME, Geddes LA, Baker LE. A simple mathematical derivation of the Stewart-Hamilton formula for the determination of cardiac output. *Med Biol Eng Comput* 1969; 7:277–281.

16. Keys JR, Hetzel PS, Wood EH. Revised equations for calculation of blood flow and central indicator dilution curves. *J Appl Physiol* 1957; 11:385–389.

17. Sapirstein LA. Regional blood flow by fractional distribution of indicators. *Am J Physiol* 1958; 193:161–168.

18. Sapirstein LA. Fractionation of the cardiac output of rats with isotopic potassium. *Circ Res* 1956; 4:689–692.

Chapter 10

Mathematical Techniques

This chapter is meant to be a back-up, in case a reader does not understand a mathematical derivation in one of the mathematical sections.

10.1. MATRIX ALGEBRA

10.1.1. *Formalism*

$$\text{If } \begin{bmatrix} a & b \\ c & d \end{bmatrix} \bullet \begin{bmatrix} A \\ B \end{bmatrix} = \begin{bmatrix} D \\ 0 \end{bmatrix}, \quad \text{then } A = \frac{(D \times d) - (0 \times b)}{(ad - cb)}.$$

To introduce matrix algebra, we start with a simple problem: The solution of two linear equations with two unknowns. The rational to introduce matrix algebra will become clear from the example given here (channel crosstalk correction) and the application in another chapter, for the integral solution in two-compartmental system.

Everyone is familiar with the solution (in x) for the linear relation: $A = a \cdot x + b$. The solution is given by: $x = \frac{A-b}{a}$.

However, the solution (in x and y) of the set of equations $A = ax + by$ and $B = cx + dy$ requires a little more, since in any one of the equations in the set, a solution in "x" leaves an unknown "y", and vice-versa.

The "easy" solution is obtained by substitution: We first solve one equation for "x", then substitute x in the second equation with the solution, which contains "y". The second equation is then reduced to one linear equation with one unknown.

$$x = \frac{A - by}{a},$$

$$B = c \cdot \frac{A - by}{a} + dy,$$

$$B = c\frac{A - by}{a} + \frac{ady}{a},$$

$$B = \frac{cA - (cb - ad)y}{a},$$

$$aB = cA - (cb - ad)y,$$

$$\frac{aB - cA}{ad - cb} = y.$$

One can then substitute the solution for y in the first equation:

$$x = \frac{A - by}{a},$$

$$x = \frac{A}{a} + \frac{b}{a} \times \frac{aB - cA}{ad - cb},$$

$$x = \frac{A(ad - cb)}{a(ad - cb)} - \frac{b(aB - cA)}{a(ad - cb)},$$

$$x = \frac{adA - bcA - abB + bcA}{a(ad - cb)}.$$

Therefore, the final solution is

$$y = \frac{a \cdot B - c \cdot A}{a \cdot d - c \cdot b},$$

$$x = \frac{d \cdot A - b \cdot B}{a \cdot d - c \cdot b}.$$

The derivation was deliberately expansive. The same solution can be easily found using matrix algebra. We start by rewriting the set of equations as follows:

$$\begin{pmatrix} a & b \\ c & d \end{pmatrix} \times \begin{pmatrix} x \\ y \end{pmatrix} = \begin{pmatrix} A \\ B \end{pmatrix}.$$

This is simply another notation for the two equations we started with.

In general, consider two matrices: the first (A) with L rows and K columns and matrix elements a_{lk} and the second (X) with K rows and M columns and matrix elements x_{km}. We could represent them as follows:

$$\begin{pmatrix} a_{11} & a_{12} & \dots & a_{1K} \\ a_{21} & a_{22} & \dots & \dots \\ \dots & \dots & \dots & \dots \\ a_{L1} & L2 & \dots & a_{LK} \end{pmatrix} \quad \text{and} \quad \begin{pmatrix} x_{11} & \dots & x_{1M} \\ \dots & \dots & \dots \\ \dots & \dots & \dots \\ x_{K1} & \dots & x_{KM} \end{pmatrix}.$$

The matrices can only be multiplied if the number of columns in the first (K) equals the number of rows in the second (K). The matrix (B) resulting from the multiplication has K rows, M columns and matrix elements b_{km}.

In the resulting matrix B, the matrix element b_{ij} is given by the sum of the multiplication of corresponding elements in row "i" of matrix A and column "j" in matrix X:

$$b_{ij} = \sum_{k=1}^{k=K} a_{ik} \cdot x_{kj}.$$

It is obvious that if one applies this rule to the matrix equation describing the two equations with two unknowns, one obtains the set of two original equations. We now define a new term, the determinant of a matrix. For a two by two matrix, the determinant is the difference of the cross-products as follows:

$$\text{Det} = \begin{vmatrix} a & b \\ c & d \end{vmatrix} = a \cdot d - c \cdot d.$$

The solution for x is obtained by substituting A and B in the first column, and making the ratio of the two determinants

$$x = \frac{\begin{vmatrix} A & b \\ B & d \end{vmatrix}}{\begin{vmatrix} a & b \\ c & d \end{vmatrix}} = \frac{A \cdot d - B \cdot b}{a \cdot d - c \cdot b},$$

and for y

$$y = \frac{\begin{vmatrix} a & A \\ c & B \end{vmatrix}}{\begin{vmatrix} a & b \\ c & d \end{vmatrix}} = \frac{a \cdot B - c \cdot A}{a \cdot d - c \cdot b}.$$

It is easy to see that the solutions for x and y are identical to the ones obtained by substitution, but the derivation is obviously simpler. In addition, if the determinant in the denominator is zero, the set of equations is ill conditioned, and the two equations describe two parallel lines: in that case there is no common solution. In a graph, the solution for two linear equations with two unknowns would lie where the lines would cross.

10.1.2. Channel Crosstalk

The most common application in nuclear medicine would be in multi-channel counting. Assume that two isotopes need to be counted. They emit gamma rays of respectively 140 and 150 keV (e.g. ^{99m}Tc and ^{123}I). Energy resolution being imperfect in nuclear medicine, the windows set at 140 ± 14 and 150 ± 15 overlap. If ^{99m}Tc alone is put in the counter, one observes that for M counts in the 140 channel, there are mM counts in the 150 channel. Conversely, if ^{123}I alone is counted, there are N counts in the 150 channel and nN in the 140 channel.

If a mixture of both is counted, channel 140 will have A counts, and channel 150 will have B counts. Which counts belong to which?

What we know is that:

$$ax + by = A.$$

$$cx + dy = B.$$

x are the counts originating from ^{99m}Tc and y from ^{123}I. We do know that if x are the total counts from ^{99m}Tc, that $c = mM/(M + mM)$ and that $a = M/(M + mM)$ or in general:

$$c = m/(1 + m).$$

$$a = 1/(1 + m).$$

$$b = n/(1 + n).$$

$$d = 1/(1 + n).$$

The coefficients are therefore known. As an example assume $m = 0.3$ and $n = 0.25$. In that case,

$$c = 0.3/1.3 = 0.23.$$

$$a = 1/1.3 = 0.77.$$

$$d = 1/1.25 = 0.8.$$

$$b = 0.25/1.25 = 0.2.$$

If $A = 100$ and $B = 200$, then the net counts for ^{99m}Tc are x and $x = \frac{Ad - Bb}{ad - cb} = \frac{100 \times 0.8 - 200 \times 0.2}{0.77 \times 0.8 - 0.23 \times 0.2} = \frac{40}{0.57} = 70$ while the net counts for ^{123}I are $y = \frac{aB - cA}{ad - cb} = 230$.

Note that the sum of the net counts of both isotopes equals $A + B$.

See Section 2.5.

10.2. LOGARITHMS AND EXPONENTIALS

In the discussion of single compartmental models and radioactive decay, we use the fact that the integral over x of dx/x is the natural logarithm of x.

$$\int_{N(0)}^{N(t)} \frac{dN}{N} = -\ln(N)|_{N(0)}^{N(t)}.$$

That in itself does not explain the nature of the logarithm. In general, since $100 = 10^2$, the logarithm on the basis of 10 of 100 is 2.

$$\log_{10}(100) = 2.$$

In the case of the natural logarithm, the base is "e", an irrational number (e is the limit of $(1 + 1/n)^n$ as n tends to infinity).[a] The usual symbol for $\log_e$ is "ln".

Exponents use the same basis. Hence (by definition),

$$\ln(e^x) = x,$$
$$e^{\ln(x)} = x. \qquad \text{(attribute 1)}$$

The interesting thing about logarithms was used in the same section:

$$\ln(a \times b) = \ln(a) + \ln(b),$$
$$\ln\left(\frac{a}{b}\right) = \ln(a) - \ln(b). \qquad \text{(attribute 2)}$$

We used attribute 2 for the transition

$$\ln(N_t) - \ln(N_0) = -\lambda t,$$
$$\ln\left(\frac{N_t}{N_0}\right) = -\lambda t,$$

and attribute 1 for the transition to

$$\frac{N(t)}{N(0)} = e^{-\lambda \cdot t}.$$

About the exponential function, we want to remember two attributes:

If $f = e^{at}$ and $g = e^{bt}$, then $fg = e^{(a+b)t}$. It follows that $f^2 = e^{2at}$, and that $\sqrt{f} = e^{at/2}$. And finally also that $f/g = e^{(a-b)t}$.

10.2.1. *Plotting Exponential Functions in Semi-Log Plots*

The product-to-sum attribute 2 is useful in illustrating exponential functions. In the simple case, we have the function

$$A(t) = A(0)e^{-\lambda t}.$$

The logarithmic transformation yields

$$\ln(A(t)) = \ln(A(0)) - \lambda t.$$

The logarithmic transformation has two characteristics. First the result is the equation of a straight line: $y = b + at$ and second, the independent variable(t) remains

---

[a]Euler gave an approximation for *e* to 18 decimal places.

Linear

Semilog

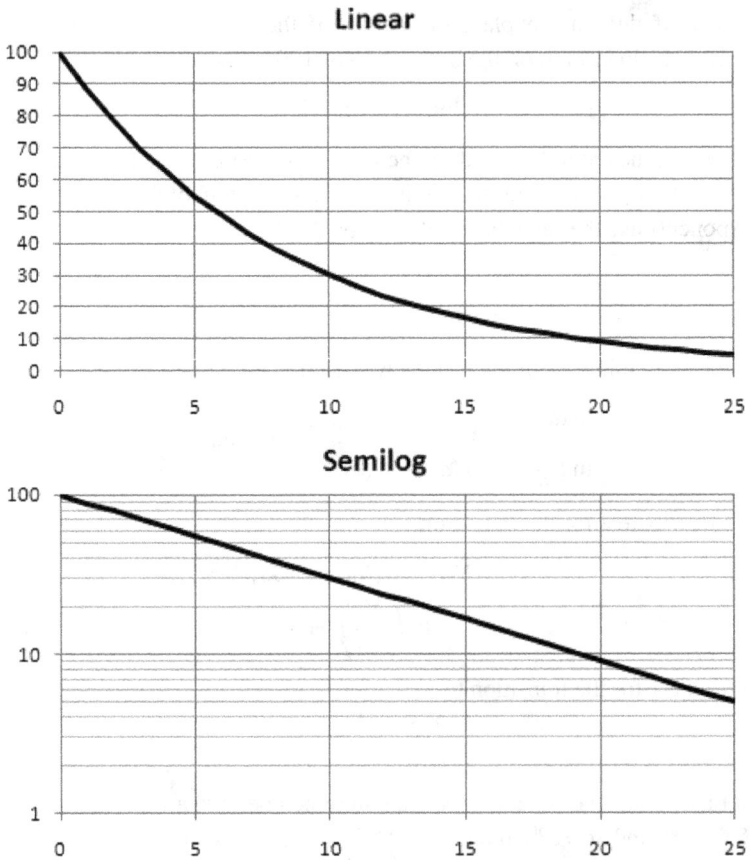

Figure 10.1   A (single) exponential on a bilinear scale and on a semi-logarithmic scale. The exponent λ in this case is 0.10. On a semi-logarithmic scale, the single exponential is a straight line.

linear, while the dependent variable ln $A(0)$ is logarithmic. Hence, the exponential function if plotted on a scale where y is logarithmic and x is linear (a semi-log plot), would appear as a straight line (Figure 10.1).

10.2.2.   *The Gamma Function*

The function described below is often quoted in the literature, and referred to as the gamma function:

$$f(t) = Kt^{\alpha}e^{-at}.$$

Specifically, $\Gamma(\alpha) = \int_0^\infty t^{\alpha-1} e^{-t} dt$.
The characteristics of Γ are as follows:

$$\Gamma(\alpha + 1) = \alpha \, \Gamma(\alpha),$$

$$\Gamma(1) = \int_0^\infty e^{-t} dt = 1,$$

and, if n is an integer, then $\Gamma(n) = (n-1)!$ where $(n-1)!$ is the product $1 \times 2 \times 3 \times \cdots \times (n-1)$.

The function has the formalism of the catenaries compartments with a single fractional turnover rate (a):

$N_n(t) = \frac{a^{n-1} t^{n-1}}{(n-1)!} Q e^{-at}$, in which the exponent α is actually an integer.

10.3. PARTIAL DERIVATIVE

A partial derivative of the product of two functions uv is $d(uv) = ud(v) + vd(u)$. We use this in the derivation of the kinetics of cathenary systems. Specifically, consider the function $N(t)e^{+at}$. The first derivative is

$$\frac{dN(t)e^{at}}{dt} = e^{at}\frac{dN(t)}{dt} + N(t)ae^{at}.$$

Consider the function: $t(1 - H(t))$. ($t = v$, $1 - H(t) = u$)
The partial derivative is

$$\frac{d[t(1 - H(t))]}{dt} = (1 - H(t))\frac{dt}{dt} + t\left[\frac{d1}{dt} - \frac{dH(t)}{dt}\right],$$

$$\frac{d[t(1 - H(t))]}{dt} = (1 - H(t)) - t\frac{dH(t)}{dt}.$$

This derivation is used in the definition of residency times.

10.4. AVERAGES

Averages are mathematical concepts, and do not really exist. If one has two observations, say 0 and 100, the average is 50, but there is no observation with a value of 50. Nevertheless, averages have uses, if one keeps that *proviso* in mind.

Everyone knows how to compute averages. If ten observations have the values 1, 2, 3, 4, 5, 6, 7, 8, 9, 10 the average is $(1+2+3+4+5+6+7+8+9+10)/10 = 5.5$. But consider the following series: 1, 2, 2, 3, 3, 3, 4, 4, 4, 4, 5, 5, 5, 6, 6, 7. The average can be computed the same way $(1+2+2+3+3+3+4+4+4+4+5+5+5+6+6+7)/16 = 4$. An alternative method is to name every value only once, but multiply it by the number of times it appears (see Table 10.1).

Table 10.1   On the left, the table shows the values, the number of times the values (frequency) appear and their product. On the right, the table shows the values and the density distribution (or normalized frequency) of those values. The density distribution sums up to 1.0 and corresponds to the frequency divided by the total number of observations. When the observations are multiplied by the normalized frequency or density distribution, the sum of the products is the average.

Value	Frequency	Product	Value	Normalized frequency	Product
1	1	1	1	0.0625	0.0625
2	2	4	2	0.1250	0.2500
3	3	9	3	0.1875	0.5625
4	4	16	4	0.2500	1.0000
5	3	15	5	0.1875	0.9375
6	2	12	6	0.1250	0.7500
7	1	7	7	0.0625	0.4375
Sum	16	64	Sum	1	4
Average $= 64/16 =$		4			

The spontaneous feeling that the average is also the most frequent occurrence comes from a familiarity with the normal distribution or bell curve (see Figure 10.2).

$$f(x) = \frac{1}{\sqrt{2\pi\sigma^2}} e^{\frac{(x-\mu)^2}{2\sigma^2}}.$$

The most frequently occurring value is the mode. The value dividing the lower 50% frequency from the upper 50% frequency is the median.

The median has the advantage, or at least characteristic, to be less sensitive to outliers (Table 10.2).

10.5. CONJUGATE COUNTING

In situations where an absolute quantification of the distribution of the tracer is desired (e.g. in dosimetry applications), people have been using conjugate counting. In conjugate counting, the images are acquired in registered anterior and posterior views (see also perfusion quantification), and (after flipping one of the images) the counts from the anterior and posterior images are combined in a geometric average. The geometric average of A and B is SQRT(AB). The goal is to avoid errors due to attenuation. Consider the situation in Figure 10.3:

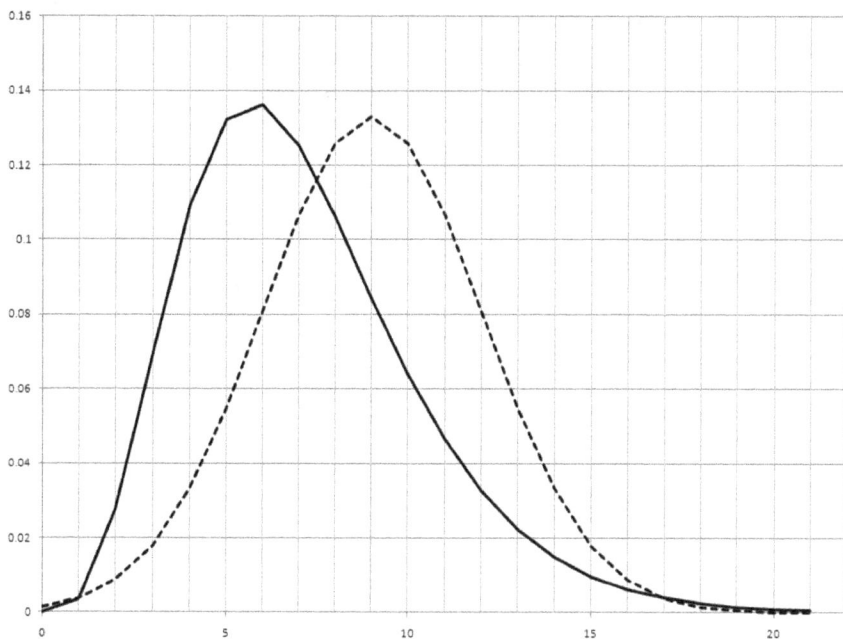

Figure 10.2 Density distribution functions. The symmetrical curve is the "normal" distribution or bell-shaped curve. The asymmetrical one is a gamma function. The area under the curves is one, by definition. In the "normal" curve, the average, mode and median are the same and equal to 9. In the asymmetrical curve, the average is 7.1, the mode is 6 and the median is 6.5. Even in the normal curve, with a standard deviation of 3, the average occurs only in 13% of the cases.

The geometric average of the anterior and posterior counts is $\sqrt{C_B C_F} = \sqrt{A^2 e^{-a(x+d-x)}} = Ae^{-ad/2}$. It follows that the attenuation effect is a function of the total body thickness at that location, but not of the position of the source.

This approach is accepted in a manner analogous of looking for lost keys under the street lamp rather than where the keys were actually lost. In reality it does not work because, because if there are two radioactive sources (A_1 and A_2) on the same line at distances x and y from the bottom, the basic equation becomes: $C_B = A_1 e^{-ax} + A_2 e^{-ay}$ and $C_F = A_1 e^{-a(d-x)} + A_2 e^{-a(d-y)}$ and the product would have cross-terms.[b]

---

[b]Because of the Swartz inequality Cauchy–Schwarz inequality (1888) (often misspelled "Schwartz"). In this case $(A + B)^*(A + B) \neq (A^2 + B^2)$.

Table 10.2   The two series differ only in the last value, which in series 2 is an outlier; the averages are different, the medians are not.

	Series 1	Series 2
	1.00	1.00
	2.00	2.00
	3.00	3.00
	4.00	4.00
	5.00	5.00
	6.00	6.00
	7.00	7.00
	8.00	8.00
	9.00	20.00
Average	5.00	6.22
Median	5.00	5.00

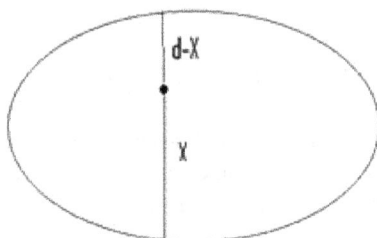

Figure 10.3   A source of activity A is imbedded in a body. The thickness of the body is d cm. The source is x cm from the bottom, and $d - x$ cm from the front. If the attenuation is homogeneous, the detector at the bottom would detect $C_B = A^{-ax}$. The detector in front would detect $C_F = A^{-a(d-x)}$, where a is the attenuation per cm.

Corrections or adaptations have been suggested, but the corrections used in PET/CT and SPECT/CT are making the approach obsolete.

10.6. FOURIER SERIES

All periodic and bounded functions can be expressed as a sum of sines and cosines. In this particular derivation, we are discussing functions with discrete values, not continuous functions (see Section 10.7.2).

Consider a function f(x) that exists in the interval $-L \leq x \geq L$:

$$f(x) = a_0 + \sum \left(a_n \cos \left(\frac{n\pi x}{L} \right) + b_n \sin \left(\frac{n\pi x}{L} \right) \right),$$

where n goes from 1 to half the number of data points or L, and a_0 is the average value of the function.

The definition of a_n and b_n is also an integral or a sum in the case of discrete data points:

$$a_n = \frac{1}{L} \sum_{j=1}^{j=2L} X(J) \cos \left(\frac{n\pi J}{L} \right),$$

$$b_n = \frac{1}{L} \sum_{j=1}^{j=2L} X(J) \sin \left(\frac{n\pi J}{L} \right).$$

An alternative expression is more useful to our purpose:

$$f(x) = \frac{a_0}{2} + \sum_{n=1}^{n=L} C_n \cos \left(\frac{n\pi x}{L} + P_n \right),$$

where $C_n = \sqrt{a_n^2 + b_n^2}$ is the amplitude (or size) of the nth harmonic and where $P_n = arctan(- b_n/a_n)$ is the phase of the nth harmonic.

If n = 1, then f(x) is the first harmonic. The number of harmonic is equal to half of the data points (Nyquist frequency) but in general, increasing the number of harmonics improves the fit (Figure 10.4). The application of the first harmonic in ventriculography is described in Section 6.2.3.2.

10.7. LINEAR TRANSFORMS

10.7.1. *Laplace Transform*

$$\Lambda_{\left(\frac{dN}{dt} \right)} = s.\Lambda_{(N)} - N(0).$$

The Laplace transform is a linear transformation (represented here by Λ). It has the strange property that the Laplacian of the derivative dN/dt of a function N is the sum of the Laplacian of the function itself $\Lambda_{(N)}$, multiplied by a constant "s", minus the initial value of the function N(0).

In the chapter of two-compartmental models, we will use it to overcome the case of an equation with a mixture of functions and their derivative.

$$\frac{dN_1}{dt} = -aN_1 + bN_2.$$

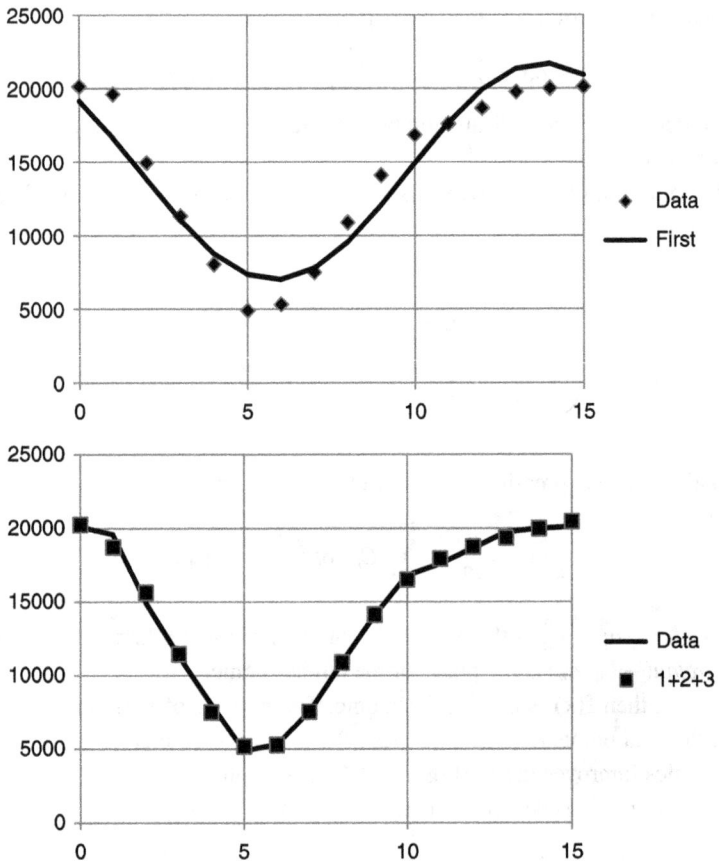

Figure 10.4 The plot on the left shows a ventricular volume curve (solid line) and the first harmonic of that curve (dotted). The fit of the first harmonic is surprisingly good but not perfect. On the right, the original data are a solid line and the dots are the fit with three harmonics. The fit is nearly perfect. The phase of the first harmonic is 0.86. A perfect symmetrical fit would have a phase of 3.14 (π), but the systole is not in the middle of the cycle.

The Laplacian is applied to both sides of the equation.

$$\Lambda_{(\frac{dN_1}{dt})} = s{\cdot}\Lambda_{(N_1)} - N_1(0),$$

$$\Lambda_{(-aN_1+bN_2)} = -a\Lambda_{(N_1)} + b\Lambda_{(N_2)}.$$

The effect is that all the terms are either the Laplacians of the function or a constant. The derivative is gone.

$$(s + a) \cdot \Lambda_{(N_1)} - b\Lambda_{(N_2)} = N_1(0).$$

It should be noted that we used the linearity of the transformation, meaning that $\Lambda_{(a+b)} = \Lambda_{(a)} + \Lambda_{(b)}$: The sum of the linear transformation of two functions is equal to the linear transformation of the sum of the two functions.

If we rearrange the terms, we obtain

$$\Lambda_{(e^{-at})} = \frac{1}{s+a}.$$

10.7.2. *Fourier Transform*

We do not intend to review all the properties and derivations of the Fourier transform, but to establish the basis of its use in imaging.

The motivation for the Fourier transform comes from the study of Fourier series (Section 10.6). In the study of Fourier series, complicated periodic functions are written as the sum of simple waves mathematically represented by sines and cosines. Due to the properties of sine and cosine, it is possible to recover the amount of each wave in the sum by an integral.

This passage from sines and cosines to complex exponentials makes it necessary for the Fourier coefficients to be complex-valued. The usual interpretation of this complex number is that it yields both the amplitude (or size) of the wave present in the function and the phase (or the initial angle) of the wave.

We may use the Fourier series to motivate the Fourier transform as follows. Suppose that f is a function which is zero outside of some interval $[-L/2, L/2]^c$ or $[-T/2, T/2]$. Then f in a Fourier series on the interval $[-T/2, T/2]$, where the "amount" (denoted by c_n) of the wave $e^{2\pi i n x / T}$ in the Fourier series of f is given by

$$\hat{f}(n/T) = c_n = \int_{-T/2}^{T/2} e^{-2\pi i n x / T} f(x) dx,$$

and f should be given by the formula

$$f(x) = \frac{1}{T} \sum_{n=-\infty}^{\infty} \hat{f}(n/T) e^{2\pi i n x / T}.$$

The main point is that if the function f(x) defines the image, and $\hat{f}(n/T)$ the Fourier transform of the image, one can return from the Fourier transform to the image function by a reverse transform.

The difference with the Fourier series, is that it applies to continuous functions. There are two principal characteristics of the transform that we will use.

---

[c] That would typically be the case for an image, that exists only within the limits of the part of the object being imaged.

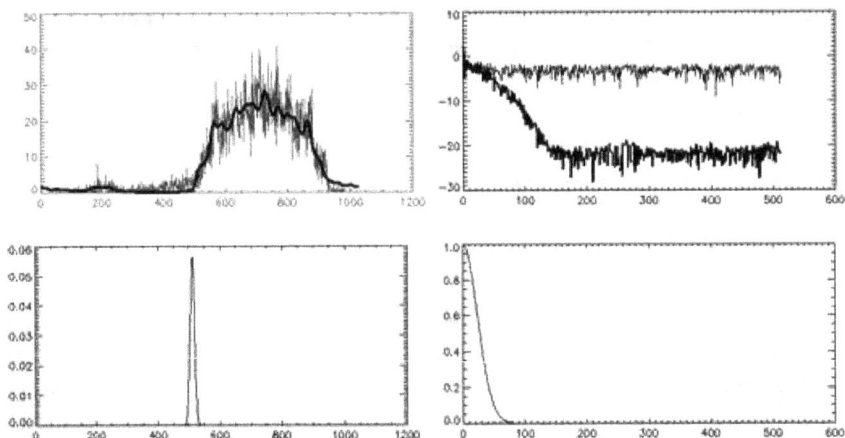

Figure 10.5 The faint tracings in the upper left quadrant represent original and noisy data. The Fourier transform of those original data is represented in the right upper quadrant, by the fainter tracings.

Linearity:
$$\text{If } h(x) = af(x) + bg(x), \quad \text{then} \quad \hat{h}(\xi) = a \cdot \hat{f}(\xi) + b \cdot \hat{g}(\xi).$$

Convolution:
$$\text{If } h(x) = (f * g) + (x), \quad \text{then} \quad \hat{h}(\xi) = \hat{f}(\xi) \cdot \hat{g}(\xi).^{\text{d}}$$

In imaging, the Fourier transform yields the contribution of frequencies to the data (see Figure 10.5). To smooth noisy data, the high frequencies are suppressed. The effect is similar to performing a convolution of the data with a filter kernel (see Sections 10.7.3 and 10.7.4).

The lower left quadrant shows the kernel of a smoothing filter, and the right lower quadrant the Fourier transform of that filter.

There would be two ways to go from the noisy tracing to the bright and smoother tracing of the left upper quadrant. One could convolute (Section 10.7.3) the filter kernel with the curve data (C*K), or multiply the Fourier transform of the curve data with the Fourier transform of the filter kernel, $\hat{C} \times \hat{K}$, and then perform an inverse transform. The bright tracings in the right upper quadrant is the result of the multiplication, in which the higher frequencies have been suppressed. The bright tracing in the left upper quadrant is the reverse transform of the result of the multiplication $\hat{C} \times \hat{K}$.

The inverse Fourier transform yields a smoother image (Figures 10.5 and 10.6).

---

[d]In this case, the symbol "*" stands for convolution.

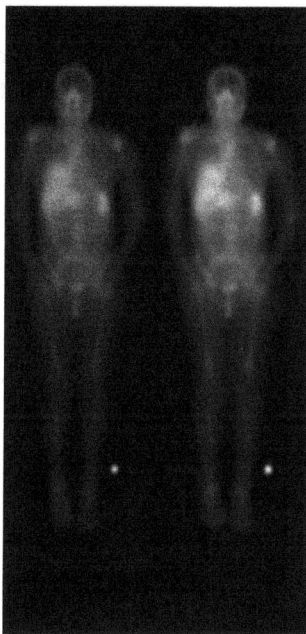

Figure 10.6 The original data on the left, the "filtered" data on the right.

10.7.3. *Convolution*

Typically, a convolution is a shift and a sum.

Consider people entering a room (e.g. a museum room) at fixed intervals in cohorts as follows: 50 enter at time 0, 300 at time 1 hour, 400 at 2 hour, 200 at 3 hour and 100 at 4 hour (see columns 1 and 2 under input time and input number) The total people entering is 1050.

The exhibit is not to everyone's taste. A fraction (0.1 or 10%) of the people do leave after 1 minute. Another fraction (0.3) leaves after 2 minutes. At 3 minutes, it is 40% and at 4 minutes, it is 0.2 or 20% (see rows 1 and 2).

The time spent in the room is randomly distributed such that: If ten people enter the room simultaneously, they will leave in cohort as follows: 3, 4, 3.

What would an observer see while watching the number of people exiting? The answer is the results of the convolution.

Consider the number leaving at time 1: They are 0.1 of those entering at time 0 or 5 (out of 50). Consider those leaving at time 2: They are 0.3 of those entering at time 0 and 0.1 of those entering at time 0. Mathematically this can be written as:

$$O(2) = T(2)E(2-1) + (T2)E(2),$$

where T is the distribution of residency times in the room and E the function describing the distribution of entering and O(I) the time of the exit. In general, we are describing a sum (Σ) of products (ExT) with a shift (I − J) (Figure 10.7 and Table 10.3):

$$O(I) = \sum_{J=0}^{J=I} T(I)E(I - J).$$

In continuous function, a convolution is represented as an integral (the sum), a product and a shift:

$$f(t) = \int_0^t h(t)c(t - \tau)d\tau.$$

In this equation, h(t) is the distribution of transit times, f(t) is the distriution of outputs and c(t − τ) the distribution of entering cohorts.

In practice, those integrations do not necessarily have an analytical form, but one can take the Fourier transform of h(t) and c(t), multiply them and take the reverse transform of the result.

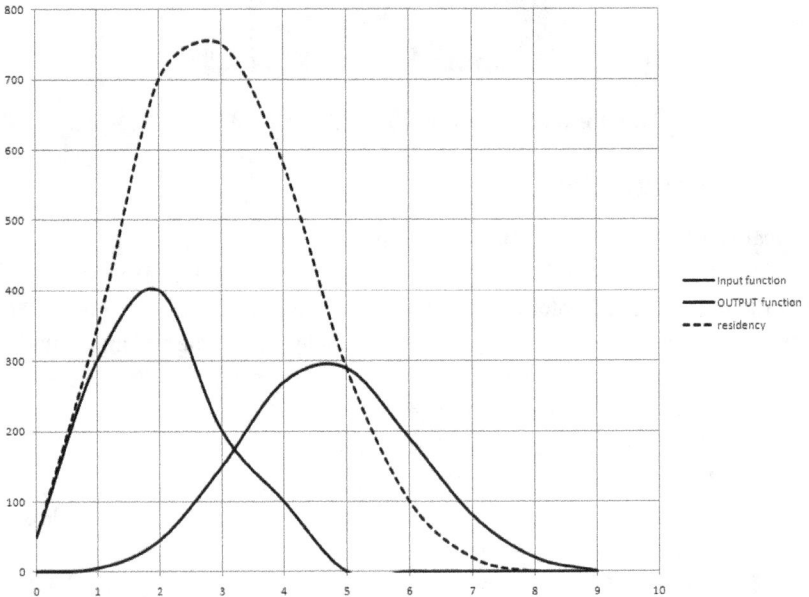

Figure 10.7 The figure illustrates the distribution of the exit patterns for five cohorts entering at different times. The output function (on the right) is characterized by a delay, compared to the input, and a widening (ranging from 1 to 9 versus 0 to 5 for the input) The middle broken curve represents the total within the system. The transfer function is the density distribution of transit times (0.1, 0.3, 0.4 and 0.2) the sum is equal to 1.0. the data are shown in Table 10.3.

Table 10.3 The table illustrates the distribution of exits of the five cohorts: A cohort of 50 enters at t = 0, 300 at t = 1 etc. 10% take 1 minute to exit, 30% take 2 etc. The effect is an output of 5 at 1 minute 45 at 2 minutes etc.

	Residency times	0	1	2	3	4	5	6	7	Sum
Input time	Input Nr	**0**	**0.1**	**0.3**	**0.4**	**0.2**	**0**	**0**	**0**	**1**
0	50	0	5	15	20	10				50
1	300		0	30	90	120	60			300
2	400			0	40	120	160	80		400
3	200				0	20	60	80	40	200
4	100					0	10	30	40	20	100
Sum and output	1050	0	5	45	150	270	290	190	80	20	1050

It is obvious from the tables and graphs, that the convolution provokes a shift. When a convolution filter is used to smooth an image, this shift is not desirable and the convolution is recentered.

10.7.4. *Smoothing and Filtering*

Smoothing image or curve data is in fact a convolution if done in an image (or curve) domain (rather than the frequency domain). The term "filtering" refers to the fact that high frequencies are filtered out or let go. Smoothing is generally used for a convolution in the image domain (Section 10.7.3), filtering is used for an operation in the frequency domain (Section 10.7.2).

Example: The kernel in this case is 0.11, 0.22, 0.33, 0.22, 0.11. The data are shown in Table 10.4. The kernel is centered on the middle value 0.33 and in the

Table 10.4 Convolution filter acting on one data point.

Data	Kernel	Product	Sum
24.6			
26.93			
28.28	0.11	3.14	
27.58	0.22	6.13	
25.73	0.33	0.33	25.6
23.78	0.2	0.22	
22.21	0.11	2.47	
21.6			

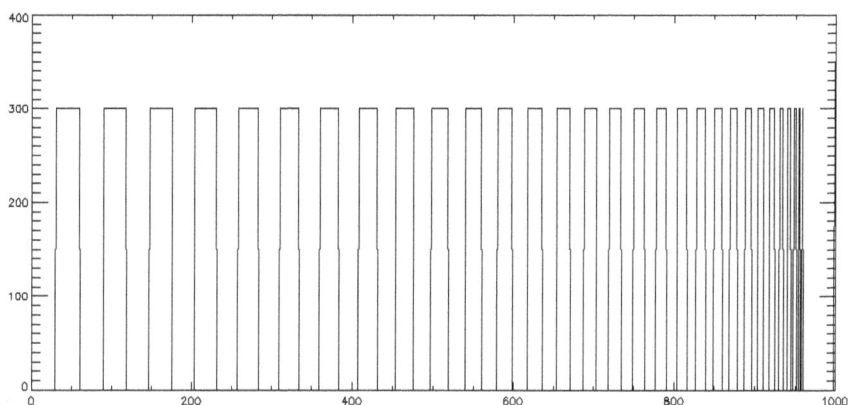

Figure 10.9 Profile of the signal. The frequency of the oscillation increases to the right of the image.

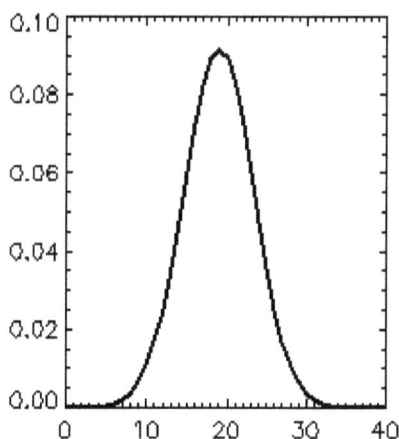

Figure 10.10 Points Spread Function.

the signal). In this case (i.e. for the PSF shown in Figure 10.9), the MTF looks like the illustrations in Figures 10.11 and 10.12.

10.7.6. *Lag Normal Function*

The gamma function was described in the catenary systems as a descriptor of arterial flow, but they lack one intuitively necessary attribute: At time zero, the model predicts that the trace is already at the last observation point.

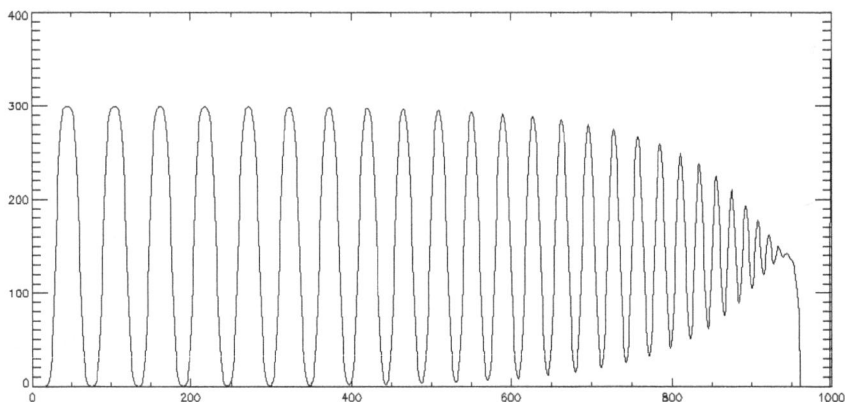

Figure 10.11 In the image the amplitude of the density oscillations decreases when the frequency increases.

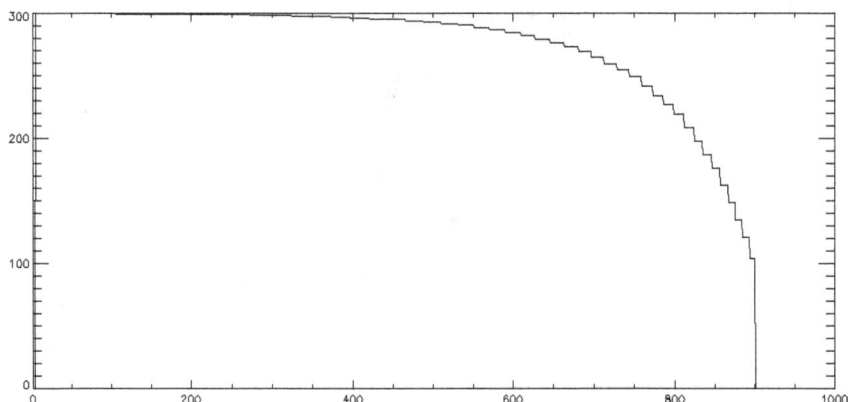

Figure 10.12 Modulation transfer function corresponding to the PSF in Figure 10.10.

Bassingthwaighte had proposed another mode, in which a time lag is allowed and a degree of mixing, which he describes as a normal function.

The mixing function and delay are expressed as

$$h_1(t) = \frac{1}{\sigma\sqrt{2\pi}} e^{-\frac{1}{2}(\frac{t-\bar{t}}{\sigma})^2}.$$

The area under the curve is unitary. The bolus in any point disappears as an exponential (again unitary):

$$h_2(t) = \frac{1}{\tau} e^{-\frac{t}{\tau}}.$$

The formulation down the line is defined by the differential equation:

$$h_3(t) = \frac{1}{\sigma\sqrt{2\pi}}e^{-\frac{1}{2}(\frac{t-\bar{t}}{\sigma})^2} - \tau\frac{dh_3(t)}{dt}.$$

There is no analytical integral solution to this differential, but it described the dispersion of the bolus and the delay of the bolus in the nth point. This analysis can be used in the description of gastric emptying studies (Section 9.2) and vascular flow models (Section 8.4.2).

Index

absorbed dose (Φ), 91
accuracy, 186
acute tubular necrosis, 10
adenosine, 119
aminophylline, 119
angioplasty, 111, 117
angiotensin-converting enzyme (ACE), 11
  inhibitor, 10, 11
anthracosis, 62
antimyosin, 114
arteriovenous malformations, 63
atrial fibrillation, 168
average life, 203
average or mean transit time, 231
average residency time $\bar{t}$, 236

Bateman equation, 209
bed rest, 174
beta-methyl iodophenyl pentadecanoic
  acid (BMIPP), 114
body surface area (BSA), 31
brachytherapy, 87
bull's eye, 123

C-11-palmitate, 114
captopril, 11
cardiac output, 28
cardiomyopathy, 174
catenary system, 207
cellularity, 115
circumferential profile, 121
compartmental analysis, 197
compartmental systems, 197
competitive system, 245

confirm coronary artery disease (CAD),
  111
congestive heart failure (CHF), 117
conjugate counting, 254
conjugate views, 63, 76
constant infusion model, 205
contingency table, 165
convoluted, 207
convolution, 261
coronary artery bypass graft (CABG), 117
coronary lesion, 111
crosstalk, 121, 161
  channel, 249
  tissue, 162
CT angiography, 50
cystouretrography, 22

decay scheme, 91
density distribution of the transit times,
  230
diffusible tracer, 111
dipyridamole, 133
doxorubin cardiotoxicity, 174
dyskinetic, 117

echocardiography, 141
effect on the exponentials, 218
effective renal plasma flow (ERPF), 3
Eisenmenger syndrome, 63
ejection fraction (EF), 162
end-diastolic count rate (EDCR), 162
end-systolic count rate (ESCR), 162
equilibrium absorbed dose constant, 89
equilibrium ECG-gated
  angiocardiography (EGNA), 164

excretion phase, 20
exercise or dipyridamole, 139
external beam radiotherapy (EBRT), 87
extraction efficiency, 5, 201
extracellular fluid (ECF) volume, 31
extraction ratio, 5
extrasystole, 168

F-18-fluorodeoxyglucose, 114
factorial, 211
FDG PET imaging, 190
filtering, 263
first harmonic analysis, 170
first order kinetics, 199
first order process, 5
first order systems, 197
first pass nuclear angiocardiography
    (FPNA), 161
first pass ventriculography, 161
fixed, 115
fluor, 95
fluorodeoxyglucose, 95
Fourier series, 256
fractional excretion rate, 201
fractional renal uptake, 218
frequency distribution, 231
furosemide, 11, 19, 20
fusion, 101

gallium, 95
gamma fit, 28
gamma function, 213
generator, 209
geometric mean, 63, 76
glomerular filtration rate (GFR), 3

half-life, 201
hibernation, 144
hydration, 19
hydronephrosis (HN), 23
hydroureteronephrosis (HUN), 23
hypokinetic, 117

infarction, 111
inhalation imaging, 48
intravenous urography (IVU), 75
inulin, 10

inverse Fourier transform, 260
iodine (^{123}I, ^{131}I, ^{125}I), 95
ischemic kidney model, 10

lag-time, 236
Laplace transform, 216
Lasix, 19
likelihood ratios are shown, 17
lung uptake, 117

matrix algebra, 247
maximum intensity projection (MIP), 78
modulation transfer function (MTF), 135
myocardial perfusion, 111

nascent urine, 4, 11
normalcy ratio, 129
Nuclear Regulatory Commission, 103

observed value, 218
operating characteristic, 72, 129, 173

para-aminohippurate (PAH), 10
partial derivative, 253
Patlak method applied to kidneys, 241
peak counts, 21
perfusion imaging, 43
phase analysis, 170
phase shifts, 165
phosphanate, 95
PIOPED, 50
PIOPED II, 60
PISAPED: Prospective, 60
plasma clearance, 5
polar transformation, 121
    3D, 123
positive inotropic response, 146
power Doppler ultrasound (PDUS), 75
pre-injection 15 minutes, 25
prevalence, 182
pulmonary arteriogram or angiogram, 50
pulmonary atresia, 64
pulmonary blood flow distribution, 64
pulmonary edema, 62
pulmonary embolism, 50

pulmonary ventilation imaging with
   krypton-81m, 46

rad, 89
radioactive decay, 199, 201
receiver operating characteristics function,
   191
redistribution image, 115
regional wall motion (RWM), 170, 173
renal cortical perfusion, 3
renal excretion rate, 3
renal glomerular function, 3
renography, 3
   captopril, 11
renovascular hypertension (RVH), 10, 75
residency time, 203
reversible defects, 139
right to left shunting, 63
risk (ischemic), 111

samarium, 95
sarcoidosis, 63
scleroderma, 63
semi-logarithmic plot, 203, 251
semiotics, 128
sestamibi, 95
single compartmental system, 199
smoothing, 263
steady state, 197
strontium, 95
substitution, 247

surgical model, 97
Swartz inequality, 255

tetralogies, 64
tetrofosmin, 95
thallium, 95
therapy with radionuclides, 87
time of peak activity, 21
tracer amount, 197
tracer kinetics, 197
transient, 115
transient defect, 139
transit time, 3
trapezoidal method, 89
two linear equations with two unknowns,
   247
two-compartmental system, 214

ultrasound (US), 72
uptake ratio, 21

valvular disease, 174
ventilation imaging, 44
ventricular function, 161
ventriculography, 161
verification bias, 129, 186
vesicoureteral reflux, 22
viability, 111, 115
voxel, 78

xenon-133, 44